Pocket Reference for
Pediatric Primary Care

Pocket Reference for
Pediatric Primary Care

Catherine E. Burns, PhD, RN, CPNP, FAAN
Professor
Primary Care Nurse Practitioner Specialty
Oregon Health Sciences University School of Nursing
Portland, Oregon

Margaret A. Brady, PhD, RN, CPNP
Professor
California State University Long Beach, Department of Nursing
Pediatric Nurse Practitioner
Miller Children's Hospital
Long Beach, California

Ardys M. Dunn, PhD, RN, PNP
Associate Professor
University of Portland School of Nursing
Portland, Oregon

Nancy Barber Starr, MS, RNC, CPNP
Pediatric Nurse Practitioner
Aurora Pediatric Associates
Aurora, Colorado

W.B. SAUNDERS COMPANY
A Harcourt Health Sciences Company
Philadelphia • London • New York • St. Louis • Sydney • Toronto

W.B. SAUNDERS COMPANY
A Harcourt Health Sciences Company

The Curtis Center
Independence Square West
Philadelphia, Pennsylvania 19106

Library of Congress Cataloging-in-Publication Data

Pocket reference for Pediatric primary care / Catherine E. Burns . . . [et al.].

p. cm.

Includes bibliographical references and index.

ISBN 0–7216–8466–1

1. Pediatrics—Handbooks, manuals, etc. 2. Pediatric nursing—Handbooks, manuals, etc. I. Burns, Catherine E. II. Pediatric primary care. [DNLM: 1. Pediatrics—United States—Handbooks. 2. Primary Health Care—United States—Handbooks. WS 39 P7395 2001]

RJ45.P525 2001 618.92—dc21

DNLM/DLC

00–037159

Vice President, Nursing Editorial Director: Sally Schrefer

Acquisitions Editor: Barbara Nelson Cullen

Associate Developmental Editor: Kara L. Johnson

Manuscript Editor: Amy Norwitz

Production Manager: Paul Nigel Harris

Illustration Specialist: Lisa Lambert

POCKET REFERENCE FOR PEDIATRIC PRIMARY CARE   ISBN 0-7216-8466-1

Printed in the United States of America.

Last digit is the print number: 9   8   7   6   5   4   3   2   1

This book is dedicated to
the infants, children, and adolescents and their families
about whom the book was written,
wishing them health, loving support, and happiness,
the real goals of this book.

CONTRIBUTORS

We acknowledge the contributions of the authors who wrote content for the main text. While the content presented herein is an extraction of material and ideas from the main text, only the four main authors, Catherine E. Burns, Margaret A. Brady, Ardys M. Dunn, and Nancy Barber Starr, wrote specifically for this book.

We hope that this reference meets a specific need of clinicians and students as they work to care for the children.

Jean Betschart, MSN, MN, CPNP, CDE
Adjunct Faculty, Department of Health Promotion and Development, University of Pittsburgh School of Nursing; Pediatric Nurse Practitioner, Department of Diabetes, Endocrinology, and Metabolism, Children's Hospital of Pittsburgh, Pittsburgh, Pennsylvania
Endocrine and Metabolic Diseases

Patricia Billings, RN, MPH, CRNP
Physicians Center, Twin Falls, Idaho
Developmental Management of School-Age Children and Adolescents

Catherine Blosser, CPNP
Pediatric Nurse Practitioner, Multnomah County Health Department, Portland, Oregon
Complementary Therapies

Margaret A. Brady, PhD, RN, CPNP
Professor, California State University Long Beach, Department of Nursing, Pediatric Nurse Practitioner, Miller Children's Hospital, Long Beach, California
Role Relationships; Approaches to Disease Management; Infectious Diseases; Atopic Disorders and Rheumatic Diseases; Respiratory Disorders; Musculoskeletal Disorders; Common Injuries

Jeanette M. Broering, MS, RN, MPH, CPNP

Director, Data Quality Assurance, Urology Outcomes Research Group, Department of Urology, University of California, San Francisco, San Francisco, California

Sexuality

Catherine E. Burns, PhD, RN, CPNP, FAAN

Professor, Primary Care Nurse Practitioner Specialty, Oregon Health Sciences University School of Nursing, Portland, Oregon

Recommendations for Preventive Care; Child Assessment in Pediatric Primary Care; Developmental Management of School-Age Children and Adolescents; Activities and Sports for Children and Adolescents; Sleep and Rest; Cognitive-Perceptual Patterns; Neurological Disorders; Musculoskeletal Disorders; Genetic Disorders; Environmental Health; Appendix C: Normal Laboratory Values; Appendix D: Healthy People 2010 Objectives: Draft for Public Comment; Child and Adolescent Focused Objectives

Melanie A. Canady, MSN, RN, CPNP

Adjunct Clinical Faculty, East Carolina University, Greenville; Certified Pediatric Nurse Practitioner, Partners in Pediaric Healthcare, Craven County Health Department-Child Health Clinic, New Bern, North Carolina

Appendix A: Medications

Jeffrey A. Dean, DDS, MSD

Associate Professor of Pediatric Dentistry and Orthodontics, Director of Advanced Education Program in Pediatric Dentistry, Indiana University School of Dentistry; Active Staff Member, Riley Hospital for Children, Indianapolis, Indiana

Dental and Oral Diseases

Barbara Jones Deloian, PhD, RN, CPNP

Assistant Professor, Adjunct, University of Colorado Health Sciences Center School of Nursing; Pediatric Nurse Practitioner, Program Evaluator, Child Development Unit/Nursing Research, The Children's Hospital, Denver, Colorado

Developmental Management in Pediatric Primary Care; Developmental Management of Infants, Toddlers, and Preschoolers

Ardys M. Dunn, PhD, RN, PNP

Associate Professor, University of Portland School of Nursing, Portland, Oregon

Health Perception and Health Management Pattern; Nutrition; Elimination; Sexuality; Environmental Health; Appendix B: Growth Grids

Connie Evers, MS, RD, LD
Portland, Oregon
  Nutrition

Judith W. Fisher, RN, FNP, MHS
Multnomah County Health Department, School-Based Clinics, Portland, Oregon
  Developmental Management of School-Age Children and Adolescents

Jan Freitas-Nichols, MSN, RN, CPNP
Primary Faculty, School of Nursing; Director of Children's Services, Doernbecher Children's Hospital, Oregon Health Sciences University, Portland, Oregon
  Cardiovascular Problems

Mark H. Goodman, MD
Adjunct Professor of Nursing, California State University, Long Beach, Long Beach, California; Associate Clinical Professor of Pediatrics, University of California, Irvine, College of Medicine, Irvine, California; Attending Physician, Miller Children's Hospital, Long Beach, California
  Infectious Diseases; Respiratory Disorders

Steven Goodstein, MS, MT (ASCP)
Assistant Professor, Oregon Health Sciences University, Portland, Oregon
  Appendix C: Normal Laboratory Values

Pamela J. Hellings, PhD, RN, CPNP
Professor and Chair, Department of Primary Care, Oregon Health Sciences University School of Nursing, Portland, Oregon
  Breastfeeding

Gail M. Houck, PhD, RN
Associate Professor, Division of Children, Adolescents, and Families School of Nursing, Oregon Health Sciences University School of Nursing, Portland, Oregon
  Coping and Stress Tolerance

Sheila M. Kodadek, PhD, RN
Oregon Health Sciences University School of Nursing, Portland, Oregon
Family Assessment in Pediatric Primary Care

Margaret MacDonald, EdD, RN, CPNP
Pediatric Nurse Practitioner, Multnomah County Health Department,
Portland, Oregon
Cultural Perspectives for Primary Health Care; Eye Problems

Diane F. Montgomery, MSN, RN, CPNP
Assistant Professor of Pediatrics, University of Texas-Houston Medical
School, Houston, Texas
Perinatal Conditions

Mary A. Murphy, PhD, RN, CPNP
Instructor, Department of Pediatrics and Clinical Associate Professor,
University of Colorado Health Sciences Center School of Nursing,
Denver, Colorado
Developmental Management of Infants, Toddlers, and Preschoolers

Deborah K. Parks, MSN, RN, PNP
Associate Professor of Pediatrics and Director, Division of Nurse
Practitioners, University of Texas-Houston Medical School,
Houston, Texas
Perinatal Conditions

Ann M. Petersen-Smith, MS, RN, CPNP
Clinical Faculty, University of Colorado Health Sciences Center; Clinical
Faculty, Regis University; Pediatric Nurse Practitioner, Emergency
Department, The Children's Hospital, Denver, Colorado
Ear Disorders; Gastrointestinal Disorders

Charles Poland II, DDS
Associate Professor, Pediatric Dentistry, Indiana University School of
Dentistry; Private Practice, Pediatric Dentistry, Indianapolis, Indiana
Dental and Oral Diseases

Kathleen C. Shelton, MN, RN, CPNP
Examiner, CARES (Child Abuse Response and Evaluation Services)
Northwest, Portland, Oregon
Cognitive-Perceptual Patterns

Nancy Barber Starr, MS, RNC, CPNP
Pediatric Nurse Practitioner, Aurora Pediatric Associates, Aurora,
Colorado
Self-Perception; Eye Problems; Genitourinary Disorders; Gynecological
Conditions; Dermatological Diseases

Martha K. Swartz, MS, RN, CS, PNP
Associate Professor, Yale University School of Nursing; Pediatric Nurse
Practitioner, Yale-New Haven Hospital, New Haven, Connecticut
Hematological Diseases

Linda Wildey
Adjunct Clinical Faculty, University of Cincinnati, College of Nursing
and Health; Associate Director of Training, Division of Adolescent
Medicine, Children's Hospital Medical Center, Cincinnati, Ohio
Developmental Management of School-Age Children and Adolescents

Robert J. Yetman, MD
Professor and Director, Division of Community and General Pediatrics,
University of Texas-Houston Medical School, Houston, Texas
Perinatal Conditions

PREFACE

This book is designed as a companion to *Pediatric Primary Care: A Handbook for Nurse Practitioners,* second edition. We have created this book at the recommendation of students, faculty, and practitioners who identified the need for a portable reference of commonly used information, including important reference materials. We have expanded on their initial ideas to prepare this reference book for ambulatory pediatric care. Experienced clinicians as well as students will undoubtedly find it useful because no one commits to memory all the norms and values, medications, and other information needed for pediatric care. Rather, clinicians learn where to find needed information quickly and easily during a busy day.

ORGANIZATION

Following the organization of the main text, the first unit of this pocket reference provides information about the standards for child health care, assessment models, an outline of family structures, and information about cultural perspectives on health care. The second unit provides information about the development of infants, preschoolers, school-age children, and adolescents. In the third unit, management of health and the functional health patterns of children are addressed. These include mental health problems, learning problems, and issues such as child abuse; a variety of chapters on nutrition, breastfeeding, elimination, sports activities, and sleep and rest round out this important unit. The fourth unit addresses diseases and disorders in all body systems. Finally, the appendices provide important information about medications used in pediatric care, growth grids, and common laboratory values.

Many new tables have been created for this *Pocket Reference* to summarize important content from the main text, as neither the focus of the book nor the size allows for detailed information to be presented. Because of the slightly later publication date, the *Pocket Reference* may contain more recently published material than is found in the main text. For example, this book has the March 2000 version of the American Academy of Pediatrics *Recommendations for Pediatric Preventive Care* and the growth grids published in summer 2000 by the Centers for Disease Control and Prevention.

ACKNOWLEDGMENTS

This book is derived from its companion text, *Pediatric Primary Care: A Handbook for Nurse Practitioners,* second edition. As such, all the people acknowledged in the main text should also be acknowledged here: the contributors to the first edition, the expert consultants, and the technical support people.

We are especially indebted to Catherine Blosser, PNP, Portland, Oregon, who provided us with many hours of library and resource help, good cheer, and advice as a practicing PNP.

We also want to especially acknowledge our family and friends, whose support gave us the time and energy to put to the task of preparing both books. We especially recognize

- Jerry Burns, Jennifer and Jill, and other family and friends of Catherine Burns
- Marvin, Malcolm, and Philip Dunn, and other family and friends of Ardys Dunn
- Mary, Martha, Greg, and Katie, and other family and friends of Margaret Brady
- Jon and Jonah Starr, in memory of John T. Barber, and APA colleagues of Nancy Barber Starr

CONTENTS

UNIT 3

Approaches to Health Management

Pediatric Primary Care Foundations

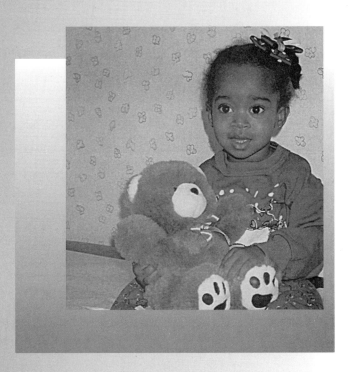

CHAPTER 1

Recommendations for Preventive Care

▬▬▬ INTRODUCTION

Preventive child health care in the United States is guided by standards and recommendations from experts in the field of pediatrics and public health. When the standards are consistently used by all primary care providers, the health of the entire pediatric population is maintained or improved. Thus, the use of appropriate guidelines for all children needs to be incorporated into the organization of health care services in all agencies and by all providers working with children. Of course, the care given each child needs to be modified according to individual factors, but efforts to meet the standards need to be made over time. National guidelines are constantly updated to reflect the changing health care problems of the population, so delivery of services also needs to be modified periodically.

Two sets of guidelines are presented in this section, but others are available from the U.S. Public Health Service and other organizations. Some special sets of guidelines have been developed for children with chronic diseases and conditions such as Down syndrome. The American Academy of Pediatrics (AAP) is a resource for most disease guidelines.

▬▬▬ CHILD HEALTH CARE RECOMMENDATIONS

Recommendations for Preventive Pediatric Health Care from the American Academy of Pediatrics

The AAP provides significant leadership in the development and modification of guidelines for care of children with many conditions (American Academy of Pediatrics Committee on Practice and Ambulatory Medicine, 2000). Table 1-1 represents the AAP's current health care recommendations.

TABLE 1-1

Recommendations for Preventive Pediatric Health Care (RE9535)

Committee on Practice and Ambulatory Medicine, American Academy of Pediatrics (2000)

Each child and family is unique; therefore, these **Recommendations for Preventive Pediatric Health Care** are designed for the care of children who are receiving competent parenting, have no manifestations of any important health problems, and are growing and developing in satisfactory fashion. **Additional visits may become necessary** if circumstances suggest variations from normal.

These guidelines represent a consensus by the Committee on Practice and Ambulatory Medicine in consultation with national committees and sections of the American Academy of Pediatrics. The Committee emphasizes the great importance of **continuity of care** in comprehensive health supervision and the need to avoid **fragmentation of care.**

Part I: Prenatal to 10 Years

AGE [5]	Prenatal [1]	Newborn [2]	INFANCY [4] 2–4 d [3]	By 1 mo	2 mo	4 mo	6 mo	9 mo	12 mo	EARLY CHILDHOOD [4] 15 mo	18 mo	24 mo	3 yr	4 yr	5 yr	MIDDLE CHILDHOOD [4] 6 yr	8 yr	10 yr
HISTORY																		
Initial/Interval	●	●	●	●	●	●	●	●	●	●	●	●	●	●	●	●	●	●
MEASUREMENTS																		
Height and Weight		●	●	●	●	●	●	●	●	●	●	●	●	●	●	●	●	●
Head Circumference		●	●	●	●	●	●	●	●	●	●	●						
Blood Pressure													●	●	●	●	●	●
SENSORY SCREENING																		
Vision		S	S	S	S	S	S	S	S	S	S	S	O[8]	O	O	O	O	O
Hearing		O[7]	S	S	S	S	S	S	S	S	S	S	S	O	O	O	O	O

DEVELOPMENTAL/
BEHAVIORAL ASSESSMENT [8]
PHYSICAL EXAMINATION [10]
PROCEDURES—GENERAL [10]
Hereditary/Metabolic Screening[11]
Immunization[12]
Hematocrit or Hemoglobin[13]
Urinalysis
PROCEDURES—PATIENTS AT
RISK
Lead Screening[16]
Tuberculin Test[17]
Cholesterol Screening[18]
ANTICIPATORY GUIDANCE [21]
Injury Prevention[22]
Violence Prevention[23]
Sleep Positioning Counseling[24]
Nutrition Counseling[25]
DENTAL REFERRAL [26]

Table continued on following page

5

T A B L E 1–1 *Continued*

Part II: 11 to 21 Years

ADOLESCENCE [4]

AGE [5]	11 yr	12 yr	13 yr	14 yr	15 yr	16 yr	17 yr	18 yr	19 yr	20 yr	21 yr
HISTORY											
Initial/Interval	●	●	●	●	●	●	●	●	●	●	●
MEASUREMENTS											
Height and Weight	●	●	●	●	●	●	●	●	●	●	●
Blood Pressure	●	●	●	●	●	●	●	●	●	●	●
SENSORY SCREENING											
Vision	S	O	S	S	O	S	S	O	S	S	S
Hearing	S	O	S	S	O	S	S	O	S	S	S
DEVELOPMENTAL/ BEHAVIORAL ASSESSMENT [8]	●	●	●	●	●	●	●	●	●	●	●
PHYSICAL EXAMINATION [9]	●	●	●	●	●	●	●	●	●	●	●
PROCEDURES— GENERAL [10]											
Immunization [12]	●	●	●	●	●	●	●	●	●	●	●
Hematocrit or Hemoglobin [13]	←———		●[14]	——————————————————————→							
Urinalysis	←————————————————					●[15]	———————————→				
PROCEDURES— PATIENTS AT RISK											
Tuberculin Test [17]	★	★	★	★	★	★	★	★	★	★	★
Cholesterol Screening [18]	★	★	★	★	★	★	★	★	★	★	★
STD Screening [19]	★	★	★	★	★	★	★	★	★	★	★
Pelvic Exam [20]	★	★	★	★	★	★	★	★←——	★[20] ——	★ —→	★
ANTICIPATORY GUIDANCE [21]	●	●	●	●	●	●	●	●	●	●	●
Injury Prevention [22]	●	●	●	●	●	●	●	●	●	●	●
Violence Prevention [23]	●	●	●	●	●	●	●	●	●	●	●
Nutrition Counseling [25]	●	●	●	●	●	●	●	●	●	●	●

Footnotes:
  1. A prenatal visit is recommended for parents who are at high risk, for first-time parents, and for those who request a conference. The prenatal visit should include anticipatory guidance, pertinent medical history, and a discussion of benefits of breastfeeding and planned method of feeding per AAP statement "The Prenatal Visit" (1996).
  2. Every infant should have a newborn evaluation after birth. Breastfeeding should be encouraged and instruction and support offered. Every breastfeeding infant should have an evaluation 48–72 hours after discharge from the hospital to include weight, formal breastfeeding evaluation, encouragement, and instruction as recommended in the AAP statement "Breastfeeding and the Use of Human Milk" (1997).
  3. For newborns discharged in less than 48 hours after delivery per AAP statement "Hospital Stay for Healthy Term Newborns" (1995).
  4. Developmental, psychosocial, and chronic disease issues for children and adolescents may require frequent counseling and treatment visits separate from preventive care visits.

T A B L E 1–1 *Continued*

5. If a child comes under care for the first time at any point on the schedule, or if any items are not accomplished at the suggested age, the schedule should be brought up to date at the earliest possible time.

6. If the patient is uncooperative, rescreen within 6 months.

7. All newborns should be screened per the AAP Task Force on Newborn and Infant Hearing statement "Newborn and Infant Hearing Loss: Detection and Intervention" (1999).

8. By history and appropriate physical examination: if suspicious, by specific objective developmental testing. Parenting skills should be fostered at every visit.

9. At each visit, a complete physical examination is essential, with infant totally unclothed, older child undressed and suitably draped.

10. These may be modified, depending upon entry point into schedule and individual need.

11. Metabolic screening (e.g., thyroid, hemoglobinopathies, PKU, galactosemia) should be done according to state law.

12. Schedule(s) per the Committee on Infectious Diseases, published annually in the January edition of *Pediatrics*. Every visit should be an opportunity to update and complete a child's immunizations.

13. See AAP *Pediatric Nutrition Handbook* (1998) for a discussion of universal and selective screening options. Consider earlier screening for high-risk infants (e.g., premature infants and low-birth-weight infants). See also "Recommendations to Prevent and Control Iron Deficiency in the United States. *MMWR.* 1998:47(RR-3):1–29.

14. All menstruating adolescents should be screened annually.

15. Conduct dipstick urinalysis for leukocytes annually for sexually active male and female adolescents.

16. For children at risk of lead exposure consult the AAP statement "Screening for Elevated Blood Levels" (1998). Additionally, screening should be done in accordance with state law where applicable.

17. TB testing per recommendations of the Committee on Infectious Diseases, published in the current edition of *Red Book: Report of the Committee on Infectious Diseases.* Testing should be done upon recognition of high-risk factors.

18. Cholesterol screening for high-risk patients per AAP statement "Cholesterol in Childhood" (1998). If family history cannot be ascertained and other risk factors are present, screening should be at the discretion of the physician.

19. All sexually active patients should be screened for sexually transmitted diseases (STDs).

20. All sexually active females should have a pelvic examination. A pelvic examination and routine Pap smear should be offered as part of preventive health maintenance between the ages of 18 and 21 years.

21. Age-appropriate discussion and counseling should be an integral part of each visit for care per the AAP *Guidelines for Health Supervision III* (1998).

22. From birth to age 12, refer to the AAP injury prevention program (TIPP*) as described in *A Guide to Safety Counseling in Office Practice* (1994).

23. Violence prevention and management for all patients per AAP Statement "The Role of the Pediatrician in Youth Violence Prevention in Clinical Practice and at the Community Level" (1999).

24. Parents and caregivers should be advised to place healthy infants on their backs when putting them to sleep. Side positioning is a reasonable alternative but carries a slightly higher risk of SIDS. Consult the AAP statement "Positioning and Sudden Infant Death Syndrome (SIDS): Update" (1996).

25. Age-appropriate nutrition counseling should be an integral part of each visit per the AAP *Handbook of Nutrition* (1998).

26. Earlier initial dental examinations may be appropriate for some children. Subsequent examinations as prescribed by dentist.

Table continued on following page

T A B L E 1–1 *Continued*

Key: ● = to be performed
★ = to be performed for patients at risk
S = subjective, by history
O = objective, by a standard testing method
← ● → = the range during which a service may be provided, with the dot indicating the preferred age.
NB: Special chemical, immunologic, and endocrine testing is usually carried out upon specific indications. Testing other than newborn (e.g., inborn errors of metabolism, sickle disease) is discretionary with the physician.

The recommendations in this statement do not indicate an exclusive course of treatment or standard of medical care. Variations, taking into account individual circumstances, may be appropriate.

Recommendations for Preventive Adolescent Health Care from the American Medical Association

The American Medical Association developed the *Guidelines for Adolescent Preventive Services* (GAPS) to address the health care needs of this high-risk population. These are listed in Table 1–2 (Elster and Kuznets, 1994).

T A B L E 1–2

American Medical Association Guidelines for Adolescent Preventive Services (GAPS)

I. Recommendations for delivery of health services
   Recommendation 1: From ages 11 to 21, all adolescents should have an annual routine health visit.
   Visits should address biomedical and psychosocial aspects of health with a preventive focus. A complete physical examination should be performed during three of these visits—11–14 years, 15–17 years, and 18–21 years—unless more frequent examinations are warranted by clinical signs or symptoms.
   Recommendation 2: Preventive services should be age and developmentally appropriate and sensitive to individual and sociocultural differences.
   Recommendation 3: Physicians should establish office policies regarding confidential care for adolescents and how parents will be involved in that care. These policies should be made clear to adolescents and their parents.

T A B L E 1–2 *Continued*

American Medical Association Guidelines for Adolescent Preventive Services (GAPS)

II. Recommendations for health guidance

Recommendation 4: Parents or other adult caregivers of adolescents should receive health guidance at least once during early adolescence, middle adolescence, and late adolescence.

Normative adolescent development (physical, sexual, and emotional), signs and symptoms of disease and emotional stress, parenting behavior that promotes healthy adolescent adjustment, benefits of discussing health-related behavior with their adolescents, planning family activities, and acting as a role model should be discussed with parents or caregivers.

Caregivers or parents should be advised of methods for helping their adolescents avoid potentially harmful behavior such as monitoring and managing the use of motor vehicles, avoiding weapons in the home, removing weapons and potentially lethal medications from homes of adolescents with suicidal intent, and monitoring social and recreational activities to restrict sexual behavior and tobacco, alcohol, and other drug use.

Recommendation 5: All adolescents should receive health guidance annually to promote a better understanding of their physical growth, psychosocial and psychosexual development, and the importance of becoming actively involved in decisions about their health care.

Recommendation 6: All adolescents should receive health guidance annually to promote the reduction of injuries, including avoidance of the use of alcohol or drugs while operating motor vehicles or where impaired judgment may lead to injury, and the use of safety devices, including safety belts, helmets, and appropriate sports protective devices.

Recommendation 7: All adolescents should receive health guidance annually about dietary habits, including the benefits of a healthy diet and ways to achieve a healthy diet and safe weight management.

Recommendation 8: All adolescents should receive health guidance annually about the benefits of exercise and should be encouraged to engage in safe exercise regularly.

Recommendation 9: All adolescents should receive health guidance annually regarding responsible sexual behavior, including abstinence. Latex condoms to prevent STDs and appropriate methods of birth control should be made available with instructions on how to use them effectively. Counseling should include effectiveness of abstinence; HIV transmission, dangers, and prevention by latex condoms; and sensible sexual behavior for those who are not sexually active, as well as for those who are using condoms and birth control appropriately.

Recommendation 10: All adolescents should receive health guidance to promote avoidance of tobacco, alcohol, abusable substances, and anabolic steroids.

Table continued on following page

T A B L E 1–2 *Continued*

American Medical Association Guidelines for Adolescent Preventive Services (GAPS)

III. Recommendations for screening

Recommendation 11: All adolescents should be screened annually for hypertension according to the National Heart, Lung, and Blood Institute Second Task Force on Blood Pressure Control in Children.

Recommendation 12: Selected adolescents should be screened to determine their risk for hyperlipidemia and adult coronary disease, as per the protocol developed by the Expert Panel on Blood Cholesterol Levels in Children and Adolescents. High-risk adolescents include those with serum cholesterol levels greater than 240 mg/dl who are older than 19 years and those with an unknown family history or parents or grandparents with coronary artery disease.

Recommendation 13: All adolescents should be screened annually for eating disorders and obesity by determining weight and stature and asking about body image and dieting patterns.

Recommendation 14: All adolescents should be asked annually about their use of tobacco products, including cigarettes and smokeless tobacco. A pattern of use and a cessation plan should be provided to those who use tobacco.

Recommendation 15: All adolescents should be asked annually about the use of alcohol and other abusable substances and their use of over-the-counter or prescription drugs for nonmedical purposes, including anabolic steroids.

Recommendation 16: All adolescents should be asked annually about involvement in sexual behavior that may result in unintended pregnancy and STDs, including HIV infection.

Recommendation 17: Sexually active adolescents should be screened for STDs.

Recommendation 18: Adolescents at risk for HIV infection should be offered confidential HIV screening with the ELISA and confirmatory tests. Risk factors include intravenous drug use, STD infection, residence in a high-prevalence area, more than one sexual partner in the past 6 months, exchange of sex for drugs or money, male gender and engaging in sex with another male, or a sexual partner at risk for HIV infection.

Recommendation 19: Female adolescents who are sexually active or any female 18 years or older should be screened annually for cervical cancer by use of a Papanicolaou test.

Recommendation 20: All adolescents should be asked annually about behavior or emotions that indicate recurrent or severe depression or a risk of suicide.

Recommendation 21: All adolescents should be asked annually about a history of emotional, physical, or sexual abuse.

Recommendation 22: All adolescents should be asked annually about learning or school problems.

T A B L E 1-2 *Continued*

American Medical Association Guidelines for Adolescent Preventive Services (GAPS)

> *Recommendation 23:* Adolescents should receive a tuberculin skin test if they have been exposed to active tuberculosis, have lived in a homeless shelter, have been incarcerated, have lived in or come from an area with a high prevalence of tuberculosis, or are currently working in a health care setting.

IV. Recommendations for immunizations

> *Recommendation 24:* All adolescents should receive prophylactic immunizations according to the guidelines established by the federally convened Advisory Committee on Immunization Practices.

ELISA = enzyme-linked immunosorbent assay; HIV = human immunodeficiency virus; STD = sexually transmitted disease.

From Elster A, Kuznets N: AMA Guidelines for Adolescent and Preventive Services (GAPS). Baltimore, Williams & Wilkins, 1994.

REFERENCES

American Academy of Pediatrics Committee on Practice and Ambulatory Medicine: Recommendations for preventive pediatric health care. Pediatrics 2000.

Elster A, Kuznets N: AMA Guidelines for Adolescent Preventive Services (GAPS). Baltimore, Williams & Wilkins, 1994, pp 347-480.

CHAPTER 2

Child Assessment in Pediatric Primary Care

▒▒▒ INTRODUCTION

Assessment of the child is the basis for all care—preventive, acute, and chronic. Effective clinicians use the history, physical examination, specific laboratory studies, other tests, and their observations of the child's behavior and interactions with family and others to identify problems and develop appropriate management plans. Contextual elements including the family, cultural background, and community will significantly affect health care decisions made by the child, family, and health care provider and need to be incorporated into the assessment process. Keep in mind that not all data need to be, or indeed can be, collected in one visit. Subjective data may be derived from written health histories, the interview, review of past records, and other sources.

Assessment of the individual client is addressed in the two assessment models below. Assessment of the *family unit* and the *culture of the family* are addressed in the following two chapters.

▒▒▒ ASSESSMENT MODELS

General Assessment Model Incorporating Disease, Daily Living, and Development of the Child

The general assessment model presented in Figure 2-1 incorporates both nursing and medical perspectives on assessment, leading to diagnoses that may be disease-, daily living-, or development-oriented, whereas the more common classic history that most clinicians are familiar with tends to best support decisions in the disease domain.

Problem-Oriented History for Adolescents

Because adolescents are seen independent of their parents and are at high risk for a variety of conditions, a special history form for this age group is recommended. Specific areas need to be adapted to the developmental level, family, culture, and community of the teenager being assessed, as shown in Figure 2-2.

F I G U R E 2–1
Problem-Oriented Health Record for Nurse Practitioners with Consideration of Disease, Daily Living, and Developmental Domains

I. PRELIMINARY INFORMATION
Date:
Name:
Birth date:
Record no:
Corrected age for preterm infant younger than
   2 yr:
Caregiver's name:
Address:
Phone:
Informant, relationship to patient, reliability as historian:

Referral source:

II. DATABASE: SUBJECTIVE INFORMATION
   A. Contextual information
      1. Family/household profile
         People in the home:
         Home environment description:
         Family care issues (time, energy, needs of other family
            members, emotional stresses):
         Family structure issues (marital status):
         Family financial issues:
      2. School/employment:
      3. Agencies involved:
   B. Chief complaint (number each one and then record the subjec-
         tive history for each, according to number)
      1. Concerns:
      2. Present problem history:
                        Illustration continued on following page

F I G U R E 2–1 *Continued*
Problem-Oriented Health Record for Nurse Practitioners with Consideration of Disease, Daily Living, and Developmental Domains

II. DATABASE: SUBJECTIVE INFORMATION Continued
   C. Disease history database
      1. Medical history
         Prenatal:
         Perinatal—birth weight, length, head circumference:
         Past diseases profile:
         Current health problems:

DIAGNOSIS	DATE	PROVIDER	CURRENT STATUS
1.			
2.			
3.			

         Operations/hospitalizations:
         Injuries:
         Allergies:
         Growth:
         Immunizations:
         Medication:
      2. Review of systems
         General:
         Skin:
         Head:
         EENT:
         Respiratory:
         Cardiovascular:
         GU:
         GI:
         MS:
         Neurological:
         Endocrine:
         Hematological:
      3. Family history of diseases
         Mother and father (age, health):
         Mother's pregnancy history:
         Familial diseases:
         Genogram if appropriate:

F I G U R E 2–1 *Continued*

Problem-Oriented Health Record for Nurse Practitioners with Consideration of Disease, Daily Living, and Developmental Domains

II. DATABASE: SUBJECTIVE INFORMATION Continued
  D. Daily living problems database
    1. Health maintenance/health perceptions
       Primary care provider:
         Last visit:
       Dentist:
         Last visit:
       Knowledge and skills for caregiving (self-care):
       Safety measures
         Car:
         Smoke alarm:
         Occupational:
         Guns locked:
         Other:
       Home and health management/resource issues:
    2. Nutrition
       Diet—breakfast, lunch, dinner:
       Supplements:
       Feeding strategies/patterns:
       Restrictions—calories, other:
    3. Activities
       Amount and type of activities:
       Play:
       Limitations/equipment:
    4. Sleep
       Number of hours:
       Disturbances:
    5. Elimination habits
       Urinary:
       Bowel:
    6. Role relationships
       Family patterns:
       Parenting patterns:
       Peers/social support:
       Communication
         Verbal:
         Nonverbal:

Illustration continued on following page

F I G U R E 2–1 *Continued*

Problem-Oriented Health Record for Nurse Practitioners with Consideration of Disease, Daily Living, and Developmental Domains

II. *DATABASE: SUBJECTIVE INFORMATION* Continued

       7. Coping/temperament and discipline
          Substance abuse—alcohol, drugs, tobacco:
       8. Cognitive/perceptual problems
          Cognitive disturbances:
          Hearing deficit:
          Vision deficit:
          Kinesthetic disturbances:
       9. Self-perception/self-concept
          Role identity:
          Self-concept, self-esteem, body image:
     10. Sexual and menstrual patterns:
     11. Values and beliefs/religious patterns:
   E. Developmental issues/problems database
       1. Motor development
          Gross motor development—past milestones and current
            skills:
          Fine motor development—past milestones and current
            skills:
       2. Language development—past milestones and current skills:
       3. Cognitive development—past milestones and current skills:
       4. Social development—past milestones and current skills:
       5. Development test scores:

III. *DATABASE: OBJECTIVE INFORMATION*

  A. Physical examination

Age:	Sex:	Height:	Weight:
HC:	BP:		TPR:

     1. General appearance:
     2. Skin:
     3. Head:
     4. Eyes:
     5. Ears:
     6. Nose:
     7. Mouth:
     8. Neck:
     9. Chest/breasts:
   10. Lungs:
   11. Heart:
   12. Abdomen:
   13. Genitalia:
   14. Anus/rectum:

Problem-Oriented Health Record for Nurse Practitioners with Consideration of Disease, Daily Living, and Developmental Domains

III. DATABASE: OBJECTIVE INFORMATION Continued
    15. MS:
    16. Neurological
       Motor
         Tone:
         Strength:
       Reflexes:
       Cranial nerves:
       Responsiveness:
       Extraneous movements:
       Gait/position:
       Cerebellar, including coordination, balance, nystagmus:
       Primitive reflexes (sensory function):
  B. Screening/laboratory data:
    1. Hct:
    2. Hearing:
    3. Vision:
    4. TB:
    5. Metabolic/newborn screens:
    6. Other:
  C. Data from other disciplines—Physical therapy, occupational therapy, speech therapy, audiology, social work, physician, other:

IV. PROBLEM LIST (USE CLASSIFICATION LIST FOR DIAGNOSES)
Include all chief complaints and problems identified by the nurse practitioner. Categorize all problems identified according to the following groups:
Diseases
Daily living problems
Developmental problems

V. PLAN
For each problem, describe plans according to diagnostic, therapeutic, and/or educational activities:
A. Disease problems
B. Daily living problems
C. Developmental problems
D. Disposition/return appointments

BP = blood pressure; EENT = ear, eye, nose, throat; GI = gastrointestinal; GU = genitourinary; HC = head circumference; Hct = hematocrit; MS = musculoskeletal; TB = tuberculosis; TPR = temperature, pulse, respiration.

From Burns C: A new assessment model and tool for nurse practitioners. J Pediatr Health Care 6:76–79, 1992.

F I G U R E 2-2

Problem-Oriented History for Adolescents

I. DATABASE: SUBJECTIVE INFORMATION

A. Contextual information
1. With whom do you live?
2. In the past year, have there been any changes in your immediate family
such as:
Marriage, separation, divorce
Serious illness or injury
Loss of job
Move/change of address
Change of school
Births, deaths
Other
3. What languages are spoken in your home?

B. Chief complaint

C. Past medical history
1. In the past year, have you had any injury or illness that made you miss school or cut down on activities, or that required medical care?
2. Have you been hospitalized in the past year?
3. Do you have any illnesses or medical conditions?
4. Are you taking any medications?
5. Have you been exposed to tuberculosis in the past year?
6. Have you stayed overnight in a homeless shelter, jail, or detention center in the past year?
7. Girls only: Have you had a period? Date of last one?

D. Review of systems
1. Do you have any concerns about
Height/weight
Blood pressure
Headaches/migraines
Eyes/vision
Hearing/ears/earaches
Nose
Frequent colds
Mouth/teeth (Frequency of tooth brushing, flossing)
Neck/back
Chest pain
Coughing/wheezing
Breasts
Heart
Stomach
Nausea/vomiting
Diarrhea/constipation
Skin (rash, acne, sore, use of sunscreen)

F I G U R E 2–2 *Continued*

Problem-Oriented History for Adolescents

I. DATABASE: SUBJECTIVE INFORMATION Continued

Muscle or joint pain
Frequent or painful urination
Sexual organs/genitals
Menstruation/periods
Future plans/job
Physical or sexual abuse
Masturbation
Cancer or dying
Other (explain)

II. FUNCTIONAL HEALTH DATABASE

A. Health maintenance/health perception
1. Do you usually wear a helmet for rollerblade, bicycle, skateboard, motorcycle, or all-terrain vehicle use?
2. Do you usually wear a seat belt when riding in a car, truck, or van?
3. In the past year, have you been in a car when the driver has been drinking or using drugs?
4. Do you use electric tools or heavy equipment at work or home?
5. Do you have questions or concerns about avoiding accidents or injuries?

B. Nutrition
1. Do you eat from the four food groups almost every day?
2. Do you have any diet/food/appetite concerns?
3. Are you eating in secret?
4. Are you satisfied with your eating patterns?
5. Do you prefer a change in your current weight?
6. Have you tried to lose weight or control weight by vomiting, taking diet pills or laxatives, or starving yourself?
7. Do you have concerns about your weight?

C. Activities
1. Do you watch television or play video games more than 2 hours per day?
2. Are you involved with exercises that make you sweat and breathe hard at least three times per week?
3. What do you do after school?
4. Do you have physical problems that limit your exercise?
5. Do you have questions or concerns about exercise or physical activity?

D. Sleep
1. Do you have trouble sleeping?
2. Do you have trouble with tiredness?

E. Elimination habits
1. Do you sometimes wet the bed?

Illustration continued on following page

F I G U R E 2–2 *Continued*

Problem-Oriented History for Adolescents

II. FUNCTIONAL HEALTH DATABASE Continued

   F. Role relationships

     1. Do you have at least one friend you really like and feel you can talk to?

     2. Do parents or guardian usually listen to you and take your feelings seriously?

     3. Do you and your parents or guardian do things together on a regular basis such as eating meals, attending religious activities, performing chores or errands, playing sports, or watching television?

     4. Is there a lot of tension or conflict in your home?

     5. Do you have questions or concerns about family or friends?

   G. Coping/temperament and discipline

     1. Alcohol

         In the past year, did you or friends get drunk or high on alcoholic beverages?

         Have you ever consumed alcohol and then done any of the following: driven a vehicle, gone swimming or boating, gotten in a fight, used tools or equipment, done something you later regretted?

         In the past year, have you ridden in a car driven by someone who was drinking or using drugs?

         Have you been criticized or gotten in trouble because of drinking?

         Do you have any questions or concerns about alcohol?

     2. Drugs

         Do you or your friends ever use marijuana or street drugs?

         Some drugs can be bought at a store without a doctor's prescription. Do you ever use nonprescription drugs to get to sleep, stay awake, calm down, or get high?

         Have you ever used steroids or supplements without a doctor telling you to do so?

         Do you have any questions or concerns about drugs or drug use?

     3. Tobacco

         Do you or your friends ever smoke cigarettes or use smokeless tobacco?

         Does anyone you live with smoke cigarettes or use smokeless tobacco?

         Do you have any questions or concerns about cigarettes or other tobacco products?

F I G U R E 2–2 *Continued*

Problem-Oriented History for Adolescents

II. FUNCTIONAL HEALTH DATABASE Continued

  4. Emotions

    Have you had fun during the past 2 weeks?

    In general, are you happy with the way things are going for you these days?

    During the past few weeks, have you often felt sad or down with nothing to look forward to?

    Have you ever seriously thought about killing yourself, made a plan to kill yourself, or actually tried to kill yourself?

    Do you think counseling would help you or someone in your family?

    Do you have any questions or concerns about physical, sexual, or emotional abuse?

  5. Weapons/violence

    Do you or does anyone you live with have a gun, rifle, shotgun, or other firearm in your home?

    In the past year, have you ever carried a gun, knife, razorblade, club, or other weapon?

    Have you been in a physical fight during the past 3 months?

    Are guns or violence a problem in your neighborhood?

    When you are angry, do you ever get violent?

    Do you have any questions or concerns about violence or your safety?

 H. Cognitive/perceptual problems

  In general, do you like school? Why?

  Are your grades this year better or worse than the year before?

  What are your usual grades?

  Have you ever had to repeat a grade in school?

  Do you cut classes or skip school?

  How many days of school have you missed this year?

  Have you ever been suspended or dropped out of school?

  Do you have any questions or concerns about school or your learning?

 I. Self-perception/self-concept

  1. Do you have any concerns about the size or shape of your body or your physical appearance?

  2. What do you like about yourself?

  3. What do you do best?

  4. If you could, what would you change about your life or yourself?

Illustration continued on following page

Problem-Oriented History for Adolescents

II. FUNCTIONAL HEALTH DATABASE *Continued*
 J. Sexual and menstrual
  1. Do you date?
  2. Do you or your friends have sexual intercourse?
  3. Do you think you might be gay, lesbian, homosexual, or bisexual?
  4. Have you ever been told that you have a sexually transmitted disease such as gonorrhea, genital herpes, chlamydia, trichomonas, syphilis, hepatitis, genital warts, AIDS, or HIV infection?
  5. Do you have any questions or concerns about sex or relationships?
  6. Are you worried about getting pregnant (girls) or do you worry about getting someone pregnant (boys)?
  7. Have you ever been forced to do something sexual that you didn't want to do?
  8. Do you practice abstinence?
  9. Do you want information or supplies to prevent pregnancy or sexually transmitted diseases, including HIV?
 K. Values and beliefs/religious
  1. Are you involved with any religious groups or activities on a regular basis?

III. DEVELOPMENT DATABASE
Throughout the history, listen for data that allow you to assess the following areas (see Developmental Management of Adolescents, Chapter 8):
 A. Motor development
  1. All teens should be active and skilled in a variety of physical activities and sports.
  2. Fine motor development should also be mature. Special arts/crafts or occupational activities may be learned.
 B. Cognitive development
  1. Early adolescents are still concrete and generally present rather than future oriented. Questions can be answered quite literally.
  2. Middle adolescents can use and understand if-then statements. They are able to understand long-term consequences and think of the future. They might challenge many ideas and rules with their newfound skills in logic and reasoning.
  3. Late adolescents are able to consider options before making decisions, engage in sophisticated moral reasoning, and use principles to guide their decisions.

F I G U R E 2–2 *Continued*

Problem-Oriented History for Adolescents

III. *DEVELOPMENT DATABASE* Continued
  C. Social development
    1. Early adolescents are egocentric in thinking. They can vacillate between childish and mature behavior, especially around their parents. Their peers are usually of the same sex. Group activities are the norm.
    2. Middle adolescents are concerned with their identity within society and less concerned with their sexual identity unless they are struggling with recognizing their homosexuality. They tend to distance themselves from parents, spend less time at home, and increasingly challenge parental control. Cliques or friends prevail, with only a few close friends. Physical intimacy can occur during this stage, and romantic partners are common.
    3. Late adolescents have distanced themselves from parents and then re-established relationships with family on a new basis of independence. Romantic, emotional intimacy appears.
  D. School/vocational development
    1. Early adolescents are usually adjusting to the expectations of middle school. Setting priorities and completing homework independently can be a challenge. Future goals are often unrealistic and change frequently.
    2. Middle adolescents are entering high school and beginning to develop an awareness that their performance in school will affect their future options for work and/or college. They do not usually have specific ideas about future vocations in mind.
    3. Late adolescents are making decisions about vocations, college, working, or entering the military.

Adapted from American Medical Association, Department of Adolescent Health: *Guidelines for Adolescent Preventive Services (GAPS) User's Manual.* Chicago, American Medical Association, 1994; other sources.

CHAPTER 3

Family Assessment in Pediatric Primary Care

Families have more effect on their children's development and well-being than any other entity. It is in the family that children can develop positive feelings of security and self-esteem and gain knowledge for independent living. Families offer health protection, promotion, and care; they transmit cultural values and beliefs and provide a safe, healthful, developmentally appropriate environment that cannot be fully duplicated by other units of society.

When the family is healthy—members support one another so that all are adequately cared for, respected, and included—children are more likely to grow to their full potential. If the family is dysfunctional, long-term effects that may never be overcome will be seen in children.

Family assessment is an important part of caring for children. It is essential that clinicians assess and manage the family issues of the children for whom they care. Table 3-1 provides a framework for basic family assessment that may uncover family problems. As for any other pediatric health care problem, if issues are identified, they must be explored and a diagnosis, management plan, and evaluation established.

T A B L E 3–1

Family Assessment Topics

ASSESSMENT AREA	ASSESSMENT TOPICS
Family composition	Persons identified as family members
	Household members and relationships
Current family situation	Recent major stresses or family changes
	Anticipated changes for the near future
Extended family context	Birth dates of grandparents
	Birthplaces of grandparents
	Description of grandparents' families
	Current location of grandparents or date/cause of death(s)
	Development of relationships and marriage of grandparents
Demographic data	Births, deaths, adoptions, marriages
	Separations, divorces
	Significant illnesses or family events
	Culture/ethnicity, religion
	Education, occupations
Historical perspectives	Knowledge of timing and repetition of significant family events or behaviors such as teen pregnancies, abuse, and alcoholism
Family relationships/parenting	Decision-maker(s) related to health care of children
	Parenting style of each parent
	Primary source of enjoyment in each child (what does the family appreciate about the child?)
	Family activities and frequency
	Processes for major family decisions
	Primary family support person for the child
	Family support processes
	Family adaptation processes
	Family nurturing processes for development of each member
	Source of parenting support for parent and reason for choice of that support person
Divorced family areas	Residence of each parent
	Custodial and visitation agreements
	Frequency and quality of contact child has with each parent
	Child's adaptation to the divorce

CHAPTER 4

Cultural Perspectives for Primary Health Care

Culture affects the way families and children perceive and interact with the world at large. Health perspectives and beliefs, health habits, and decision-making about health care all are affected by a family's culture. When families appear "noncompliant" or use health care resources in what appear to be inappropriate ways, cultural differences should be considered as a possible factor. Health care providers bring their own cultural values and beliefs to their work, and their culture may conflict with that of their clients. Communication with patients and families can be impaired if the patient's cultural perspectives are not valued and understood by the clinician.

Table 4-1 provides information about some cultural characteristics of major U.S. population groups. To avoid stereotyping, the clinician must validate each family's perspectives in relation to the generally understood characteristics of the cultural group as a whole. Age, education, length of time in the United States, experiences and life events, and other factors may significantly modify beliefs and health care practices. Failure to validate cultural perspectives with families can result in misunderstanding and, ultimately, less than optimal health care outcomes.

A few selected questions can help the clinician understand the family's essential health beliefs in relation to a problem at hand. These questions are listed in Table 4-2.

Communication with patients and families is disrupted when the clinician and family do not speak the same language. Use of interpreters familiar with both languages is essential to bridge the communication gap. Working effectively with interpreters will maximize the clinician's effectiveness. Some ideas for working with interpreters are listed in Table 4-3.

TABLE 4-1
Cultural Perspectives of Major U.S. Population Groups

GROUP	CULTURAL IDENTITY	FAMILY STRUCTURE	TIME/SPATIAL PERSPECTIVES	HEALTH PERSPECTIVES	LANGUAGE/ COMMUNICATION STYLE
White, middle-class American	Blend of European cultures. Strong work ethic. Entrepreneurism. Individualism vs. collectivistic, community views.	Nuclear or single-parent family most common. Divorce with joint custody common. Day care for working-parent families.	Time conscious, future oriented. Desire personal space.	Scientific perspectives common vs. divine intervention. Primary prevention valued. Illness in child strains working-parent households.	Verbal cues most important. Touch acceptable. Privacy and confidentiality important.
Poor American	May affiliate with African-American, Hispanic, Native-American, or white cultures.	Single-mother household most common. Runaway teenagers may have no family unit.	Present orientation. Spatial needs vary.	Fatalistic view of health and illness. Folk healers or remedies may be used. Health care often delayed.	Hostility, mistrust of larger society makes communication difficult.

Table continued on following page

T A B L E 4-1 Continued

Cultural Perspectives of Major U.S. Population Groups

GROUP	CULTURAL IDENTITY	FAMILY STRUCTURE	TIME/SPATIAL PERSPECTIVES	HEALTH PERSPECTIVES	LANGUAGE/ COMMUNICATION STYLE
African-American	Black identity with diversity by social class, age, sex, socialization, life experiences.	50% female-headed households. Extended family important with strong kinship ties.	Middle class is time conscious, future oriented. Lower class tends to be more present oriented. Spatial needs vary with greater space for dominant culture.	Life is a continuous mind/body process. Nature's forces may bring illness. Scientific perspectives common to many.	Black English common. Nonverbal cues and context important.
Hispanic	Fastest-growing minority, with many young families. Identity varies with country of origin. Collectivism more important than individualism.	Large, extended families.	Present to future oriented. Close spatial distances.	Health or illness related to divine forces. May not use preventive services. Use of folk healers and remedies common.	Nonverbal cues and context important. Usually Spanish languages with variations by country of origin. Modesty, privacy, politeness valued.

| Asian-American | Five distinct ethnic groups (Chinese, Japanese, Korean, Vietnamese, Pacific Islander) plus others. Most value harmony with nature, family heritage, consideration of others. Achievement and education important. Collectivism more important than individualism. | Family-centered. May be male dominated. Extended family important. | Future orientation increases with assimilation into U.S. culture. Space needs tend to be modest. | Health is a balance with nature. Evil spirits may cause illness. Folk healers and remedies may be used. Scientific perspectives prevail among more acculturated and higher socioeconomic status. | Verbal communication is formal with context; nonverbal cues important. Politeness valued. Privacy important. |

Table continued on following page

T A B L E 4–1 *Continued*

Cultural Perspectives of Major U.S. Population Groups

GROUP	CULTURAL IDENTITY	FAMILY STRUCTURE	TIME/SPATIAL PERSPECTIVES	HEALTH PERSPECTIVES	LANGUAGE/ COMMUNICATION STYLE
Native-American	Identity is with the tribe. Value harmony with nature. Emotional attachments to land and nature may be strong. Collectivism more important than individualism.	Large, extended families on reservations. Elders revered. Autonomy, self-initiation, cooperation highly valued.	Present orientation with reverence for the past. Time not measured with detail. Family zone very private.	Health is a balance with nature. Illness caused by imbalance or a manifestation of bad thoughts or anger. Folk healers and remedies common.	Nonverbal cues and context important. Slow, deliberate communication with participation of family members. Minimal eye contact preferred.

Russian-American	Identity with specific country. Strong work ethic, individualistic. Religious expression varies.	Extended, multigenerational families. Patriarchal.	Future orientation with reverence for the past. Time valued.	Low expectations for health care services and experiences with authoritarian providers. May use folk remedies along with professional advice.	Russian most common, but many have a second language. Open communication in family but less eye contact and openness in public.
Arab-American	Identity is with the specific country.	Family and close friends share intense devotion to one another. Patriarchal. Extended family. Mistrust of those outside the family circle must be overcome.	Present orientation. Time may not be measured with detail. Close spatial distances acceptable.*	Western medicine respected, but other disease etiologies may be considered related to divine wishes, Evil Eye, and others.	Context and nonverbal cues important. Relationships to be established before important ideas are communicated. Sexual topics are extremely private and not easily discussed.

*Spatial distance = distance between people in social situations.

31

T A B L E 4–2

Identifying Family Perspectives on Health Areas

- What is the problem called?
- What does the family believe is happening and why?
- What aspects of the problem are important to the family?
- Why do you think the problem started when it did?
- What do you think the problem does?
- How severe is the problem?
- What treatment should the patient receive?
- What results do you hope for?
- What do you fear most about the illness?
- How has the problem affected the family?
- What are the family's goals for health care?
- How can the problem be avoided in the future?
- What relief measures have been tried?
- Who has been consulted for help (besides dominant culture health care providers)?
- What has helped in the past?

Includes some items from Kleinman A: The Illness Narratives: Suffering, Healing, and the Human Condition. New York, Basic Books, 1988.

TABLE 4-3

Interpreter's and Provider's Roles

INTERPRETER'S ROLE

■ Be familiar with the client's culture as well as language. Act as a "cultural broker" as much as possible, helping both the client and clinician to understand the other's views, beliefs, and goals for the child.

■ Sit or stand behind provider so that provider can maintain eye contact with client. Sit behind a screen if privacy is required.

■ Ensure that the provider is apprised of whole statements from client, including seemingly extraneous data.

■ Facilitate the process of explaining pathophysiology, instructions for home management, assessment of patient, and parental level of understanding.

■ Write instructions for the family in their language, and review them again before the family leaves.

PROVIDER'S ROLE

■ Do not use family member as interpreter, if possible.

■ Don't rely on the interpreter entirely. Simple, courteous phrases can set a positive tone. Having some knowledge of the language can facilitate evaluation of the interpreter's work and allow preparation of responses as the client's comments are spoken.

■ Prepare the interpreter by prefacing the dialogue with goals and issues to be addressed in the conversation.

■ Stop after about 30 seconds of speech to allow the interpreter time to translate.

■ Address the client, not the interpreter.

■ Speak slowly and clearly. Avoid jargon. Avoid double negatives, and use short declarative statements.

■ Don't expect the length of interpreter remarks to match the phrases to be translated.

■ Express ideas in several different ways.

■ Don't expect perfection.

Management of Development

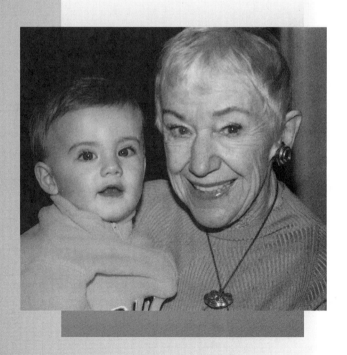

CHAPTER 5

Developmental Management in Pediatric Primary Care

The development of young children is a delight to behold. They change and learn quickly, with novel behaviors emerging almost daily. Understanding the expected behaviors at any age as well as the predicted trajectory for change is essential for the primary care provider's work with children and their families. Development is complex, affected by temperament as well as genetic, environmental, social, physiological, and cultural factors. The clinician needs to understand interactions among the various factors to know whether the child is progressing normally or is experiencing difficulties that merit intervention. Parents need to understand their child's development to maximize the effectiveness of their parenting behaviors, to interpret the cues their child is giving about needs and desires, to communicate their affection, and to plan for the next stage. Table 5-1 compares the developmental stages of children as presented by the early developmental theorists Freud (1938) Kohlberg (1969), Piaget (see Ginsburg and Potter, 1969), and Erikson (1964).

Characteristics of temperament, outlined in Table 5-2, strongly influence the interactions children have with their environment, parents, siblings, other children, and adults. By assessing for and discussing characteristics of temperament, the nurse practitioner can help parents understand and adapt to their child's unique qualities.

Parent-child interactions can be put at risk by stressors faced by the family. The nurse practitioner must be alert to signs that parents are having difficulty fulfilling their role or that children are not receiving the care needed for optimum growth and development. Table 5-3 outlines red flags related to parenting that warrant more in-depth assessment by the pediatric provider. Red flags relating to children in specific age groups are found in following chapters.

Continued on page 42

TABLE 5-1

Comparison of Early Developmental Theorists

AGE	FREUD	KOHLBERG		PIAGET		ERIKSON	
		Stages	Stages/Substages	Characteristics		Psychological Crisis	Themes
0–12 mo	Oral stage	"Amoral," preconventional level	1: Punishment and obedience	Sensorimotor stage	Innate infant reflexes	Trust vs. mistrust	To get; to give in return
				1. Reflexive stage: 0–1 mo			
				2. Primary circular stage: 1–4 mo	Repetitive responses		
				3. Secondary circular stage: 4–8 mo	Outward-directed behaviors		
				4. Coordination of secondary circular stage: 8–12 mo	Object permanence and goal-directed behaviors		
12–18 mo				5. Tertiary circular reactions stage: 12–18 mo	Causality and object permanence through several steps	Autonomy vs. shame	To hold on; to let go
18–36 mo	Anal stage	Stages 1 and 2, conventional level	2: Instrumental realistic orientation	6. Mental combinations stage: 18–24 mo	Memory used for problem-solving		

Age	Freud	Kohlberg		Piaget		Erikson	Purpose
3–6 yr	Oedipal stage	Stages 1–3	3: Interpersonal acceptance of "nice" girl and "good" boy social concept	Preoperational stage 1. Preconceptual stage: 2–4 yr	Increased use of symbols, especially language; representational thought, egocentrism, assimilation, and symbolic play	Initiative vs. guilt	To make things; to play
				2. Intuitive stage: 4–7 yr	Increased symbolic functioning, language, decreasing egocentricity, imitation of reality		
6–11 yr	Latency stage	Stages 2–5	4: The "law and order" orientation 5: Social contract and utilitarian orientation	Concrete operational stage	Flexible thought: understands rules of reversibility and decentration, conservation, and identity Declining egocentrism: ability to understand another's perspective Logical reasoning: understands concepts of relation, ordering, conservation; able to classify objects Social cognition: improved sense of equality and justice	Industry vs. inferiority	To make things; to complete

Table continued on following page

39

TABLE 5-1 Continued
Comparison of Early Developmental Theorists

	KOHLBERG		PIAGET		ERIKSON	
AGE	FREUD	Stages	Stages/Substages	Characteristics	Psychological Crisis	Themes
12–17 yr	Adolescence (Oedipus complex) Stages 4-6	6: Universal ethical principle orientation	Formal operational stage	Development of logical thinking, the ability to work with abstract ideas; able to synthesize and integrate concepts into larger schemes	Identity vs. role confusion	To be oneself; to share being oneself or not being oneself
17-30 yr	Young adult Stages 4-6		Formal operational stage		Intimacy vs. isolation	To lose and find oneself in another

T A B L E 5–2

Characteristics of Temperament

TEMPERAMENT CHARACTERISTIC	DESCRIPTION
Activity	What is the child's activity level? Is the child moving all the time he or she is awake, some of the time, or rarely?
Rhythmicity	How predictable is the child's sleep/wake pattern, feeding schedule, and elimination pattern?
Approach/withdrawal	What is the child's response when presented with something new such as a new toy, an experience, or new person? Does he or she immediately approach or turn away?
Adaptability	How quickly does the child get used to new things? Quickly or not at all?
Threshold of response	How much stimulation does the child require for calming? A quiet voice and touch or more intense, loud voice or firm grasp?
Intensity of reaction	Are the child's responses (crying or laughing) very subtle or extremely intense?
Quality of mood	Is the child's mood usually outgoing, happy, joyful, pleasant or unfriendly, withdrawn, or quiet?
Distractability	How easily is the child distracted by outside disturbance such as a phone ringing, TV, siblings?
Attention span and persistence	How long will the child continue to play with a particular toy or engage in a certain activity? Does this continue even when there are distractions?

T A B L E 5–3

Parenting Red Flags

MODERATE CONCERN	EXTREME CONCERN
Disinclination to separate from child, or prematurely hastening separation	Extreme depression and withdrawal; rejection of child
Signs of despondency, apathy, or hostility	Intense hostility; aggression toward child
Fearful, dependent, apprehensive	Uncontrollable fears, anxieties, guilt
Disinterested in or rejecting of infant or child	Complete inability to function in family role
Overly critical, mocking, and censuring of child; tendency to undermine child's confidence	Severe moralistic prohibition of child's independent strivings
Inconsistent in discipline or control; erratic in behavior	Domestic abuse or violence in the home
Very restrictive and overly moralistic environment	Self-destructive behaviors: alcohol or drug abuse

REFERENCES

Erikson E: Insight and Responsibility. New York, Norton, 1964.

Freud S: An Outline of Psychoanalysis. London, Hogarth, 1938.

Ginsburg H, Opper S: Piaget's Theory of Intellectual Development. Englewood Cliffs, NJ, Prentice-Hall, 1969.

Kohlberg L: Stage and sequence: The cognitive-development approach to socialization. *In* Goslin D (ed): Handbook of Socialization: Theory and Research. New York, Rand McNally, 1969, pp 347–480.

CHAPTER 6

Developmental Management of Infants, Toddlers, and Preschoolers

Development of young children proceeds in several areas at once. Children's maturation is generally assessed in four major fields: fine and gross motor, cognitive, language, and social. The major milestones of motor development are summarized in Table 6-1.

Acquisition of speech and language is a major achievement for toddlers and preschoolers; precursors for their language skills occur in infancy. *Speech* and *language* are not synonymous terms, the former referring to the production of sounds and the latter to development of a system of communication with others. Major milestones for both are given in Table 6-2. The development of language primarily depends on cognitive development. Understanding and using a system of rules to guide word construction and modification, sentence construction, nonverbal communication, and all the nuances of learning to communicate with others requires more of the infant and young child than any other cognitive task. Cognitive development is essential to language development.

The development of speech sounds is quite predictable. Understanding which sounds should be pronounced clearly at which ages helps the clinician identify the child with true speech problems and/or reassure the parents who have many questions. Figure 6-1 gives information about the median age of customary sound acquisitions. Intelligibility is an associated area that must be assessed. Table 6-3 provides some guidelines in this area.

Assuming that the clinician has a good understanding of developmental milestones, it is useful when evaluating children's development to consider behaviors that are outside normal limits. Table 6-4 summarizes some of the developmental behaviors outside normal limits for infants, and Table 6-5 provides similar information for toddlers and preschoolers.

TABLE 6-1

Fine Motor and Gross Motor Developmental Milestones for Infants and Preschoolers

AGE	FINE MOTOR MOVEMENT	ORAL MOVEMENT	GROSS MOTOR MOVEMENT
Birth	Flexion	Suckling tongue movements, extension-retraction of tongue, up and down jaw movements, low approximation of lips	Momentary head control when held sitting
1 mo	Extension, nondirected swipes	Rooting	Turns head when prone
4 mo	Directed swipes, corralling, reaching		Sits with support, rolls over, head steady in sitting
4–5 mo	Ulnar-palmar grasp		"Swims" in prone position, no head lag
6–7 mo	Radial-palmar grasp, raking	Sucking with negative oral cavity pressure, rhythmical jaw movements, firm approximation of lips	Sits independently, rocks on hands and knees, free headlift in supine
7–8 mo	Radial digital grasp	Phasic bite reflex, rhythmical bite and release pattern	Supports weight standing, bounces when held
7–9 mo	Scissors grasp	Munching, early chewing	Sits alone well, may crawl
9–10 mo	Voluntary release		Cruises, pivots while seated, pulls to stand
12 mo	Picks up pellet with pincer grasp	Chewing with spreading/rolling tongue movements, tongue lateralization, rotary jaw movements, controlled sustained bite	Walks with one hand held, stands alone momentarily

Age		
18 mo	Makes tower of four cubes, imitates scribbling, dumps pellet, puts blocks in large holes, drinks from cup with little spilling, can take off socks	Directed throwing, walks well independently, climbs into adult chair
24 mo	Makes tower of seven cubes, does circular scribbling, folds paper once imitatively, turns doorknobs, turns pages one at a time, unbuttons or unzips large fasteners, puts on coat with assistance	Throws overhand, runs well, kicks ball, up and down stairs 2 feet/step
30 mo	Makes tower of nine cubes, makes vertical and horizontal strokes, imitates circle, buttons large button, uses fork in fist, twists jar lids	Jumps off ground with both feet
36 mo	Makes tower of 10 cubes, imitates bridge of three cubes, copies circle, snips with scissors, can brush teeth but not well, puts shoes on feet	Broad jumps, walks up stairs alternating feet, may pedal tricycle, balance one foot 2–3 sec
48 mo	Copies bridge from model, copies cross and square, cuts curved line with scissors, dresses self, strings small beads	Pedals tricycle, runs smoothly, hops on one foot, catches large ball
60 mo	May print name; copies triangle, opens lock with key, bathes self, cuts out simple shapes, pours from small pitcher	Walks downstairs alternating feet, catches bounced ball, skips, stands on one foot 7–8 sec

Data from many developmental tests.

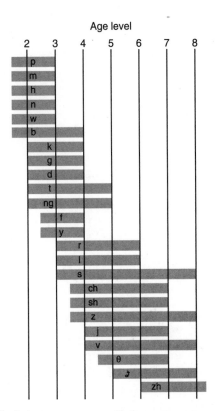

F I G U R E 6-1
Average age estimates for development of consonant sounds from ages 1 to 7 years. (From Van Riper C, Erickson RL: Speech Correction: An Introduction to Speech Pathology and Audiology, 9th ed, p 98. Needham Heights, MA. © 1996 by Allyn & Bacon. Reprinted by permission.)

TABLE 6–2

Speech and Language Milestones: Areas for Assessment

AGE	RECEPTIVE LANGUAGE	EXPRESSIVE LANGUAGE
0–3 mo	Attends to voice, turns head or eyes Startles to loud sounds Quiets in response to voice Smiles, coos, gurgles to voice	Undifferentiated but strong cry Coos and gurgles Single-syllable repetition /G/, /K/, /H/, and /NG/ appear
3–6 mo	Actively seeks sound source May look in response to name Responses may vary to angry or happy voice	Increased babbling, vocal play Laughs Increased repetitive babbling (gaga) Vocalizes to toys Spontaneous smile to verbal play Increased intensity and nasal tone Vocalizes to removal of toy Experiments with own voice
6–9 mo	May look at family member when named Inhibits to "no" Begins interest in pictures when named Individual words begin to take on meaning	Babbles tunefully Increased sound combinations Uses /M/, /N/, /B/, /D/, /T/ Initiates sounds such as click or kiss Uses nonspecific "mama" and "dada"
9–12 mo	Will give toy on request Understands simple commands Turns head to own name Understands "hot," "where's . . .?" Responds with gestures to "bye-bye"	Increased imitating efforts Has one word with specific reference Accompanies vocalizations with gestures Jargon increases Imitates animal sounds
12–18 mo	Follows simple one-step commands Understands new words weekly Increased interest in named pictures Differentiates environmental sounds Points to familiar objects and body parts when named Understands simple questions Begins to distinguish "you" from "me"	All vowels, many consonants present Increased use of true words Jargon is sentence-like Shows "no" behavior Names a few pictures 10+ words Can imitate nonspeech sounds (cough, tongue click)

Table continued on following page

T A B L E 6-2 *Continued*

Speech and Language Milestones: Areas for Assessment

AGE	RECEPTIVE LANGUAGE	EXPRESSIVE LANGUAGE
18–24 mo	Follows two-step commands Vocabulary increases rapidly Enjoys simple stories Recognizes pronouns	Names some body parts Imitates two-word combinations Dramatic increase in vocabulary Speech combines jargon and words Names self Answers some questions Begins to combine words
24–30 mo	Understands prepositions "in" and "on" Seems to understand most of what is said Understands more reasoning ("when you are done, then . . .") Identifies object when given function (wear on feet, cook on)	Jargon reduced Two- to three-word sentences Repeats two digits Increased use of pronouns Asks simple questions Joins in songs and nursery rhymes
30–36 mo	Listens to adult conversations Understands preposition "under" Can categorize items by function Begins to recognize colors Begins to take turns Understands "big/little," "boy/girl"	Can repeat simple phrases and sentences Answers questions (wear on feet, to bed) Repeats three digits Uses regular plurals Can help tell simple story
36–42 mo	Understands fast Understands prepositions "behind" and "in front" Responds to simple three-part commands Increasing understanding of adjectives and plurals Understands "just one"	Understands and answers (cold, tired, hungry) Mostly three- to four-word sentences Gives full name Begins rote counting Begins to relate events Lots of questions, some beginning prepositions ("on," "in")

T A B L E 6–2 *Continued*

Speech and Language Milestones: Areas for Assessment

AGE	RECEPTIVE LANGUAGE	EXPRESSIVE LANGUAGE
42–48 mo	Recognizes coins Begins to understand future and past tenses Understands number concepts—more than one	Uses prepositions Tells stories Can give function of objects Repeats larger than six-word sentences Repeats four digits Gives age Good intelligibility
48–60 mo	Responds to three-action commands	Asks "how" questions Answers verbally to questions like "How are you?" Uses past and future tenses Can use conjunctions to string words and phrases together

Data from D. Anderson, Ph.D., Speech Pathologist, Portland, OR, using items from a variety of developmental tests.

T A B L E 6–3

Speech Intelligibility Milestones

AGE	GENERAL INTELLIGIBILITY
1–2 yr	Words used may be no more than 25% intelligible to unfamiliar listener Jargon near 18 mo is nearly 100% unintelligible Improvement noted at 21–24 mo
2–3 yr	Words about 65% intelligible by 2 yr; 70–80% in context by 3 yr Many individual sounds faulty, but total context generally understood Some incomprehensibility due to faulty sentence structure
3–4 yr	Speech usually 90–100% in context Individual sounds still faulty, and some trouble with sentence structure
4–5 yr	Speech is intelligible in context, although some sounds still faulty
5–6 yr	Good intelligibility

T A B L E 6-4

Developmental Red Flags: Newborns and Infants
Part I: Psychosocial, Emotional, Cognitive, Visual, Language, and Hearing Skills

AGE	PSYCHOSOCIAL/EMOTIONAL SKILLS	COGNITIVE AND VISUAL ABILITIES	LANGUAGE AND HEARING
Newborn/1 mo	Diffuse nonverbal cues Poor state transitions Irritable Withdrawn or depressed Lack of consistent, safe child care	Doll's eyes No red light reflex Poor alert state No visual tracking Not able to fix on face or object	No startle to sound or sudden noises No quieting to voice High-pitched cry Does not turn to voice, rattle, or bell No sounds, coos, or squeals
3 mo	Lack of social smile	Not visually alert	No babbling
6 mo	No smiles No response to play Solemn appearance	Does not reach for objects Does not look at caregiver	Does not respond to voice, bell, rattle, or loud noises, even with startle Lack of single or combined sounds
9 mo	Intense stranger anxiety or absent stranger anxiety Does not seek comfort from caregiver when stressed	No visual awareness No reaching out for toys No toy exploration visually or orally	Does not respond to name or voice Does not respond to any words
12 mo	No response to game playing No response to reading or interactive activities Withdrawn or solemn	Does not visually follow activities in the environment	Inability to localize to sound Not imitating speech sounds Not using two or three words Does not point

T A B L E 6-4

Developmental Red Flags: Newborns and Infants
Part 2: Physical Development, Fine Motor Skills, and Gross Motor Skills

AGE	PHYSICAL DEVELOPMENT (AUTONOMIC STABILITY/ RHYTHMICITY/SLEEP/ TEMPERAMENT)	FINE MOTOR (FEEDING/SELFCARE)	GROSS MOTOR (STRENGTH/COORDINATION)
Newborn/1 mo	Lack of return to birth weight by 2-wk exam Poor coordination of suck/swallow Tachypnea/bradycardia with feedings Poor habituation to external stimuli	Hands held fisted Absent or asymmetric palmar grasp	Asymmetric movements Hyper- or hypotonia Asymmetric primitive reflexes
3 mo	Less than 1 lb weight gain in 1 mo Head circumference increasing greater than 2 percentile lines on growth curve or showing no increase in size Continuing problems with poor suck/swallow Difficulty with regulation of sleep/wake cycle	Hands fisted with oppositional thumb No hand-to-mouth activity	Asymmetric movements Hyper- or hypotonia Does not attempt to raise head when on stomach

Table continued on following page

Developmental Red Flags: Newborns and Infants
Part 2: Physical Development, Fine Motor Skills, and Gross Motor Skills

AGE	PHYSICAL DEVELOPMENT (AUTONOMIC STABILITY/ RHYTHMICITY/SLEEP/ TEMPERAMENT)	FINE MOTOR (FEEDING/SELFCARE)	GROSS MOTOR (STRENGTH/COORDINATION)
6 mo	Less than double birth weight Head circumference showing no increase Continuation of poor feeding or sleep regulation Difficulty with self-calming	Does not reach for objects, hold rattle, hold hands together Does not grasp at clothes	Persistent primitive reflexes Does not attempt to sit with support Head lag with pull-to-sit Scissoring
9 mo	Parent control issues with feeding or sleep	Does not feed self Does not sit in high chair Does not eat solid food Does not pick up toys with one hand	Does not sit even in tripod position No lateral prop reflex Asymmetric crawl, hand movements, or other movements
12 mo	Less than triple birth weight Losing more than 2 percentile lines on growth curve for weight, length, or head circumference Poor sleep/wake cycle Extreme inability to separate from parent	Persistent mouthing Does not attempt to feed self or hold cup Not able to hold toy in each hand or transfer objects	Does not pull self to stand Does not move around the environment to explore

TABLE 6-5
Developmental Red Flags: Toddlers and Preschoolers

AGE	GROWTH/ RHYTHMICITY/ SLEEP/ TEMPERAMENT	PSYCHOSOCIAL/ EMOTIONAL SKILLS	COGNITIVE AND VISUAL ABILITIES	LANGUAGE AND HEARING	FINE MOTOR (FEEDING/SELF-CARE)	GROSS MOTOR (STRENGTH/ COORDINATION)
15 mo	No nighttime ritual Difficulty with transitions Parents express concern about temperament or control issues	Problems with attachment to caregiver	Lack of object permanence	Lack of consonant production Does not imitate words No gestures/ pointing	No self-feeding	No attempts at walking
18 mo	Poor sleep schedule Problems with control/behavior	Does not pull person to show something	Primary play: mouthing of toys No finger exploration of objects Lack of imitation	Unable to follow simple directions (e.g., "no," "jump")	Does not try to scribble spontaneously Unable to use spoon	Not yet walking or frequently falls when walking

Table continued on following page

T A B L E 6–5 Continued

Developmental Red Flags: Toddlers and Preschoolers

AGE	GROWTH/ RHYTHMICITY/ SLEEP/ TEMPERAMENT	PSYCHOSOCIAL/ EMOTIONAL SKILLS	COGNITIVE AND VISUAL ABILITIES	LANGUAGE AND HEARING	FINE MOTOR (FEEDING/SELF-CARE)	GROSS MOTOR (STRENGTH/ COORDINATION)
24 mo	Less than 4 times birth weight or falling off growth curve Poor sleep schedule Awakens at night; unable to put self back to sleep	Absent symbolic play No evidence of parallel play Displays destructive behaviors Always clings to mother	Unable to dump pellet from bottle	Use of noncommunicative speech (echolalia, rote phrases) Unable to identify five pictures Unable to name body parts No jargon History of >10 episodes of otitis media	Unable to stack four to five blocks Still eating pureed foods Unable to imitate scribbles on paper	Unable to walk downstairs holding a rail Persistent waddle walk Persistent toe-walking

Age						
30 mo	Resistance to regular bedtime Beginning behavior issues	Problems with biting, hitting playmates, parents	Does not try to get toy with stick	No two-word sentences Unable to name some body parts	Unable to feed self Unable to tower six blocks Unable to imitate circle shape Unable to imitate vertical stroke	Unable to jump in place Unable to kick ball on request
36 mo	Problems with toilet training Unable to calm self	Not able to dress self Does not understand taking turns		Unable to give full name Unable to match two colors Does not use plurals Does not know two to three prepositions Unable to tell a story Unclear consonants Unintelligible speech Unable to construct a sentence	Unable to build a tower of 10 blocks Holds crayon with fist Unable to draw circle	Unable to balance on one foot for 1 sec Toeing in causes tripping with running

Table continued on following page

TABLE 6–5 Continued
Developmental Red Flags: Toddlers and Preschoolers

AGE	GROWTH/ RHYTHMICITY/ SLEEP/ TEMPERAMENT	PSYCHOSOCIAL/ EMOTIONAL SKILLS	COGNITIVE AND VISUAL ABILITIES	LANGUAGE AND HEARING	FINE MOTOR (FEEDING/SELF-CARE)	GROSS MOTOR (STRENGTH/ COORDINATION)
48 mo	Lack of bedtime ritual Behavior concerns: withdrawn or acting out Stool holding Problems with toilet training	Unable to play games, follow rules Unable to follow limits/rules at home (e.g., put toys away) Cruelty to animals, friends Interest in fires, fire starting Persistent fears or severe shyness Inability to separate from mother	Unable to count three objects Unable to recall four numbers Unable to identify what to do in danger, fire, with a stranger Consistently poor judgment	Difficulty understanding language Problems understanding prepositions Limited vocabulary Unclear speech	Lack of self-care skills—dressing, feeding Unable to button clothes Unable to copy square	Unable to balance on one foot for 4 sec Unable to alternate steps when climbing stairs

60 mo					
Continued sleep problems Concerns with night terrors Hair pulling—scalp or eyelashes	Difficulty making and keeping friends; no friends Difficulty understanding sharing, school rules, organization of daily activities Cruelty to animals, friends Interest in fires, fire starting Bullying or being bullied Prolonged fighting, hitting, hurting Withdrawal, sadness, extreme rituals	Unable to count to 10 Unable to identify colors Difficulty following three-step command	Speech pattern not 100% understandable Cannot identify a penny, nickel, or dime	Unable to copy triangle Unable to draw a person with a body	Difficulty hopping, jumping

CHAPTER 7

Developmental Management of School-Age Children and Adolescents

School entry is a major developmental transition for young children. Success in school can set the stage for future achievement and help children feel more secure, self-confident, and positive about themselves and the world around them. It is important to ensure that children are ready to meet the demands of first grade. Table 7-1 lists basic skills the nurse practitioner and parent can assess to determine a child's school readiness.

Development of the school-age child and adolescent spans a wide range of normal. Expected milestones in physical, cognitive, and affective growth are outlined in Table 7-2. Pubertal changes and Tanner's stages of physical sexual maturity are presented in Figures 7-1, 7-2, and 7-3.

Indications that the child has failed to achieve these milestones are listed in Tables 7-3 and 7-4. These "developmental red flags" are cause for concern, further evaluation, and intervention.

T A B L E 7–1

Basic First-Grade School Readiness Skills

Language skills	Counts 10 or more objects
	Uses complete sentences of at least five words
	Uses future tense
	Gives first and last name
	Recognizes four colors
	Defines five to seven words
	Communicates needs
	Recalls parts of a story
	Follows three-part commands
	Understands number concepts
Personal and social skills	Separates easily from parent
	Dresses without supervision
	Plays interactively with other children
	Has toilet skills
	Follows instructions
	Feels support from other adults
Fine motor and adaptive skills	Copies geometrical shapes (circle, square, triangle)
	Draws a person (six parts with distinct body)
	Prints some letters
	Classifies similar objects
Gross motor skills	Hops on one foot
	Catches bounced ball
	Walks backward heel/toe
	Balances on each foot 6 sec

T A B L E 7-2

Developmental Milestones of School-Age Children and Adolescents

AGE GROUP	PHYSICAL	COGNITIVE	AFFECTIVE
School-age child	Begins pubertal changes. These may occur as early as • 8 yr for girls • 9–10 yr for boys Displays increasing interest in body and its functions; may express body image concerns Expresses sense of gender identity	Enters concrete operational stage and demonstrates • Flexible thought: understands rules of reversibility and decentration, conservation, and identity; is able to focus on multiple aspects of problems at once • Declining egocentrism: is able to understand another's perspective • Logical reasoning: understands concepts of relation, ordering; is able to classify objects • Social cognition: has improved sense of equality and justice; relative morality	Achieves Erikson's stage of Industry vs. Inferiority, leading to sense of mastery, competence, and self-esteem; is able to complete projects Develops social network of peers who accept and reward child Demonstrates positive temperament that supports successful school performance, peer interactions, and family functioning

Adolescent	Pubertal changes continue:	Enters formal operational stage:	Establishes self-identity:
	• Experiences growth from prepubescence to sexual maturity	• Develops logical thinking; is able to work with abstract ideas, synthesize and integrate concepts into larger schemes	• Functions independently of parents
	• Reaches adult parameters of height and physical growth by late adolescence	• Develops personal value system, sense of moral integrity; has orientation to a universal ethical principle	• Develops new relationships with peers and other adults
	• Becomes comfortable with own body		• Articulates plans for the future
			• Demonstrates responsibility for self, others, and community
			Develops intimate relationships:
			• Expresses respect and caring for self and other in relationship
			• Uses contraception and protection if in sexual relationship

TABLE 7-3

Developmental Red Flags: School-Age Children

AGE	PSYCHOSOCIAL/EMOTIONAL SKILL	COGNITIVE AND VISUAL ABILITIES	LANGUAGE/ HEARING	FINE MOTOR	GROSS MOTOR
6 yr	Problems with peer relationships Latchkey: stays home alone Unable to state special quality about self Flat affect, depression, withdrawn Cruelty to animals, friends Interest in fires/fire setting	School problems with grades, behavior, interest in grades Unable to sit still in class Unable to give age Watches television more than 2 hr per day Unable to name interests	Language partially unintelligible	Unable to copy + Picture of self includes less than 8 parts	Unable to catch a ball
8 yr	Lack of hobbies Lack of best friend Cruelty to animals, friends Interest in fires/fire setting Flat affect, depression, withdrawn	Unable to state days of the week Unable to add and subtract Unable to identify right and left	Unable to read simple phrases Unable to relate simple story	Unable to copy a diamond and square Unable to print name Unable to tie shoes Picture of self includes less than 12–16 parts	Unable to walk a straight line Poor coordination/ endurance/ strength

Age					
10 yr	Lack of participation in team sports or extracurricular activities at school Lacks understanding of rules Poor peer influence, interest in gangs Cruelty to animals, friends Interest in fires/fire setting Flat affect, depression, withdrawn	Lack of operational thinking: cause and effect, relationships of whole and parts, nonegocentric thinking	Problems with reading and math	Difficulty holding pencil, with penmanship/cursive writing	Problems throwing or catching
12 yr	Risk-taking behaviors: smoking, alcohol, sex Problems about sexuality Cruelty to animals, friends Interest in fires/fire setting Flat affect, depression, withdrawn	Difficulty with school work Lack of organizational skills for homework	Problems understanding/following through with verbal instructions Problems with reading comprehension	Problems getting written homework done because of difficulties holding pencil or doing paper and pencil tasks	Unable to list strengths and physical things he/she likes to do

TABLE 7-4

Developmental Red Flags: Adolescents

AGE	PHYSICAL AND SEXUAL DEVELOPMENT	PSYCHOSOCIAL DEVELOPMENT	COGNITIVE DEVELOPMENT
Early adolescence (11–14 yr)	Difficulty reading close or distant Female kyphosis/scoliosis Less than Tanner stage 2 Female short stature or lack of height spurt Poor nutrition, underweight, poor oral health, caries, malocclusion Loss of appetite Chronic disease such as heart disease, diabetes, or a family member with a chronic or lifelong illness No physical activity; overweight Sleep disturbance Sexual experimentation	Social habits: Early experimentation with drugs or alcohol (including tobacco) Relationships: Permissive or authoritarian parental style No participation in home chores History of family violence School fights No close or "best" friend Friends or siblings in gangs Cruelty to animals Sexuality: Sexual orientation worries Mood: Pervasive sad mood, feelings of hopelessness, suicidal thoughts or gestures, history of previous suicide attempt Flattened affect without expressions of joy, sorrow, or excitement Excessive worrying or rumination	Low IQ Behind in grade or failing classes Chronic absenteeism or class skipping Attention problems Lack of organizational skills for homework Disruptive behavior Unable to identify feelings Unable to control own behavior (e.g., anger, impulsivity)

Middle adolescence (15–17 yr)

Difficulty reading close or distant
Male kyphosis/scoliosis
Less than Tanner stage 4
Male short stature or lack of height spurt
Male muscular growth without testicular maturation
Male persistent gynecomastia and acne
Female primary or secondary amenorrhea
Poor nutrition, underweight, poor oral health, caries, malocclusion
Loss of appetite
Chronic disease such as heart disease, diabetes, or a family member with a chronic or lifelong illness
No physical activity; overweight
Sleep disturbance
Unprotected sexual intercourse
Multiple sexual partners

Self-concept:
Believes self to be "ugly" or "fat"; is dieting despite normal body size and shape
Negative feelings of self-worth
Does not fantasize or dream about adult career
Social habits:
Recurrent experimentation or frequent use of drugs or alcohol; blackouts
Drinking and driving
Relationships:
Excessively oppositional, defiant of all authority
Abusive dating relationships
School fights
No identified peer group
Gang association or involvement
Sexuality:
Same as early adolescence
Mood:
Same as early adolescence
Self-concept:
Same as early adolescence

Low IQ
Behind in grade or failing classes
Chronic absenteeism or class skipping
Attention problems
Disruptive behavior
Unable to differentiate emotional states from physical states
Unable to control own behavior (e.g., anger, impulsivity)
Poor judgment

Table continued on following page

T·A·B·L·E 7-4 Continued

Developmental Red Flags: Adolescents

AGE	PHYSICAL AND SEXUAL DEVELOPMENT	PSYCHOSOCIAL DEVELOPMENT	COGNITIVE DEVELOPMENT

Late adolescence (18–21 yr)	Difficulty reading close or distant
	Less than Tanner stage 5
	Poor nutrition, poor oral health, caries, malocclusion
	Loss of appetite
	Chronic disease such as heart disease, diabetes, or a family member with a chronic or lifelong illness
	No physical activity; overweight
	Sleep disturbance
	Unprotected sexual intercourse
	Multiple sexual partners
		Social habits:
		  Substance abuse
		  Drinking and driving
		Relationships:
		  Lacks intimate relationships
		  Abusive dating relationships
		  Unable to separate from peer groups
		  Unable to separate from parents
		  Gang association or involvement
		  Unable to keep a job
		Sexuality:
		  Same as early adolescence
		Mood:
		  Same as early adolescence
		Self-concept:
		  Same as early adolescence
			Low IQ
			Behind in grade or failing classes
			Dropout
			Attention problems
			Disruptive behavior
			Persistent egocentrism
			Unable to control own behavior (e.g., anger, impulsivity)
			Unable to reason or plan based on future/abstract concepts
			Poor judgment
			Chronic health care seeking for psychosomatic complaints

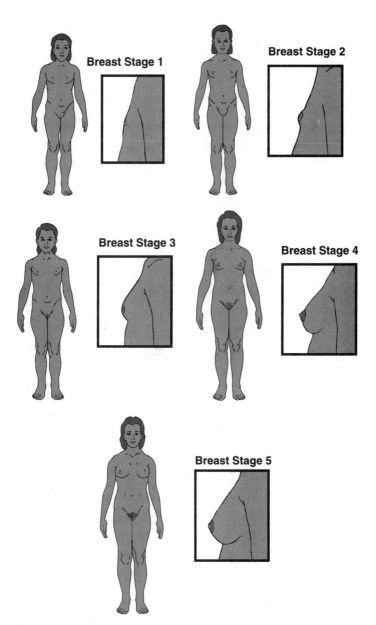

FIGURE 7–1

Tanner's stages: Female. (Reprinted with permission, The Division of Adolescent Medicine, Children's Hospital Medical Center, Cincinnati, Ohio, copyright © 1995.) *Illustration continued on following page*

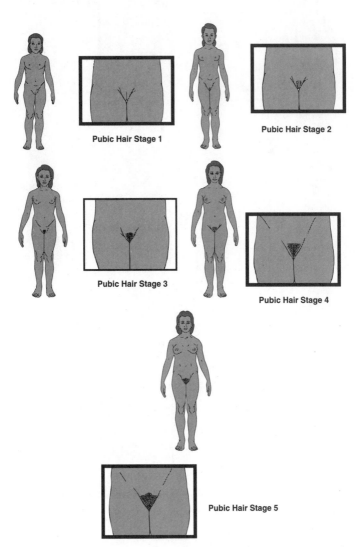

Pubic Hair Stage 1

Pubic Hair Stage 2

Pubic Hair Stage 3

Pubic Hair Stage 4

Pubic Hair Stage 5

F I G U R E 7-1 *Continued*

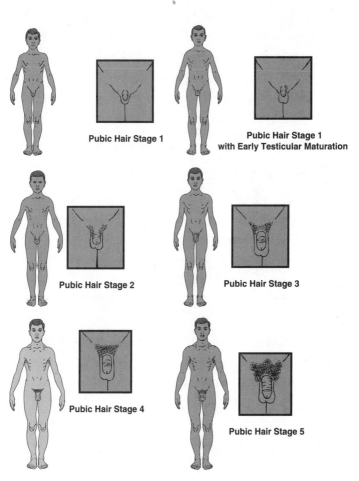

Pubic Hair Stage 1

Pubic Hair Stage 1
with Early Testicular Maturation

Pubic Hair Stage 2

Pubic Hair Stage 3

Pubic Hair Stage 4

Pubic Hair Stage 5

F I G U R E 7–2

Tanner's stages: Male. (Reprinted with permission, The Division of Adolescent Medicine, Children's Hospital Medical Center, Cincinnati, Ohio, copyright © 1995.)

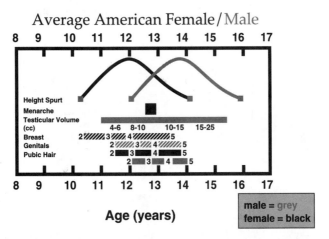

Average American Female / Male

F I G U R E 7–3

Sequence of pubertal events. Breast, genital, and pubic hair development indicate Tanner's stages 2 to 5. (Reprinted with permission, The Division of Adolescent Medicine, Children's Hospital Medical Center, Cincinnati, Ohio, copyright © 1995.)

UNIT 3

Approaches to Health Management

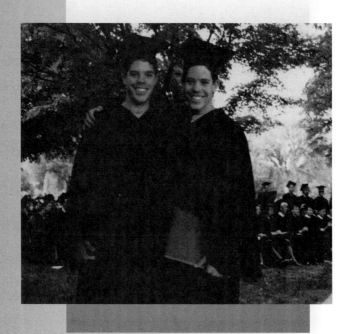

CHAPTER 8

Health Perception and Health Management Pattern

The health of children is fundamentally connected to parental, family, and community interactions. Therefore, assessment and management of growth, development, and disease processes must involve the whole child—including physical, developmental, psychological, emotional, and interactional qualities. The health supervision visit should include issues of daily living (e.g., sleep patterns, toileting, nutrition) as well as the more commonly emphasized physical concerns (Table 8-1). Issues of daily living affect health status and can be evaluated using the system of Functional Health Patterns (Gordon, 1987). Discussion of these issues during the health supervision visit emphasizes anticipatory guidance and patient-parent education.

Efforts to prevent disease and injury are integral to health maintenance. Children, because of their unique and age-specific developmental characteristics, are particularly prone to injury. Injury prevention strategies, tailored to these characteristics, are listed in Tables 8-2 through 8-5. Recommendations for use of child restraint systems, based on age, are listed in Table 8-6.

Continued on page 93

TABLE 8-1

Health Supervision Visits: Assessment of Daily Living and Functional Health Patterns

	INFANT	TODDLER	PRESCHOOL CHILD	SCHOOL-AGE CHILD	ADOLESCENT
Parent-child interaction	Assess degree of mutual and reciprocal response between infant and parents Assess emotional status of parents Assess appropriateness of parental response to infant's cues	Assess parental confidence in role Assess emotional status of parents Assess appropriateness of parental response to toddler's cues Assess degree of affection demonstrated between toddler and parents Assess parental encouragement of independence, yet active involvement with child	Assess consistency in parents' behavior Assess emotional status of parents Assess appropriateness of parental response to child's cues Assess degree to which parents provide affection, praise, emotional support, and encourage child to express feelings Assess parental encouragement of independence, yet active engagement with child	Determine whether parents express clear, consistent, but flexible expectations Assess appropriate limits set by parents Assess degree to which parents provide attention, affection, praise, approval, emotional support, and encourage child to express feelings Assess degree to which parents support independence, yet participate with child in activities Assess degree to which child demonstrates self-confidence, industriousness, cooperation, and consideration	Assess parental confidence and pleasure in role Assess open communication with mutual respect for privacy Assess parental encouragement of independence and activities with peers Assess setting of reasonable and consistent limits Assess active parental interest in adolescent's activities, friends, school performance Assess parental pride and pleasure in adolescent's achievements

Developmental assessment to determine extent to which child has achieved milestones and received emotional nurturing	See Chapters 6 and 15	See Chapters 6 and 15	See Chapters 6 and 15; look for child who is friendly, secure, cooperative, proud, and happy Conduct speech evaluation	See Chapters 7 and 15 Conduct speech evaluation	See Chapters 7 and 15
Nutrition/metabolic	Discuss choice of feeding, breastfeeding versus bottle feeding (see Chapter 10); when to introduce solids; management of feeding problems or special nutritional needs (see Chapter 9) Fluoride beginning at 6 mo as indicated according to fluoride level in water source Skin care: Apply sunscreen whenever child is exposed to sun	Discuss management of self-feeding, feeding problems, or special nutritional needs (see Chapter 9) Explain pattern of dentition, need for good oral hygiene (see Chapter 29) Continue fluoride as indicated Skin care: Apply sunscreen whenever child is exposed to sun	Discuss need for well-balanced diet Discuss parents' responsibility to provide nutritious foods, pleasant atmosphere for meals, and healthy role models for child; child's responsibility to select appropriate foods from those provided (see Chapter 9) Explain pattern of dentition, need for dental assessment (see Chapter 29) Continue fluoride as indicated Skin care: Apply sunscreen whenever child is exposed to sun	Discuss healthy food selections with child (see Chapter 9) Encourage daily dental hygiene (see Chapter 29) Continue fluoride as indicated Skin care: Apply sunscreen whenever child is exposed to sun	Discuss nutritional needs, dietary patterns Discuss body image and self-perception as they relate to eating habits (see Chapter 9) Encourage good oral hygiene, regular dental care (see Chapter 29), orthodontia Fluoride until age 16, as indicated Skin care: Apply sunscreen whenever child is exposed to sun Discuss acne management as appropriate

Table continued on following page

75

T A B L E 8-1 *Continued*
Health Supervision Visits: Assessment of Daily Living and Functional Health Patterns

	INFANT	TODDLER	PRESCHOOL CHILD	SCHOOL-AGE CHILD	ADOLESCENT
Sleep and rest: discuss sleep needs, patterns, and changes as child grows (see Chapter 13)	Discuss the importance of bedtime ritual, infant cues for sleep and wake states Instruct parents to position infant on back for sleep	Discuss the importance of bedtime ritual	Discuss typical night fears, night terrors	Discuss sleepwalking and night terrors	Discuss sleep needs during rapid growth of adolescence
Activity and exercise (see Chapter 12): discuss injury prevention (see Tables 8-2 through 8-5)	Discuss physical developmental needs and skills of infant	Discuss need to set limits and provide safe environment for expression of physical needs and developing skills	Discuss need to set limits and provide safe environment for expression of physical needs and skills Encourage child's active, pretend, and fantasy play; discourage passive activities such as watching television Discuss child's tendency to become overtired, often needing parent's help to calm down	Encourage regular physical activity Discuss bicycle, skateboard, swimming safety Discuss balance of nutrition with exercise to achieve appropriate weight gain Evaluate for scoliosis in child aged 10–12 years	Encourage regular physical activity, participation in fitness and organized sports activities Evaluate for scoliosis Evaluate for sports fitness

Elimination (see Chapter 11)	Discuss diapering, infant patterns of stooling and urination	Discuss toilet training	Discuss management of occasional "accidents" in toilet-trained child Teach good hygiene, handwashing	Discuss importance of good hygiene, handwashing Explain relationship between nutrition, exercise, and elimination	Discuss importance of good hygiene, handwashing Explain relationship between nutrition, exercise, and elimination Perform pelvic examination in sexually active girl, those with history of mother taking diethylstilbestrol (DES) Teach breast and testicular self-examination Recommend folic acid 400 µg/day for girl

Table continued on following page

TABLE 8–1 Continued

Health Supervision Visits: Assessment of Daily Living and Functional Health Patterns

	INFANT	TODDLER	PRESCHOOL CHILD	SCHOOL-AGE CHILD	ADOLESCENT
Role relationships (see Chapters 3 and 16)	Discuss infant's interaction with siblings and other family members; evaluate impact child has on family system, place of child in family	Discuss discipline strategies, interaction of toddler with siblings and other family members, impact child has on family system, place of child in family, day care needs and plans	Discuss discipline strategies, interaction of child with siblings and other family members, impact child has on family system, place of child in family, day care needs and plans, school readiness for older preschool-age child	Discuss importance of increasing child's participation in family activities, taking more responsibility for tasks in household; discuss nature of child's interaction in school and with peer group; suggest that parents encourage and participate in hobbies, reading, other activities with child and peer group	Discuss importance of increasing independence in adolescents, responsibilities at home, school, or workplace; emphasize need to keep communication open among adolescent, peers, and parents

Self-concept/self-perception (see Chapter 15)	Explain process of infant's developing an awareness of self as separate from parents and others	Explain importance of giving child positive feedback on achievements Encourage parents to relate to child in warm, loving manner; avoid harsh words and punitive parental behavior	Encourage parents to give children choices, allowing children to express selves and participate in family tasks Explain children's sense of absolutes at this age; discourage teasing and threats Encourage parents to participate in child's activities (e.g., school field trips)	Encourage parents to give child attention and positive reinforcement of choices, allowing child to express self and expecting participation in family tasks	Give adolescent opportunities to discuss changes in self and to openly ask questions about development Encourage parents to give adolescent positive attention, reinforcement for healthy choices and appropriate activities, allowing adolescent privacy, and expecting reasonable participation in family activities

Table continued on following page

T A B L E 8–1 *Continued*

Health Supervision Visits: Assessment of Daily Living and Functional Health Patterns

	INFANT	TODDLER	PRESCHOOL CHILD	SCHOOL-AGE CHILD	ADOLESCENT
Coping and stress tolerance (see Chapter 18)	Identify family support network Assess knowledge of community resources Assess knowledge of child development Identify level of parenting skills Discuss how parents' health habits (e.g., smoking, exercise, diet) may affect child	Identify family support network Assess knowledge of community resources Assess parents' knowledge of child development Identify level of parenting skills Discuss discipline styles and options Encourage parent to guide and instruct child's positive social behavior (e.g., not hitting or biting)	Identify family support network Assess knowledge of community resources Assess parents' knowledge of child development Identify level of parenting skills Discuss discipline styles and options; need to set limits Encourage parents to help child name and identify feelings and discuss ways the child can manage feelings	Identify family support network Assess knowledge of community resources Assess parents' knowledge of child development Identify level of parenting skills Discuss discipline styles and options; need to set limits Encourage parents to praise child's efforts at self-control, management of feelings Assess for depression	Identify family support network Assess knowledge of community resources Assess parents' knowledge of child development Identify level of parenting skills Discuss discipline styles and options Encourage parents to provide appropriate limits while fostering independence Discuss adolescent's emotional states related to rapid growth and changes of puberty Assess for depression

Values and beliefs	Discuss parents' expectations of self and child as family grows	Encourage parents to identify their value and belief framework Discuss how they demonstrate their beliefs to their child	Encourage parents to provide opportunities for child to express ideas, feelings, and emotions Include child in family spiritual activities	Encourage parents to provide opportunity for child to explore understanding of emotions, values, and beliefs in more formal settings (e.g., religious institutions, spiritual activities)	Explain to parents that adolescent, as part of normal process of developing self-identity, may appear to reject family values Encourage adolescent to discuss values and beliefs

TABLE 8-2

Primary Injury Prevention Related to Developmental Characteristics of Infants

50% of injury-related deaths in infants occur before 4 mo of age
40% of all injury-related deaths in infants are due to asphyxiation
20% of all injury-related deaths in infants result from motor vehicle trauma
After 4 mo of age, falls account for a significant number of injuries

AGE AND DEVELOPMENTAL CHARACTERISTICS	POTENTIAL INJURIES	STRATEGIES FOR PREVENTION
BIRTH TO 6 MO		
Poor head control at younger ages	Injury to neck	Handle child with care when picking up or moving
		Support neck of young infant
		Supervise other children when they are playing with infant
		Never jiggle or shake infant
Reflex behavior; especially strong suck reflex in early months	Aspiration of foreign objects	Keep occlusive materials, especially plastic, out of child's bed
	Suffocation	Check toys, mobiles for sharp, detachable parts, strings, or cords
		Handle child with care when picking up or moving
Skin thin and sensitive	Friction burns	Do not hold infant in lap when drinking hot beverage or smoking
	Burns	Set water heater thermostat at <120°F
	Sunburn	Use cover-up (e.g., hat) whenever child is exposed to sun; avoid exposure

Developmental abilities	Injury	Preventive measures
Poor body temperature control	Hypothermia Hyperthermia	Dress infant appropriately
Rolls, turns, and scoots	Falls	Never leave child alone in car Do not leave infant alone on bed, changing table, or other area from which infant may fall Use playpen as a safe area
	May slide between mattress and crib slats Drowning	Make sure mattress fits tightly against railings and that railings are no more than 2⅜ inches apart Place washcloth under infant in bath; stay with infant during bathing
	Motor vehicle trauma Burns	Correctly use approved child safety restraint units in cars Install smoke detectors in home and check batteries routinely
6 TO 12 MO		
Grasps and mouths objects	Aspiration of foreign objects Suffocation	Keep small, sharp objects off floor and play area, out of reach Check toys for detachable parts Keep balloons, plastic wrappers, and plastic bags out of reach
	Poisoning	Use childproof caps on medications Keep medications out of reach in locked cabinet Keep household, garden, and car products out of reach Supervise children's activity Keep syrup of ipecac in home Keep poison control numbers near telephone and alert older siblings and babysitters about them

Table continued on following page

TABLE 8-2 *Continued*

Primary Injury Prevention Related to Developmental Characteristics of Infants

50% of injury-related deaths in infants occur before 4 mo of age
40% of all injury-related deaths in infants are due to asphyxiation
20% of all injury-related deaths in infants result from motor vehicle trauma
After 4 mo of age, falls account for a significant number of injuries

AGE AND DEVELOPMENTAL CHARACTERISTICS	POTENTIAL INJURIES	STRATEGIES FOR PREVENTION
6 TO 12 MO *Continued*		
Sits, rolls, scoots, crawls, may stand while holding support, cruises, may walk	Falls	Do not use walkers
		Supervise children's activities
		Survey home for all accident hazards, sharp objects, table edges, stairs, loose rugs; remove those possible, provide protection of infant for others; use gates
	Drowning	Keep pool or water ponds behind closed and locked gates
		Never leave children alone in bath
		Use playpen as a safe area
Pulls and reaches	May pull objects down onto self	Remove tablecloths, dangling cords, appliances that may be in infant's reach
	Burns	Do not drink hot beverages or smoke when holding infant
	Electrocution	Insert plastic plugs in electrical outlets
Developing fine pincer grasp	Swallowing, aspiration, or insertion of foreign body in body orifices	Keep small objects out of reach
	Motor vehicle trauma	Correctly use approved child safety restraint units in cars
	Fire	Install smoke detectors in home and check batteries routinely
		Install carbon monoxide detectors in home

TABLE 8-3

Primary Injury Prevention Related to Developmental Characteristics of Toddlers and Preschoolers

44% of all deaths in children age 1 to 4 yr are injury related
Injuries cause more death and disability than all contagious diseases combined
Poisonings are the number one cause of injuries, followed by burns, drowning, and choking

DEVELOPMENTAL CHARACTERISTICS	POTENTIAL INJURIES	STRATEGIES FOR PREVENTION
Increased fine motor skills: Can open doors, gates, drawers, bottles, boxes Increased curiosity	Poisoning	Use childproof caps on medications; keep medicines locked in cabinet out of reach Keep household, garden, and car products locked or out of reach Keep bottle of syrup of ipecac in home Place Mr. YUK stickers on toxic materials Have telephone number of Poison Control Center readily available
Increased gross motor skills and control: Able to walk, run, climb, throw objects, ride tricycle Engages in more active play outdoors, with peers	Falls	Confine play to fenced area Supervise play, especially in areas where climbing occurs Use gates or screens to block off stair; lock windows and doors
	Sunburn Motor vehicle trauma	Use sunscreen whenever children are exposed to sun Use approved child safety restraints Provide tricycle/bicycle helmet Teach children sidewalk, street, and highway safety Never let children cross street alone or play on sidewalks near streets unsupervised
	Contusions and bites	Supervise interactive play of children Teach children how to share, control tempers; use adult interaction or distraction to stop harmful behavior or tantrum trauma

Table continued on following page

TABLE 8-3 Continued
Primary Injury Prevention Related to Developmental Characteristics of Toddlers and Preschoolers

44% of all deaths in children age 1 to 4 yr are injury related
Injuries cause more death and disability than all contagious diseases combined
Poisonings are the number one cause of injuries, followed by burns, drowning, and choking

DEVELOPMENTAL CHARACTERISTICS	POTENTIAL INJURIES	STRATEGIES FOR PREVENTION
Increased curiosity: reaches, stretches, and pulls	Burns, scalding	Turn handles of cooking utensils away from outer edge of stove Use caution in kitchen with children about Adjust hot water thermostat to 120°F Keep matches out of reach
Increased curiosity, desire to explore	Drowning	Fence swimming pools Supervise use of swimming and wading pools
Easily distracted, lacks judgment, unaware of danger of heights, water, fire, toxic materials, electricity, weapons, animals, or strangers	Other injuries	Never leave children unattended in a car or alone at home Do not allow children to play near running machinery, mowers, cars, or tools Provide plastic covers for electrical outlets; teach children safety with electrical appliances and cords Do not allow children to use pointed objects in play Do not allow children to run or walk with sticks, lollipops, or other such objects Remove weapons from the house or keep in locked cabinet, guns unloaded; store ammunition in separate, locked area Teach children to avoid strange animals, especially ones that are eating
Easily distracted, not always attentive	Abuse Choking, aspiration	Teach stranger safety Do not give foods that can be easily aspirated, such as nuts, gum, popcorn, hotdogs, grapes Supervise mealtimes and snacks

Primary Injury Prevention Related to Developmental Characteristics of School-Age Children

51% of all deaths in children age 5 to 9 yr are injury related
58% of all deaths in children age 10 to 14 yr are injury related
Motor vehicle and pedestrian accidents, burns, drowning, and choking are the most common fatal injuries
1 in 10 injury fatalities is related to motor vehicle trauma or bicycle use

DEVELOPMENTAL CHARACTERISTICS	POTENTIAL INJURIES	STRATEGIES FOR PREVENTION
Motor skills improve: Becomes more physically agile and coordinated	Motor vehicle trauma as passenger, pedestrian, or cyclist	Use approved safety restraints in car Provide bicycle helmet and insist on its use Teach importance of seatbelt and helmet use Teach bicycle safety Do not allow children to ride tricycles or bicycles with training wheels in the street Prohibit use of all-terrain vehicles Teach pedestrian safety
Is adventurous and more independent, looks for new challenges; may accept dares	Falls	Use knee pads, elbow pads, wrist support, and helmets when skateboarding
	Drowning	Teach to swim; teach rules of water safety: swim in a supervised area with a buddy, check depth before diving, use life preservers in boats
Engages in sports and strenuous exercise Enjoys physical activity Works hard to improve skills Can strain self with excessive activity	Sprains and strains, fractures, and other bodily injuries	Encourage child to be active and stay conditioned; if child is engaged in organized sports, provide supervised strength training Ensure use of properly fitted equipment for each sport and safe playing area

Table continued on following page

87

T A B L E 8-4 *Continued*

Primary Injury Prevention Related to Developmental Characteristics of School-Age Children

51% of all deaths in children age 5 to 9 yr are injury related
58% of all deaths in children age 10 to 14 yr are injury related
Motor vehicle and pedestrian accidents, burns, drowning, and choking are the most common fatal injuries
1 in 10 injury fatalities is related to motor vehicle trauma or bicycle use

DEVELOPMENTAL CHARACTERISTICS	POTENTIAL INJURIES	STRATEGIES FOR PREVENTION
Engages in group activities, subject to peer approval	Burns	Teach children dangers of flammable and toxic materials; how to handle them safely
Is curious and exploring		Supervise use of matches
Easily distracted by environment		Develop a family plan for fires
Accepts explanations and is responsive to reasoning	Poisoning	Keep hazardous materials out of reach, in locked location; supervise their use
	Choking	Teach first aid, what to do in case of burns, choking, or poisoning
		Keep Poison Control Center telephone number readily available
	Sunburn	Use sunscreen whenever children will be exposed to sun
	Abuse	Teach child to memorize telephone number and address, use of 911
		Warn child never to go with or accept things from strangers

TABLE 8-5

Primary Injury Prevention Related to Developmental Characteristics of Adolescents

Nearly 80% of all fatal injuries are related to motor vehicles
1 in 50 teens is hospitalized for motor vehicle injury every year
Sports injuries are the most common nonfatal injury
Drownings, burns, and poisoning (drugs and alcohol) are the 2nd, 3rd, and 4th leading causes of injury, respectively

DEVELOPMENTAL CHARACTERISTICS	POTENTIAL INJURIES	STRATEGIES FOR PREVENTION
Able to legally drive motor vehicles	Motor vehicle trauma as passenger, pedestrian, or cyclist	Use approved safety restraints Take driver's education classes Use bicycle helmet Encourage to learn how to maintain bicycle Teach proper use of all-terrain vehicles Reinforce pedestrian safety Emphasize danger of driving, drinking, and drug use; support peer group efforts to control inappropriate behavior
Increased physical strength and ability	Falls	Use knee pads, elbow pads, wrist support, and helmet when skateboarding Use helmet when cycling

Table continued on following page

T A B L E 8–5 Continued

Primary Injury Prevention Related to Developmental Characteristics of Adolescents

Nearly 80% of all fatal injuries are related to motor vehicles
1 in 50 teens is hospitalized for motor vehicle injury every year
Sports injuries are the most common nonfatal injury
Drownings, burns, and poisoning (drugs and alcohol) are the 2nd, 3rd, and 4th leading causes of injury, respectively

DEVELOPMENTAL CHARACTERISTICS	POTENTIAL INJURIES	STRATEGIES FOR PREVENTION
Perception of invulnerability; may take risks	Drowning	Teach to swim Reinforce rules of water safety: swim in a supervised area with a buddy, check depth before diving, use life preservers in boats and when water skiing
More participation in structured sports activities	Sprains, strains, fractures, and other bodily injuries	Encourage adolescent to stay active and conditioned, engage in supervised strength training
Use of complex equipment, tools, weapons	Burns Bodily injury Choking	Teach first aid and cardiopulmonary resuscitation: what to do in the event of injuries, burns, choking, or poisonings Teach gun safety
Strong peer influence	Poisoning (drug and alcohol abuse)	Teach dangers of drug and alcohol use
Need for independence and peer approval Able to problem solve, reason, and think abstractly		Provide an opportunity to discuss values, perceptions, fears, and needs related to high-risk behaviors; discuss how adolescent deals with anger and violence, as well as how to prevent trauma related to violence; encourage healthy options

Vehicle Child Restraint Systems: Recommendations for Use

AGE OF CHILD	WEIGHT OF CHILD	TYPE OF RESTRAINT
Infant <1 yr	Up to about 20 lb	Child restraint system (CRS) designed for infant; rear-facing; always in back seat, as automatic air bag for front passenger seat may strike child with injury-causing, even fatal, force; seated upright
Toddlers	20–40 lb	CRS designed for toddler; always in back seat; facing forward, although earlier research indicates serious or fatal neck injuries in children <18 mo riding in this position despite their weight (Fuchs et al., 1989), and a 13-yr study by Volvo demonstrated few injuries in children <5 yr riding in a rear-facing position (Carlson et al., 1989)
Preschool and early elementary school-age children	40–60 lb	Booster seat, without shield, used with seatbelt that has lap/shoulder belt Booster seat, with shield, used with seatbelt that has lap belt only

Table continued on following page

91

TABLE 8-6 Continued
Vehicle Child Restraint Systems: Recommendations for Use

AGE OF CHILD	WEIGHT OF CHILD	TYPE OF RESTRAINT
Older children	>60 lb	Adult lap/shoulder restraint that fits correctly: child sits with buttocks against the seat back, lap belt lies low and tight across the top of the thighs, shoulder strap crosses the shoulder and chest (not the neck or face) with no slack Lap belt alone if shoulder strap is unavailable
CHILDREN WITH SPECIAL NEEDS		
Very small infants	<7 lb	If child is in infant seat, have close-fitting harness and no shield Maximum distance from crotch strap to back of seat is 5.5 inches; height of harness straps should be <10 inches
Children with physical disabilities		If child is too small for seat, use car bed with restraints that allow child to lie flat The Spelcast child restraint, modified to hold a child weighing <40 lb in a hip spica cast The modified E-Z-On Vest restrains a child who must lie flat

Adapted from Stewart (1993) and National Highway Traffic Safety Administration (1996).

REFERENCES

Carlsson G, Norin H, Yslander L: Rearward facing child seats: The safest car restraint for children? Proceedings of the 33rd Annual Association for the Advancement of Automotive Medicine, 1989.

Fuchs S, Barthel MJ, Flannery AM, et al: Cervical spine fractures sustained by young children in forward-facing car seats. Pediatrics 84:348-354, 1989.

Gordon M: Nursing Diagnosis: Process and Application. New York, McGraw-Hill, 1987.

National Highway Traffic Safety Administration: Size and Weight Guide for Child Safety Seats. NHTSA Facts. Washington, DC, U.S. Department of Transportation, 1996.

Stewart DD: Child passenger safety: Current technical issues for advocates and professionals. Fam Comm Health 15(4):12-27, 1993.

CHAPTER 9

Nutrition

Good nutrition is the foundation of good health. When caring for children, nurse practitioners must be able to assess nutritional status as well as understand the relationship among nutrition, growth and development, and disease states.

▬ NUTRITIONAL ASSESSMENT

Anthropometric measures are used to gauge adequate nutritional intake (Table 9-1 and Appendix B). When a child experiences a nutritional deficit, the first parameter affected is weight; if the deficit is chronic, vertical height gain will slow, followed by changes in developmental capacity, especially cognitive and neurological abilities.

The trajectory of a child's growth should be plotted accurately on standardized growth grids (see Appendix B), and the pattern should be consistent over time. Generally, rapid change (either an increase or decrease) or a variation across two or more lines on the growth grid is cause for concern. Consider the phenotypes of parents and siblings when evaluating a particular child's status because some children are genetically programmed to be smaller or larger than the norm for their age. Also, the growth pattern of children with special conditions (e.g., those with Down syndrome) will not be accurately measured using standard grids.

If they are well-nourished, children who were born prematurely or small for gestational age experience "catch-up" growth in the first years of life. Table 9-2 identifies estimated caloric intake required, and Table 9-3 lists suggestions for increasing energy intake to meet the extra growth needs of these children.

T A B L E 9-1

Average Weight and Height Gains in Infancy Through Adolescence

AGE	WEIGHT	HEIGHT
INFANT (mo)		
0–3	Average weekly gain 210 g (8 oz)	Average monthly gain 3.5 cm
3–6	Average weekly gain 140 g (5 oz); birth weight doubles by 4–6 mo	Average monthly gain 2.0 cm
6–12	Average weekly gain 85–140 g (3–5 oz); birth weight triples by 1 yr	Average monthly gain 1.2–1.5 cm
TODDLER (yr)		
1–3	Average yearly gain 2–3 kg (4.4–6.6 lb)	Average yearly gain: 1–2 years: 12 cm 2–3 years: 6–8 cm Height at 2 yr: approximately half of adult height
PRESCHOOL-AGE CHILD (yr)		
3–6	Average yearly gain 1.8–2.7 kg (4–6 lb)	Average yearly gain 6–8 cm
SCHOOL-AGE CHILD (yr)		
6–12	Average yearly gain 1.8–2.7 kg (4–6 lb)	Average yearly gain 5 cm
PREADOLESCENT/ ADOLESCENT (yr)		
Girl, 10–14	Average total gain 17.5 kg (38.5 lb)	Average yearly gain 6–8.3 cm 95% of adult height achieved by onset of menarche
Boy, 12–16	Average total gain 23.7 kg (52.1 lb)	Average yearly gain 6–9.5 cm 95% of adult height achieved by 15 yr

Adapted from Behrman RE, Kliegman RM, Arvin AM (eds): Nelson Textbook of Pediatrics, 15th ed. Philadelphia, WB Saunders, 1996.

T A B L E 9–2

Estimating Catch-Up Growth Requirements*

Catch-up growth requirement (kcal/kg/d)	=	Calories required for weight age (kcal/kg/d)	×	Ideal weight for age (kg)
				Actual weight (kg)

1. Plot the child's height and weight on the NCHS growth charts.
2. Determine at what age the present weight would be at the 50th percentile (weight age).
3. Determine recommended calories for weight age using the table below.

	WEIGHT		RECOMMENDED
AGE	kg	lb	INTAKE kcal/kg/d
0.0–6 mo	6	13	108
6–12 mo	9	20	98
1–3 yr	13	29	102
4–6 yr	20	44	90
7–10 yr	28	62	70
Boys			
11–14 yr	45	99	55
15–18 yr	66	145	45
19–24 yr	72	160	40
Girls			
11–14 yr	46	101	40
15–18 yr	55	120	38
19–24 yr	58	128	38

4. Determine the ideal weight (50th percentile) for the child's present age.
5. Multiply the value obtained in (3) by the value obtained in (4).
6. Divide the value obtained in (5) by actual weight.

*Guidelines are used to estimate catch-up growth requirements: Precise individual needs vary and are mediated by medical status and diagnosis.

Based on National Academy of Sciences: Recommended Dietary Allowances, 10th ed. Washington, DC, National Academy of Sciences, 1989.

NCHS = National Center for Health Statistics.

From Rathbun JM, Peterson KE: Nutrition in failure to thrive. *In* Grand RJ, Sutphen JL, Dietz WH (eds): Pediatric Nutrition. Boston, Butterworths, 1987.

T A B L E 9-3

Suggestions for Increasing Energy Intake

- Use readily available economical foods that are familiar to the child.
- Fortify milk by adding 1 c nonfat dry milk powder to 1 qt of whole milk. Drink or use to prepare cooked cereals, creamed soups, pancakes, pudding, milkshakes (do *not* use with children younger than 2 yr of age).
- Add additional margarine or cheese to potatoes, vegetables, casseroles, rice, pasta, cooked cereals, etc.
- Encourage high-calorie snacks such as fruit juice, dried fruits, nuts, bananas, cheese cubes, pudding or custard, cereal with whole milk, fruit yogurt (alone or as a dip for fruit), cheese or peanut butter on crackers, olives, sliced or mashed avocado (as a dip for vegetables or crackers).
- Add instant breakfast mixes to whole milk.
- Use commercially prepared formula with high caloric content.
- Use commercial liquid supplements such as Pediasure or Pediasure with fiber (Ross Laboratories) for children with lactose intolerance.
- Establish regular times for meals and snacks, 2 to 4 hr apart. Do not allow the child to nibble continually on small amounts of food.
- Keep mealtimes relaxed and pleasant. Avoid scolding, nagging, or force feeding.
- Allow the infant or child to provide cues regarding hunger and satiety.

All children require certain nutrients to achieve optimal growth. The food pyramids in Figures 9-1 and 9-2 reflect current recommendations for basic nutritional intake in omnivorous and vegetarian diets.

▓▓▓ VEGETARIAN DIETS

Vegetarians are categorized into one of three groups:

- *Vegans,* or strict vegetarians, who eat only foods of plant origin
- *Lacto-vegetarians,* who include milk and dairy products in their diet as well as all plant-based foods
- *Lacto-ovo-vegetarians,* who consume eggs, dairy products, and all plant-based foods in their diet

Although most vegetarian diets can provide all essential nutrients, vitamin B_{12}, in the form of a supplement or in a supplemented food (such as fortified soy milk), is required for the child eating a vegan diet because bioavailable vitamin B_{12} is present only in animal-based foods. Children eating vegan diets can also require supplemental zinc, iron, calcium, and vitamin D (Table 9-4).

Text continued on page 104

MILK & MILK PRODUCTS	MEAT & MEAT ALTERNATIVES	VEGETABLES	FRUITS	BREADS & CEREALS
Supplies: **Calcium,** riboflavin, protein	Supplies: **Iron, protein,** niacin, thiamine, zinc, B₁₂	Supplies: **Folic acid, vitamins A and C,** fiber	Supplies: **Folic acid, vitamins A and C,** fiber	Supplies: **Fiber, complex carbohydrate,** thiamine, iron, niacin
Amount recommended: 2–3 servings each day	Amount recommended: 2–3 servings each day	Amount recommended: 3–5 servings each day	Amount recommended: 2–4 servings each day	Amount recommended: 6–11 servings each day
★ ★ ★ ★	★ ★ ★ ★	★ ★ ★ ★	★ ★ ★ ★	★ ★ ★ ★
nonfat plain yogurt, nonfat milk, nonfat cream cheese, 1% milk, buttermilk, low-fat cheese, 2% milk	fish, shellfish, poultry (light meat, skinless), turkey, ham, beef (round and sirloin, well trimmed), pork (tenderloin, well trimmed), veal (leg and shoulder, well trimmed), lentils	red and green bell peppers, bok choy, spinach, leaf lettuce, broccoli, carrots, cauliflower	papaya, strawberries, kiwi, orange, grapefruit, orange juice, cantaloupe, mandarin oranges, mango	barley, bulgur, bran or whole grain cereals, popcorn (air-popped or lite microwave), whole grain breads, oatmeal, whole grain pasta, corn or whole wheat tortilla
★ ★ ★	★ ★ ★	★ ★ ★	★ ★ ★	★ ★ ★
part-skim ricotta cheese, whole milk, regular-fat cheese, low-fat chocolate milk, low-fat fruit yogurt, nonfat frozen yogurt	beef (rib, chuck, flank, and ground), ham (lean), tofu, veal and lamb (leg and loin), poultry (dark meat with skin), pork (loin and rib), Canadian bacon, poultry sausage, dried beans and peas, eggs	cabbage, chard, asparagus, kale, vegetable juice, brussels sprouts, iceberg lettuce, sweet potato, tomato, snow peas, zucchini, okra, winter squash, green beans	honeydew, raspberries, apricots, rhubarb, pineapple, watermelon, pineapple juice, blueberries	brown rice, bran muffin, whole grain crackers, soft pretzel or breadstick, English muffin, enriched pasta, popcorn (oil-popped)
★ ★	★ ★	★ ★	★ ★	★ ★
pudding, custard, low-fat frozen yogurt, ice milk	hot dogs, pork sausage, chicken nuggets, fish sticks, nuts and seeds	beets, cucumber, celery, jicama, artichoke, peas, mushrooms	peach, banana, plum, cherries, frozen fruit juice bar, canned fruit	flour tortilla, bagel, enriched breads, enriched rice, pancakes, waffles, graham crackers, saltines, sweetened cereal, dry pretzels or breadsticks
★	★	★	★	★
milkshake, cottage cheese, ice cream, nonfat sour cream	peanut butter, bologna	eggplant, corn, avocado, potato	pear, apple, dried fruit, grapes, raisins	cornbread, fruit or nut bread, biscuit, stuffing, croissant

Sometimes Foods: Alcoholic beverages, bacon, bouillon, butter, cakes, candy, coffee, cookies, condiments, snack crackers, cream, regular-fat cream cheese, doughnuts, french fries, fruit-flavored drinks, gelatin dessert, gravy, honey, jam, jelly, margarine, mayonnaise, nondairy creamer, olives, onion rings, pickles, pies, potato chips, salad dressings, sauces, seasonings, sherbet, soft drinks, sour cream, sugar, tea, tortilla chips, vegetable oils

F I G U R E 9–1

Pyramid plus. (Adapted from Nutrition Education Services/Oregon Dairy Council, 1994.)

How Many Servings Do You Need Each Day?
Use these ranges as your guide for how much food to eat each day. Choose the lower or higher number of servings based on your calorie needs. If you eat more or less than one serving, count as partial servings. For children under age 5, a serving is ¼-½ of a standard serving. However to get enough calcium, all children need a total of at least 2 standard servings of milk or milk products each day.

SOMETIMES FOODS

Sometimes foods provide little or no nutrition and are often high in fat, sugar, salt, and calories. They should be eaten in moderation and not in place of servings from the five food groups.

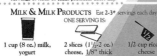

MILK & MILK PRODUCTS Eat 2-3* servings each day
ONE SERVING IS:

1 cup (8 oz.) milk, yogurt   2 slices (1½-2 oz.) cheese, 1/8" thick   1/2 cup ricotta cheese

2 cups cottage cheese   1½ cups frozen yogurt, ice milk or ice cream

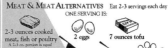

MEAT & MEAT ALTERNATIVES Eat 2-3 servings each day
ONE SERVING IS:

2-3 ounces cooked meat, fish or poultry
A 2-3 oz. portion is equal in size to a deck of cards   2 eggs   7 ounces tofu

1 cup cooked dried peas or beans   1/2 cup nuts or seeds   4 tablespoons peanut butter

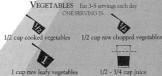

VEGETABLES Eat 3-5 servings each day
ONE SERVING IS:

1/2 cup cooked vegetables   1/2 cup raw chopped vegetables

1 cup raw leafy vegetables   1/2 - 3/4 cup juice

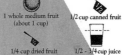

FRUITS Eat 2-4 servings each day
ONE SERVING IS:

1 whole medium fruit (about 1 cup)   1/2 cup canned fruit

1/4 cup dried fruit   1/2 - 3/4 cup juice

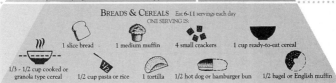
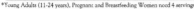

BREADS & CEREALS Eat 6-11 servings each day
ONE SERVING IS:

1 slice bread   1 medium muffin   4 small crackers   1 cup ready-to-eat cereal

1/3 - 1/2 cup cooked or granola type cereal   1/2 cup pasta or rice   1 tortilla   1/2 hot dog or hamburger bun   1/2 bagel or English muffin

*Young Adults (11-24 years), Pregnant and Breastfeeding Women need 4 servings   © 1994. Nutrition Education Services / Oregon Dairy Council.

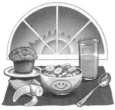
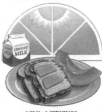
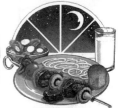

MILK = 1/2 SERVING
MEAT = 0 SERVINGS
VEGETABLES = 0 SERVINGS
FRUITS = 2 SERVINGS
BREADS & CEREALS = 2 SERVINGS

MILK = 2 SERVINGS
MEAT = 1 SERVING
VEGETABLES = 1/2 SERVING
FRUITS = 1 SERVING
BREADS & CEREALS = 2 SERVINGS

MILK = 1 SERVING
MEAT = 1 SERVING
VEGETABLES = 2 ½ SERVINGS
FRUITS = 0 SERVINGS
BREADS & CEREALS = 2 SERVINGS

F I G U R E 9-1 *Continued*

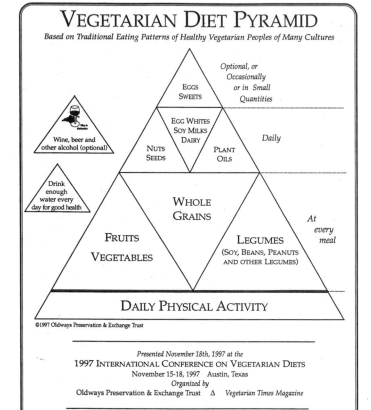

FIGURE 9-2

Vegetarian food pyramid. (© 1997 Oldways Preservation & Exchange Trust.)

TABLE 9-4

Vitamins and Minerals at Risk for Deficit in Strict Vegetarian (Vegan) Diets

VITAMINS AND MINERALS AT RISK FOR DEFICIT	USUAL SOURCES	ALTERNATIVE SOURCES IN VEGAN DIET
Vitamin D	Animal products: egg yolk, butter, liver, salmon, sardines, tuna; sunlight	Fortified cereals, milk, or margarine; sunlight (20-30 min/d, 2-3 times per wk)
Vitamin B_{12}	Animal products only: meat, fish, eggs, dairy products	Fortified soy milk, fortified soy-based meat substitutes, nutritional yeast, fortified cereals, vitamin supplements
Riboflavin	Milk and meat are best sources; also in eggs, dried yeast, grains, dark-green leafy vegetables, avocado, broccoli	Brewer's yeast, wheat germ, beans, almonds, soybeans, tofu, dark-green leafy vegetables, avocado, broccoli, orange juice
Calcium	Milk is best source; also in some fruits, nuts, dark-green leafy vegetables	Fortified soy milk, dried fruits, almonds, sunflower, filberts, whole sesame seeds, green leafy vegetables (avoid spinach, Swiss chard, beet greens, whose oxalic acid hinders calcium absorption)
Iron	Iron in meat sources is more bioavailable than iron in plants; lentils, beans (cooked black, soy, garbanzo, lima) are good sources	All legumes, almonds, pecans, dates, prunes, raisins, fortified cereals, white or brown rice; absorption is enhanced by ascorbic acid-rich foods
Zinc	Meats, animal products, seafood (especially oysters), eggs; found in whole grains, brown rice, nuts, spinach; however, best plant sources also contain phytic acid, which inhibits zinc absorption	Whole grains, brown rice, almonds, wheat germ, tofu, pecans, spinach

T A B L E 9-5
Iron-Rich Foods

	HIGH LEVELS (>5 mg/serving)	MODERATE LEVELS (2-4 mg/serving)	LOW LEVELS (<2 mg/serving)
Breads, grains, cereals, seeds	Almonds (1 cup, whole, oil roasted)	Bagel (1, egg or plain)	Biscuits (1 each)
	Cashews (1 cup, dry roasted)	Bread, Indian fry (1 piece)	Bread (1 slice, whole wheat)
	Fortified cereals	Breadstick (10, plain, without salt)	Egg noodles (1 cup, cooked)
	Mixed nuts (1 cup, dry roasted with peanuts)	Filberts (1 cup, dried)	English muffin (1 each)
	Brown glutinous rice (1 cup, cooked)	Gingerbread (1 piece)	Pancakes (1 each)
	Sunflower seeds (1 cup, dry roasted)	Muffin (1 wheat)	Peanut butter (2 tbsp)
	Watermelon kernels (1 cup, dried)	Peanuts (1 cup, dried)	
	Wheat germ (1 cup, toasted)	White rice (1 cup, enriched, regular, cooked)	
		Waffles (2 each)	
		Walnuts (1 cup, dried)	
Fruits	Apricot (1 cup, dried halves)	Avocado (1 whole)	Apple (1 medium, unpeeled)
		Currants (1 cup, dried Zante)	Apple juice (1 cup)
		Fig (10 each, dried)	Banana (1 medium)
		Pear (10 each, dried halves)	Dried mixed fruit (2 oz)
		Prune juice (1 cup)	Orange (1 medium)
		Raisins (1 cup)	Orange juice (1 cup)

Vegetables	Kidney beans (1 cup, cooked, fresh) Lentils (1 cup, cooked) Soybeans (1 cup, cooked) White beans (1 cup, cooked) Spinach (1 cup, cooked)	Black beans (1 cup, cooked) Garbanzo beans (1 cup, cooked) Refried beans (1 cup, canned) Beet greens (1 cup, cooked) Potatoes (1 medium, with skin, baked) Snow peas with pods (1 cup, raw or cooked)	Kidney beans (1 cup, canned) Green beans (1 cup, raw or cooked) Broccoli (1 cup) Carrots (1 cup) Corn (1/2 cup) Lettuce (1 cup) Peas (1 cup, fresh, cooked) Potato chips (1 oz) Spinach (1 cup, raw) Sweet potatoes (1 cup, fresh, boiled, mashed) Tomatoes (1 cup fresh) Tomato juice (1 cup, canned) Turnip greens (1 cup, cooked)
Meats, poultry, fish, other protein sources	Beef heart meat (1/2 cup, cooked) Beef liver (3 oz, simmered) Clams (3.5 oz, 5 each, or 1 cup) Oysters (6 each, or 1 cup, Eastern) Veal liver (3 oz, simmered)	Ground beef (3.5 oz, cooked, lean) Catfish (1 piece, floured, fried) Tuna (1 cup, canned, water packed)	Roast beef (3 oz, lean) Chicken (1 cup, dark or light meat) Egg (one, whole) Halibut (1 piece, baked or broiled) Ham (1 cup, roasted) Bacon (3 pieces, cooked) Pork (3 oz, lean shoulder roast)

Adapted from Hands ES: Food Finder: Food Sources of Vitamins & Minerals, 3rd ed. Salem, OR, ESHA Research, 1995.

▉ IRON DEFICIENCY

Children may lack any dietary nutrient, but iron deficiency is a common problem seen by the pediatric provider. In fact, iron deficiency anemia is the most common hematological disease in children (Behrman et al., 1996). At high risk are premature infants, infants exclusively breastfed after 4 months of age, and adolescents experiencing rapid growth and menstruation. To prevent iron deficiency anemia,

- Children under 10 years should take in 8 to 10 mg of iron daily; older children and adolescents need 12 to 30 mg of iron daily, depending on weight, age, and gender
- Iron supplements should be given to all premature infants
- From 4 months of age, infants who are breastfed exclusively should receive iron supplements
- Infants should be introduced to solid foods by 6 months
- Bottle-fed infants should receive iron-fortified formula
- Children's diets should contain adequate iron-rich foods (Table 9-5).

▉ EATING DISORDERS: ANOREXIA, BULIMIA, AND OBESITY

Eating disorders represent a significant problem in the pediatric population, and the primary care provider must be alert to early signs. Even children as young as 6 to 8 years of age may be heard expressing concern that they are "too fat." Adolescent girls are particularly prone to anorexia and bulimia. Table 9-6 lists several questions that can be used to quickly assess for a possible eating disorder. Obesity and overweight are more common eating disorders, often requiring long-term management. Calculation of body mass index (BMI) helps the primary care provider determine whether a child is overweight (see Table 9-7). Table 9-8 outlines guidelines to assist the primary care provider treating children who are overweight. To help prevent eating problems, anticipatory guidance of children should include a discussion of healthy nutrition, exercise, fitness, and a positive body image.

T A B L E 9–6
Quick Assessment Tool for Eating Disorders

	YES	NO
1. Do you spend most of your time thinking about food?	—	—
2. Do you panic if you gain a pound or two?	—	—
3. Do you ever eat uncontrollably?	—	—
4. Do you feel guilt and remorse after eating?	—	—
5. Do you ever fast or restrict your diet?	—	—
6. Do you vomit or use laxatives to control your weight?	—	—
7. Are your periods irregular, or have you stopped menstruating?	—	—
8. Do you have a strict exercise regimen?	—	—
9. Do you panic if you are unable to exercise as much as you'd like?	—	—

From Decker SD: Eating disorders. *In* Johnson BS (ed): Psychiatric-Mental Health Nursing: Adaptation and Growth, 4th ed. Philadelphia, JB Lippincott, 1997, p. 700.

T A B L E 9–7
Calculation of Body Mass Index*

AGE	EXPECTED PARAMETERS
≤14 yr	19–20
15 yr	25
≥16 yr	28

*Body mass index (BMI) = weight (in kg) divided by the square of the height (in meters).

T A B L E 9–8

Guidelines for Managing Childhood Obesity

- Do not put child on a diet. Instead, gradually modify the entire family's eating habits. For example, serve fruit as a substitute for dessert, switch to nonfat or 1% milk, experiment with low-fat recipes and methods of food preparation, and use reduced-fat margarine, salad dressings, and other low-fat condiments. Serve nutrient-dense foods that reflect the food guide pyramid, including whole grains, fruits, vegetables, lean protein foods, and low-fat dairy products.
- Do not force children to clean their plates. They should eat only until they are full.
- Schedule and enforce regular times for meals and snacks. Do not skip meals. Do not allow children to nibble throughout the day.
- Have low-calorie, nutritious snacks readily available, such as air-popped popcorn, pretzels, low-fat yogurt, frozen fruit juice bars, skim milk, low-sugar cereals, fresh fruit, and raw vegetables.
- Do not have high-calorie snacks readily available (e.g., potato chips, cookies, cakes, pies, ice cream, candy, pop, and doughnuts).
- Promote physical activity. Make daily exercise a priority. Encourage family participation, individual exercise, and team sports and structured activities with peers.
- Limit television viewing. Children who watch 4 or more hours of television per day are twice as likely as other children to become obese. Children are more sedentary when they watch television, and frequent food advertising has been linked to increased snacking.
- Scale back television watching slowly, replacing time with activities, hobbies, or chores.
- Praise and reward children for the progress they make in reaching nutrition, activity, self-esteem, or weight goals. Emphasize the uniqueness of each child, pointing out special talents, abilities, and positive qualities.

REFERENCES

Behrman RE, Kliegman RM, Arvin AM: Nelson Textbook of Pediatrics, 15th ed. Philadelphia, WB Saunders, 1996.

Decker SD: Eating disorders. *In* Johnson BS (ed): Psychiatric-Mental Health Nursing: Adaptation and Growth, 4th ed. Philadelphia, JB Lippincott, 1997, p 700.

Hands ES: Food Finder: Food Sources of Vitamins & Minerals, 3rd ed. Salem, OR, ESHA Research, 1995.

National Academy of Sciences: Recommended Dietary Allowances, 10th ed. Washington, DC, National Academy of Sciences, 1989.

Nutrition Education Services/Oregon Dairy Council: Pyramid Plus. Portland, OR, National Education Services, 1994.

Oldways Preservation & Exchange Trust: Vegetarian Diet Pyramid. Vegetarian Times, 1997.

Rathbun JM, Peterson KE: Nutrition in failure to thrive. *In* Grand RJ, Sutphen JL, Dietz WH (eds): Pediatric Nutrition. Boston, Butterworths, 1987, pp 627–643.

CHAPTER 10

Breastfeeding

Breast milk is the ideal food for newborns and infants, and every mother should be encouraged to breastfeed. There are many benefits of breastfeeding, including

- Natural immunity for the infant, contributing to fewer infections
- Lower exposure to allergens
- Decreased incidence of sudden infant death syndrome
- Closer bonding between mother and infant
- Convenience
- Lower cost

Although breastfeeding is recommended for a minimum of 12 months (American Academy of Pediatrics, 1997), receiving breast milk for any length of time is beneficial.

ESTABLISHING BREASTFEEDING

New mothers often have questions about breastfeeding—how to get started; what problems to look for; how to tell if the baby is getting enough to eat. The primary care provider is in an ideal position to answer these questions and to facilitate breastfeeding.

Establishing a proper latch-on is one of the first skills the mother and newborn learn. Figure 10-1 illustrates proper latch-on, with the infant's tongue cupping the nipple and areola and the top and bottom lips flanged out.

Without use of a precision scale, it is impossible to determine the exact amount of breast milk babies ingest. Fortunately, infants tell us in many less quantitative ways whether breastfeeding is effective and if they are getting enough milk. Table 10-1 lists behaviors that, if present, indicate that the infant is adequately nourished.

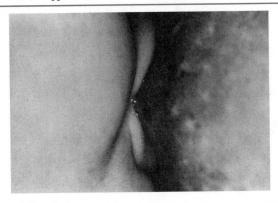

F I G U R E 10–1
Infant properly latched on the breast with lips flanged outward. (Photo courtesy of UNICEF.)

Breastfed infants tend to weigh less than their formula-fed counterparts, but after the mother's breast milk comes in in the first week of life, they gain 0.5 to 1 oz per day (4 to 7 oz per week). Their birth weight is regained by 2 weeks, doubled by 5 to 6 months, and tripled by 12 months.

BREASTFEEDING PROBLEMS

A number of problems can interfere with effective breastfeeding, and early intervention by the nurse practitioner can ensure that breastfeeding continues with the infant receiving optimal nourishment. Table 10–2 identifies some common breastfeeding problems and their management strategies.

T A B L E 10–1
Criteria to Assess Effective Breastfeeding

- Infant feeding cues: active rooting and sucking when hungry; satiation after feeding
- Audible swallowing that sounds like a "glug" or air blowing out of the baby's nose
- Smooth suck-swallow pattern
- Active, alert, content infant
- Developmental appropriateness
- Age-appropriate height and head circumference
- Good skin turgor and color
- At least six wet diapers and several stools per day

T A B L E 10–2

Common Breastfeeding Problems and Management Strategies

PROBLEM	MANAGEMENT STRATEGIES
Flat or inverted nipples	Prenatal: • Use breast shells during third trimester. Consult with obstetrician or nurse midwife before use Postpartum: • Use football-hold position for feeding • Wear breast shells between feedings • Massage nipple and apply cold cloth or ice before feeding
Sore nipples	• Establish correct latch-on and positioning for feeding • Rub a few drops of colostrum or hindmilk on nipples after feeding and air dry • Expose nipples to air or sunlight for brief periods • Use breast shell to prevent clothing from rubbing against nipples • Nurse for shorter, more frequent feedings • Nurse from less sore side first; pump breast if nipple is too sore • Use mild analgesic as needed
Severe engorgement	• Apply wet heat: hot shower; hot, wet packs (can wrap breast in wet disposable diaper) • *Gently* massage entire breast • Use electric pump with intermittent suction, minimum setting • Express small amount of milk before feeding to soften the areola • Nurse frequently, especially while the milk supply is being established
Mastitis	• Treat 10–14 d with antibiotic that covers *Staphylococcus aureus* • Rest • Use analgesic as needed • Nurse frequently; pump breast if nursing is too painful; the breast milk is *not* infected and is fine for the infant • Apply wet heat • Increase fluids • Do not wean abruptly because this can lead to abscess formation

Table continued on following page

T A B L E 10–2 *Continued*

Common Breastfeeding Problems and Management Strategies

PROBLEM	MANAGEMENT STRATEGIES
Nipple confusion	• Avoid offering bottle nipples and pacifiers for first 4–6 weeks • Ensure correct latch-on and positioning so infant can suck correctly; may need to "retrain" infant to suck • Do not use nipple shields • If supplements are given, use an eyedropper, spoon, syringe, or cup, or 5-F feeding tube taped to the breast so that the nipple, areola, and feeding tube are in the infant's mouth
Breast milk jaundice	• Continue breastfeeding unless infant has signs of pathological jaundice
Thrush	• Rub nystatin (1 ml [1,000,000 units]) on lesions in infant's mouth after feeding and cleaning the mucosa • Apply nystatin to mother's nipples after feeding and cleaning the skin
Poor weight gain	• Assess thoroughly to determine cause • History of infant and maternal factors • Breastfeeding technique • Provide instruction, support, and reinforcement for use of correct technique • Refer for treatment of physical or organic causes • Provide immediate infusion of calories if infant has lost too much weight and does not have the energy to adequately suck • If supplements are given, use an eyedropper, spoon, syringe, or cup or 5-F feeding tube taped to the breast so that the nipple, areola, and feeding tube are in the infant's mouth

TABLE 10-3

Breastfeeding and Returning to Work: Advice for Mothers

BEFORE RETURNING TO WORK

Practice pumping
Begin freezing milk
Introduce a bottle to your baby at 3 to 4 wk of age
Offer a bottle 1 or 2 times a week

STORAGE OF BREAST MILK

Refrigerate milk for only 24–48 hr
Freeze milk in refrigerator freezer for a maximum of 3 mo; deep-freeze for a
    maximum of 6 mo
Store milk in plastic baby bottles or disposable milk bags
Label with date and baby's name
Transport milk in cooler bag or container with ice/gel pak

HOW TO INCREASE MILK SUPPLY

Relax and avoid fatigue
Pump an extra time per day or add another feeding
Massage breasts before nursing
Have a picture of your baby at the pump
Play relaxing music or taped sounds of baby while pumping

RETURNING TO WORK

Pump 2–3 times a day, depending on the infant's age
Plan on 15–30 min per pumping session
Wear clothes to hide leaks and offer easy access to breasts

FEEDING BREAST MILK

Warm or thaw milk in warm water
Do not microwave because milk will heat unevenly and present a risk for
    burns
Refrigerate milk for no more than 24 hr after thawing
Can refeed milk once if the entire bottle is not finished
Refeed leftover milk at next feeding
Do not refeed leftover milk if baby has thrush
Do not add milk to a bottle that has already been used

GENERAL IMPORTANT REMINDERS

Wash hands before and after pumping
Clean pump parts with dish detergent after each use
Have care provider wash hands before and after feeding breast milk

Adapted from Humphrey N: Breastfeeding. Working moms can make it work. Adv Nurs
Pract 2:22, 1994.

Mothers who return to work should be encouraged to continue breastfeeding as long as possible. Table 10-3 outlines issues to be considered as the primary care provider and mother plan how to best integrate working and breastfeeding.

REFERENCES

American Academy of Pediatrics: Breastfeeding and the use of human milk. Pediatrics 100(6):1035–1039, 1997.

Humphrey N: Breastfeeding: Working moms can make it work. ADVANCE for Nurse Practitioners 2(6):22, 1994.

CHAPTER 11

Elimination

Healthy children demonstrate a wide range of "normal" elimination patterns. The nurse practitioner can provide parents and children with anticipatory guidance about toileting and toilet training, as well as help families manage problems related to elimination.

Children are capable of voluntary bladder and bowel control by about 18 to 24 months of age, but toilet-training readiness is a function of a number of factors, outlined in Table 11-1. The task of achieving toilet training, usually complete by age 4, requires a great deal of

TABLE 11-1

Guidelines for Assessing Toilet-Training Readiness

Child's physical skills	Has voluntary sphincter control
	Stays dry for 2 hr, may wake from naps still dry
	Is able to sit, walk, and squat
	Assists in dressing self
Child's cognitive skills	Recognizes urge to urinate or defecate
	Understands meaning of words used by family in toileting
	Understands what toilet is for
	Understands connection between dry pants and toilet
	Is able to follow directions
	Is able to communicate needs
Child's interpersonal skills	Demonstrates desire to please parent
	Expresses curiosity about use of toilet
	Expresses desire to be dry and clean
Parental skills	Expresses desire to assist child with training
	Recognizes child's cues of readiness
	Has no compelling factor that will interfere with training (e.g., new job, move, family loss)

patience, sensitivity, humor, and understanding on the part of parents. Advice and support from the nurse practitioner may be essential factors that make this a positive experience for both child and parent. Guidelines for managing toilet training are noted in Table 11-2.

After an age when voluntary control should be established, some children experience problems with involuntary control of either stool (encopresis) or urine (enuresis or dysfunctional bladder). These conditions present a challenge to the child, family, and nurse practitioner and can involve significant emotional impact. The child is often shunned by peers, teachers, and even family members. Changing the offensive behaviors can be extremely difficult, requiring a long-term plan with focused, conscientious actions on the part of parents and the child. Table 11-3 outlines a recommended protocol for management of constipated encopresis.

T A B L E 11–2

Management of Toilet Training

Keep child as clean and dry as possible:
  Change diapers frequently
  Introduce training pants when child stays dry for several hours. Use them during the day, and diaper at night
Talk to child about toilet training:
  Praise child for coming to you to have diaper changed
  Explain connection between being clean and dry and using toilet
  Encourage child to use toilet from time to time during the day, especially before going out to play, going on a trip, before naps, and at bedtime
Teach child how to use toilet:
  Allow child to observe while parents or older siblings use toilet
  Demonstrate how to sit on toilet, use toilet paper, flush, and wash one's hands
Provide practice time for child:
  Provide a potty chair or portable toilet seat for a regular toilet
  Allow child to sit on potty chair with clothes or diaper on
  Encourage child to use potty chair while parent uses regular toilet
  Have child sit on toilet without diapers for 5 to 10 minutes at a time
  Schedule practice sessions for times a child usually urinates or defecates
Provide a comfortable, safe-feeling environment:
  Seat child facing backward on a regular toilet or provide a footstool to rest the feet on
  Never flush the toilet when child is sitting on it
  Stay with child for safety reasons
Give consistent, positive feedback:
  Praise child for trying, as well as for success
  Never demand performance
  Never make child sit on toilet if child resists
  Be understanding of child's refusal to use toilet
  Ignore or minimize undesired behavior
  Never scold or punish a child for wetting or soiling

TABLE 11-3
Management of Children With Constipated Encopresis

TREATMENT PHASE	TREATMENT PROGRAM	COMMENTS
Catharsis	In the home: four 3-d cycles (12 d total): Day 1: Fleet enema (adult size) Day 2: Bisacodyl (Dulcolax) suppository Day 3: Bisacodyl tablet Day 13: Bisacodyl tablet Return to clinic Follow-up abdominal radiograph to confirm catharsis	Catharsis may need to occur in the hospital if: Retention is severe Home compliance is poor Parents prefer admission Parents should not administer enemas for psychological reasons Goal of catharsis is to empty the bowel. The child may have soft stools for several days after catharsis; parents and patient should be informed that ongoing maintenance is essential for the bowel to return to fully normal functioning. Initial improvement can be falsely reassuring and may contribute to poor compliance to maintenance regimen
Maintenance	Stool softener (e.g., mineral oil), starting at 2 tbsp bid. Titrate dose to facilitate soft stools without mineral oil leakage Daily multivitamin to counteract possible decreased absorption of fat-soluble vitamins Oral laxatives (e.g., milk of magnesia, senna concentrate [Senokot]) may be substituted for or used alternately with stool softener Toilet sitting at least twice a day for 10 min each time Increased activity, increased fluids (other than milk), increased fiber in diet	Goals of maintenance: No soiling Regular, soft bowel movements (at least every other day) Increased ability to sense the urge to defecate Toilet sitting should be scheduled at times the child is most likely to have a bowel movement (e.g., on wakening, after meals)
Follow-up	Regular visits (every 4–10 wk), depending on severity and need of family Telephone availability to discuss progress and adjust doses Counseling or referral as appropriate for psychosocial and developmental issues Continued education of normal bowel function	Goals of follow-up visits: Monitor compliance Provide encouragement and support Detect and treat relapse early if it occurs

Adapted from Levine MD, Carey WB, Crocker AC: Developmental-Behavioral Pediatrics, 3rd ed. Philadelphia, WB Saunders, 1999.

Treatment of functional enuresis (i.e., nonorganic) takes several approaches. Preschool and early school-age children often wet their beds during sleep, and functional enuresis is usually self-limited. As a result, aggressive treatment should be delayed until the child is 6 to 8 years of age. Strategies for use with the 6-year-old or older child are listed in Table 11–4. Successful treatment has been correlated with positive family functioning and requires active involvement of both parents and children.

Table 11–5 presents guidelines for bladder retraining for children with dysfunctional voiding or pediatric unstable bladder, in which

TABLE 11–4
Management of Enuresis in Children

STRATEGY	COMMENTS
ENURESIS ALARM	Behavioral modification. An electric alarm with a bell or buzzer wakes the child when he or she begins to wet. Initially, the child learns to wake and use the toilet when stimulated by the buzzer; subsequently, he or she associates the beginning of urination with waking and toileting.
MOTIVATIONAL THERAPY	Family provides encouragement and reinforcement (e.g., a "star chart," rewards, and praise) for positive behaviors. Children should be seen by the primary care provider every 2 weeks. Provider support is essential. The method assumes that children will take responsibility for the problem and for learning how to resolve it. Emotionally time-consuming; requires a high level of healthy communication between parents and children.
BLADDER CONTROL TRAINING	Directed toward "training" the bladder to hold greater quantities of urine, assuming that stretching the bladder leads to an increased threshold before the bladder is stimulated to empty. Children are taught to • Be more sensitive to cues of a full bladder • Control stopping and starting the urinary stream as they urinate • Postpone urinating until they "can't hold it any longer"

T A B L E   11–4   *Continued*

Management of Enuresis in Children

STRATEGY	COMMENTS
DRUG THERAPY	Children taking medications on a regular basis should have a drug "holiday" every 3 months to assess the need for continued pharmacotherapy. After 1 month without wetting, medications can be tapered over a 2–4-wk period.
• Imipramine hydrochloride Initially, 25 mg daily 1 hr before bedtime. After 1 wk, can increase to 50 mg for children 6–12 yr; 75 mg for children over 12 yr	Not recommended for children under 6 yr of age. Has serious side effects; has been fatal in some cases. Administer with great care. Use least amount effective. Tricyclic antidepressant with an as yet unknown mechanism of action.
• Desmopressin acetate (DDAVP) Oral: 0.2-mg tablets once daily at bedtime; can be adjusted up to maximum of 0.6 mg/d	Not recommended for children under 6 yr of age. Often effective in children with family history of enuresis. When switching from nasal spray to tablets, give first oral dose 24 hr after last intranasal dose.
Nasal spray or solution: 20 µg (2 sprays) or 0.2 ml solution intranasally at bedtime; can be adjusted up to 40 µg or down to 10 µg/d	When using nasal spray, administer one-half dose per nostril. Changes in nasal mucosa (e.g., with upper respiratory infection) may compromise absorption; administer an antihistamine or decongestant 30–60 min before using, or consider oral form. Caution must be taken with patients who are hypertensive or have a potential for fluid electrolyte imbalance (e.g., children with cystic fibrosis susceptible to hyponatremia) Manufacturer recommends that treatment beyond 7 d should include electrolyte studies.
• Oxybutynin chloride 5 mg bid, maximum 5 mg tid	Not recommended for children under 5 yr of age.

T A B L E 11–5

Bladder Retraining for Dysfunctional Voiding

- Establish a schedule for voiding. Have child go to bathroom every 2–4 hr, whether urgency is felt or not.
- Void with relaxation. Have child take a deep breath and relax sphincter when exhaling. Use a straw to breathe through. Have child try grasping his or her fingers together and pulling them apart.
- Void to completion. Teach child to use the Credé maneuver or manual pressure over the suprapubic area to complete voiding.
- Double void. After the child voids completely, have him or her wait on the toilet 2–3 min and attempt to void again.

children have difficulty starting micturition, preventing leaking, or completely emptying the bladder.

REFERENCE

Levine MD, Carey WB, Crocker AC: Developmental-Behavioral Pediatrics, 3rd ed. Philadelphia, WB Saunders, 1999.

CHAPTER 12

Activities and Sports for Children and Adolescents

Helping children to be active is important to their health and well-being. The nurse practitioner working with children and adolescents around sports issues must try to help clients and families find a balance between the health benefits of exercise and fitness and the risks of injuries.

■■■■ SPORTS PREPARTICIPATION ASSESSMENT

The preparticipation assessment allows the provider to assess the young person's health risks for participation in a variety of sports. It also offers an opportunity for discussion related to health maintenance and promotion because the athlete wants to be at optimal performance levels. Previous trauma, cardiovascular, musculoskeletal, chronic diseases, and other health problems are risk factors for participation. Table 12-1 summarizes the health history for sports participation recommended by the American Academy of Pediatrics and other organizations. Figure 12-1 provides suggestions for the musculoskeletal assessment of athletes for participation in various sports. It does not replace the general physical examination that should also be completed.

■■■■ CLASSIFICATION OF SPORTS AND HEALTH CONDITIONS FOR SPORTS PARTICIPATION RISK ASSESSMENT

Tables 12-2 and 12-3 are used together after the health of the athlete is assessed. These two tables assist the NP to make decisions about risks of participation in contact, limited contact, or noncontact sports. Table 12-2 classifies most sports by collision risks. Table 12-3 identifies medical conditions and recommendations for level of participation in various collision and noncollision sports as classified in Table 12-2.

Text continued on page 134

T A B L E 12-1

Sports Preparticipation History Questions

1. Have you had a medical illness or injury since your last checkup or sports physical?
2. Have you ever been hospitalized overnight?
3. Are you currently taking any prescription or nonprescription (over-the-counter) medications or pills or using an inhaler?
   Have you ever taken any supplements or vitamins to help you gain or lose weight or improve your performance?
4. Do you have allergies (e.g., to pollen, medicine, food, or stinging insects)?
5. Have you ever passed out during or after exercise?
   Have you ever been dizzy during or after exercise?
   Have you ever had chest pain during or after exercise?
   Do you get tired more quickly than your friends do during exercise?
   Have you ever had racing of your heart or skipped heartbeats?
   Have you had high blood pressure or high cholesterol?
   Have you ever been told you had a heart murmur?
   Has any family member or relative died of heart problems or of sudden death before age 50?
   Have you had a severe viral infection (e.g., myocarditis or mononucleosis) within the past month?
   Has a physician ever denied or restricted your participation in sports for any heart problems?
6. Do you have any current skin problems (e.g., itching, rashes, acne, warts, fungus, or blisters)?
7. Have you ever had a head injury or concussion?
   Have you ever been knocked out, become unconscious, or lost your memory?
   Have you ever had a seizure?
   Do you have frequent or severe headaches?
   Have you ever had numbness or tingling in your arms, hands, legs, or feet?
   Have you ever had a stinger, burner, or pinched nerve?
8. Have you ever become ill from exercising in the heat?
9. Do you cough, wheeze, or have trouble breathing during or after activity?
   Do you have asthma?
   Do you have seasonal allergies that require medical treatment?

T A B L E   12–1

Sports Preparticipation History Questions Continued

10. Do you use any special protective or corrective equipment or devices that are not usually used for your sport or position (e.g., knee brace, special neck roll, foot orthoses, retainer on your teeth, hearing aid)?

11. Have you had any problems with your eyes or vision?
    Do you wear glasses, contacts, or protective eyewear?

12. Have you ever had a sprain, strain, or swelling after injury?
    Have you broken or fractured any bones or dislocated any joints?
    Have you had any other problems with pain or swelling in muscles, tendons, bones, or joints?
    If yes, check appropriate box and explain below:

    | _____ head | _____ elbow | _____ hip |
    | _____ neck | _____ forearm | _____ thigh |
    | _____ back | _____ wrist | _____ knee |
    | _____ chest | _____ hand | _____ shin/calf |
    | _____ shoulder | _____ finger | _____ ankle |
    | _____ upper arm | | _____ foot |

13. Do you want to weigh more or less than you do now?
    Do you lose weight regularly to meet weight requirements for your sport?

14. Do you feel stressed out?

15. Record the dates of your most recent immunizations:

    | _____ tetanus | _____ measles |
    | _____ hepatitis B | _____ chickenpox |

Females only:

16. When was your first menstrual period?
    When was your most recent menstrual period?
    How much time do you usually have from the start of one period to the start of another?
    How many periods have you had in the last year?
    What was the longest time between periods in the last year?

Adapted from American Academy of Family Physicians, American Academy of Pediatrics, American Medical Society for Sports Medicine, et al. Preparticipation Physical Evaluation, 2nd ed., p. 47. New York, McGraw-Hill, 1997.

F I G U R E   12–1

The sports preparticipation musculoskeletal examination. (Used with permission of Ross Products Division, Abbott Laboratories, Columbus, OH 43216. From For the Practitioner: Orthopaedic Screening Examination for Participation in Sports. ©1981 Ross Products Division, Abbott Laboratories.)

See illustrations on following pages

EXAMINATION PARAMETERS

- Appropriate for interscholastic, intramural, and extramural sports activities.
- A screening evaluation created to direct attention to problems but not evaluate the problems.
- Identifies the following conditions that might be adversely affected by athletic participation:
  a. Congenital problems
  b. Acquired problems

HISTORY

Questions such as the following are to be answered by the athlete and signed by BOTH the athlete and parent:

- Have you ever had an illness, condition, or injury that required you to go to the hospital, either as a patient overnight or in the emergency room or for x-rays; required an operation; caused you to see a doctor; caused you to miss a game or practice?
- Are you now or have you been under the care of a physician for any reason?
- Do you currently have any medical problems or injuries?
- Have you ever had a broken bone, joint sprain or ligament tear, muscle pull, head injury, neck injury or nerve pinch, dislocated joint, back trouble or problems?

ACTIVITY 1

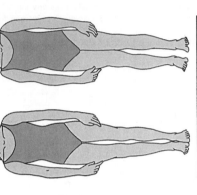

Normal   Abnormal

INSTRUCTIONS OBSERVATIONS

Stand straight with arms at sides.
Symmetry of upper and lower extremities and trunk.
Common abnormalities:
1. Enlarged acromioclavicular joint
2. Enlarged sternoclavicular joint
3. Asymmetrical waist (leg length difference or scoliosis)
4. Swollen knee
5. Swollen ankle

FIGURE 12–1

See legend on previous page

ACTIVITY 2

Normal

Abnormal

INSTRUCTIONS

Look at ceiling; look at floor; touch right (left) ear to shoulder; look over right (left) shoulder.

OBSERVATIONS

Should be able to touch chin to chest, ears to shoulders and look equally over shoulders.
Common abnormalities (may indicate previous neck injury):
1. Loss of flexion
2. Loss of lateral bending
3. Loss of rotation

FIGURE 12−1

Illustration continued on following page

123

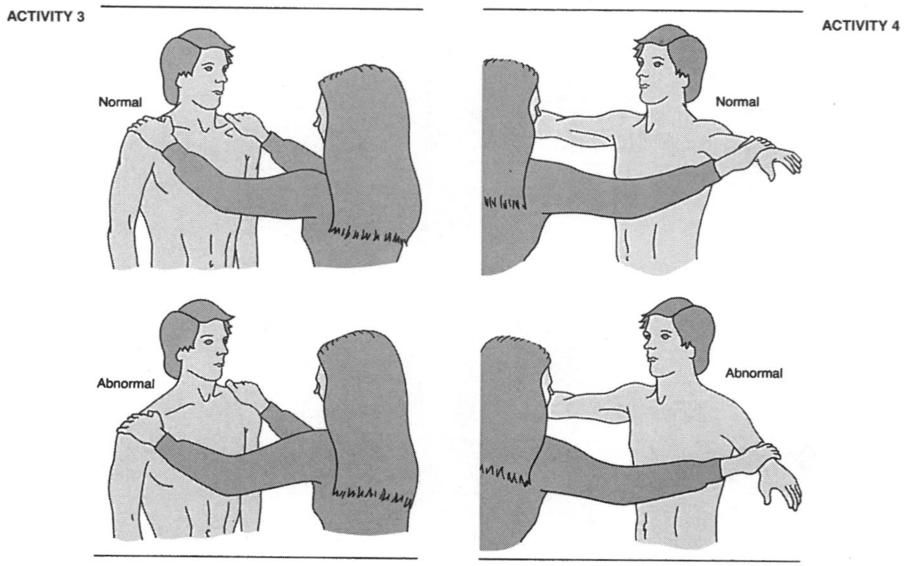

ACTIVITY 3   ACTIVITY 4

Normal   Abnormal   Normal   Abnormal

FIGURE 12-1 Continued

ACTIVITY 6

ACTIVITY 5

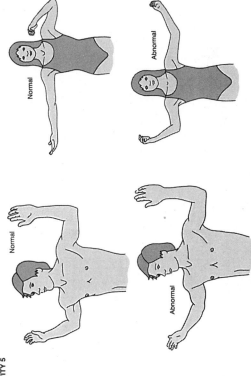

Normal

Abnormal

Normal

Abnormal

ACTIVITY 5

INSTRUCTIONS Hold arms out from sides with elbows bent (90°); raise hands back vertically as far as they will go.

OBSERVATIONS Hands go back equally and at least to upright vertical position.
Common abnormalities (may indicate shoulder problem or old dislocation):
1. Loss of external rotation

ACTIVITY 6

INSTRUCTIONS Hold arms out from sides, palms up; straighten elbows completely; bend completely.

OBSERVATIONS Motion equal left and right.
Common abnormalities (may indicate old elbow injury, old dislocation, fracture, etc.):
1. Loss of extension
2. Loss of flexion

F I G U R E 1 2 – 1 Continued

Illustration continued on following page

125

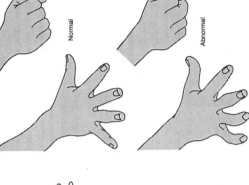

ACTIVITY 7

ACTIVITY 8

Normal

Abnormal

Normal

Abnormal

INSTRUCTIONS Hold arms down at sides with elbows bent (90°); supinate palms; pronate palms.

OBSERVATIONS Palms should go from facing ceiling to facing floor. Common abnormalities (may indicate old forearm, wrist, or elbow injury):
1. Lack of full supination
2. Lack of full pronation

INSTRUCTIONS Make a fist; open hand and spread fingers.

OBSERVATIONS Fist should be tight and fingers straight when spread. Common abnormalities (may indicate old finger fractures or sprains):
1. Protruding knuckle from fist
2. Swollen and/or crooked finger

FIGURE 12–1 *Continued*

ACTIVITY 9

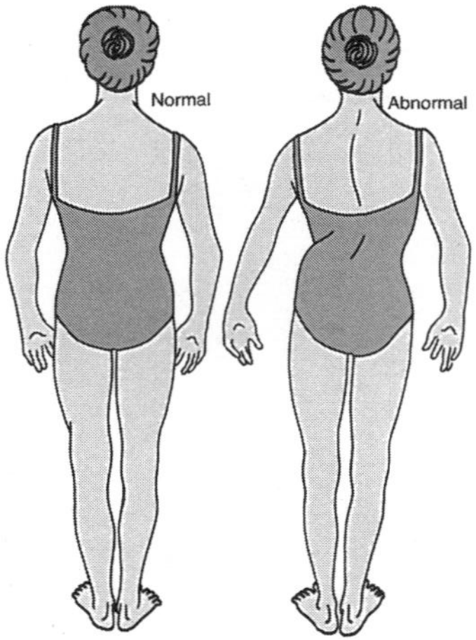

ACTIVITY 10

Normal Abnormal

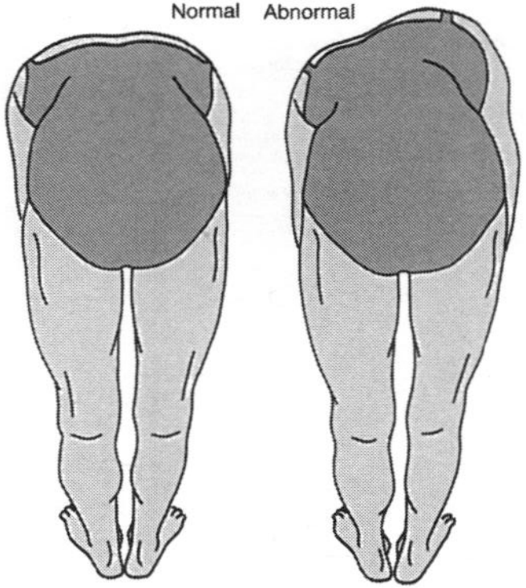

Normal Abnormal

INSTRUCTIONS

OBSERVATIONS

With back to examiner stand up straight.

Symmetry of shoulders, waist, thighs, and calves.
Common abnormalities:
1. High shoulder (scoliosis) or low shoulder (muscle loss)
2. Prominent rib cage (scoliosis)
3. High hip or asymmetrical waist (leg length difference or scoliosis)
4. Small calf or thigh (weakness from old injury)

INSTRUCTIONS

OBSERVATIONS

Bend forward slowly as to touch toes.

Bends forward straightly and smoothly.
Common abnormalities:
1. Twists to side (low back pain)
2. Back asymmetrical (scoliosis)

FIGURE 1–2–1 Continued

Illustration continued on following page

127

ACTIVITY 11

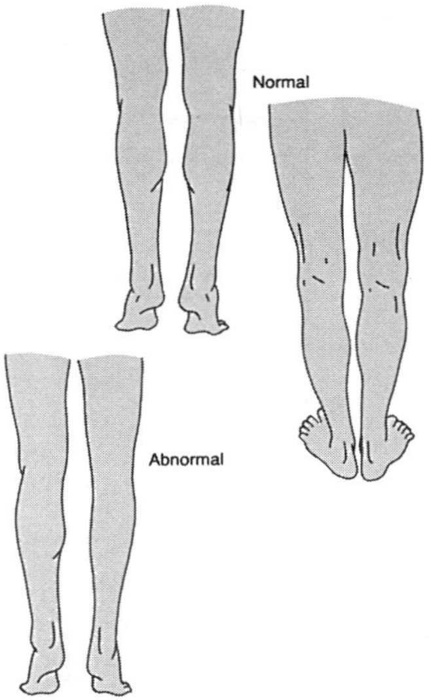

Normal

Abnormal

INSTRUCTIONS Stand on heels; stand on toes.

OBSERVATIONS Equal elevation right and left; symmetry of calf muscles.
Common abnormalities:
1. Wasting of calf muscles (Achilles injury or old ankle injury)

ACTIVITY 12

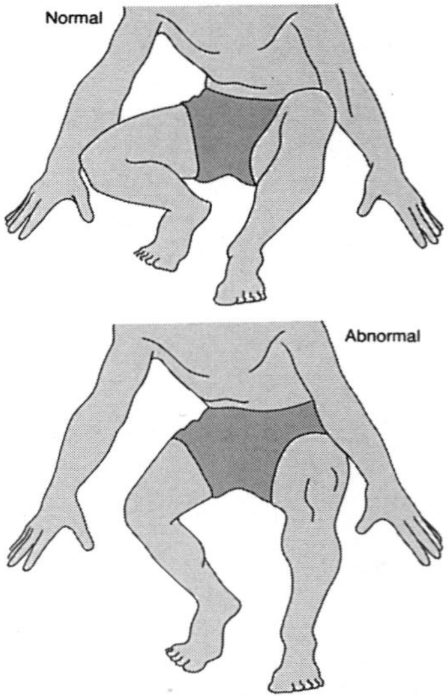

Normal

Abnormal

INSTRUCTIONS
OBSERVATIONS Squat on heels; duck walk 4 steps and stand up.
Maneuver is painless; heel to buttock distance equal left and right; knee flexion equal during walk; rises straight up.
Common abnormalities:
1. Inability to fully flex one knee
2. Inability to stand up without twisting or bending to one side

FIGURE 12–1 Continued

128

T A B L E 12–2

Classification of Sports by Contact

CONTACT/COLLISION	LIMITED CONTACT	NONCONTACT
Basketball	Baseball	Archery
Boxing*	Bicycling	Badminton
Diving	Cheerleading	Body building
Field hockey	Canoeing/kayaking	Canoeing/kayaking
Football	(white water)	(flat water)
flag	Fencing	Crew/rowing
tackle	Field	Curling
Ice hockey	high jump	Dancing
Lacrosse	pole vault	Field
Martial arts	Floor hockey	discus
Rodeo	Gymnastics	javelin
Rugby	Handball	shot put
Ski jumping	Horseback riding	Golf
Soccer	Racquetball	Orienteering
Team handball	Skating	Power lifting
Water polo	ice	Race walking
Wrestling	in-line	Riflery
	roller	Rope jumping
	Skiing	Running
	cross-country	Sailing
	downhill	Scuba diving
	water	Strength training
	Softball	Swimming
	Squash	Table tennis
	Ultimate frisbee	Tennis
	Volleyball	Track
	Windsurfing/surfing	Weightlifting

*Participation not recommended.

Used with permission of the American Academy of Pediatrics, American Academy of Pediatrics Committee on Sports Medicine. Medical conditions affecting sports participation. Pediatrics 94:757–760, 1994. Copyright 1994 by the American Academy of Pediatrics.

T A B L E 12–3

Medical Conditions and Sports Participation*

CONDITION	MAY PARTICIPATE?
Atlantoaxial instability (instability of the joint between cervical vertebrae 1 and 2)	Qualified yes
Explanation: Athlete needs evaluation to assess risk of spinal cord injury during sports participation.	
Bleeding disorder	Qualified yes
Explanation: Athlete needs evaluation.	
Cardiovascular diseases: Carditis (inflammation of the heart)	No
Explanation: Carditis may result in sudden death with exertion.	
Hypertension (high blood pressure)	Qualified yes
Explanation: Those with significant essential (unexplained) hypertension should avoid weightlifting and power lifting, body building, and strength training. Those with secondary hypertension (hypertension caused by a previously identified disease) or severe essential hypertension need evaluation.	
Congenital heart disease (structural heart defects present at birth)	Qualified yes
Explanation: Those with mild forms may participate fully; those with moderate or severe forms, or those who have undergone surgery, need evaluation.	
Dysrhythmia (irregular heart rhythm)	Qualified yes
Explanation: Athlete needs evaluation because some types of dysrhythmia require therapy or make certain sports dangerous, or both.	
Mitral valve prolapse (abnormal heart valve)	Qualified yes
Explanation: Those with symptoms (chest pain, symptoms of possible dysrhythmia) or evidence of mitral regurgitation (leaking) on physical examination need evaluation. All others may participate fully.	
Heart murmur	Qualified yes
Explanation: If the murmur is innocent (does not indicate heart disease), full participation is permitted. Otherwise, the athlete needs evaluation (see "Congenital heart disease" and "Mitral valve prolapse" listed earlier).	
Cerebral palsy	Qualified yes
Explanation: Athlete needs evaluation.	
Diabetes mellitus	Yes
Explanation: All sports can be played with proper attention to diet, hydration, and insulin therapy. Particular attention is needed for activities that last 30 min or more.	
Diarrhea	Qualified no
Explanation: Unless disease is mild, no participation is permitted, because diarrhea may increase the risk of dehydration and heat illness (see "Fever" listed later).	

T A B L E   12–3

Medical Conditions and Sports Participation* Continued

CONDITION	MAY PARTICIPATE?
Eating disorders: Anorexia nervosa, bulimia nervosa	Qualified yes
Explanation: These patients need both medical and psychiatric assessment before participation may be allowed.	
Eyes: Functionally one-eyed athlete, loss of an eye, detached retina, previous eye surgery, or serious eye injury	Qualified yes
Explanation: A functionally one-eyed athlete has a best corrected visual acuity of <20/40 in the worse eye. These athletes would suffer significant disability if the better eye was seriously injured as would those with loss of an eye. Some athletes who have previously undergone eye surgery or had a serious eye injury may have an increased risk of injury because of weakened eye tissue. Availability of eye guards approved by the American Society of Testing Materials (ASTM) and other protective equipment may allow participation in most sports, but this must be judged on an individual basis.	
Fever	No
Explanation: Fever can increase cardiopulmonary effort, reduce maximum exercise capacity, make heat illness more likely, and increase orthostatic hypotension during exercise. Fever may rarely accompany myocarditis or other infections that may make exercise dangerous.	
Heat illness: History of	Qualified yes
Explanation: Because of the increased likelihood of recurrence, the athlete needs individual assessment to determine the presence of predisposing conditions and to arrange a prevention strategy.	
HIV infection	Yes
Explanation: Because of the apparent minimal risk to others, all sports may be played that the state of health allows. In all athletes, skin lesions should be properly covered, and athletic personnel should use universal precautions when handling blood or body fluids with visible blood.	
Kidney: Absence of one	Qualified yes
Explanation: Athlete needs individual assessment for contact, collision, and limited contact sports.	
Liver: Enlarged	Qualified yes
Explanation: If the liver is acutely enlarged, participation should be avoided because of risk of rupture. If the liver is chronically enlarged, individual assessment is needed before collision, contact, or limited contact sports are played.	
Malignancy	Qualified yes
Explanation: Athlete needs individual assessment.	

Table continued on following page

T A B L E   12–3

Medical Conditions and Sports Participation* Continued

CONDITION	MAY PARTICIPATE?
Musculoskeletal disorders	Qualified yes
Explanation: Athlete needs individual assessment.	
Neurological disorders: History of serious head or spine trauma, severe or repeated concussions, or craniotomy	Qualified yes
Explanation: Athlete needs individual assessment for collision, contact, or limited contact sports and also for noncontact sports if there are deficits in judgment or cognition. Research supports a conservative approach to management of concussion.	
Convulsive disorder: Well controlled	Yes
Explanation: Risk of convulsion during participation is minimal.	
Convulsive disorders: Poorly controlled	Qualified yes
Explanation: Athlete needs individual assessment for collision, contact, or limited contact sports. Avoid the following noncontact sports: Archery, riflery, swimming, weightlifting, power lifting, strength training, or sports involving heights. In these sports, occurrence of a convulsion may be a risk to self or others.	
Obesity	Qualified yes
Explanation: Because of the risk of heat illness, obese persons need careful acclimatization and hydration.	
Organ transplant recipient	Qualified yes
Explanation: Athlete needs individual assessment.	
Ovary: absence of one	Yes
Explanation: Risk of severe injury to the remaining ovary is minimal.	
Respiratory: Pulmonary compromise, including cystic fibrosis	Qualified yes
Explanation: Athlete needs individual assessment, but generally all sports may be played if oxygenation remains satisfactory during a graded exercise test. Patients with cystic fibrosis need acclimatization and good hydration to reduce the risk of heat illness.	
Asthma	Yes
Explanation: With proper medication and education, only athletes with the most severe asthma have to modify their participation.	

T A B L E   12–3

Medical Conditions and Sports Participation* Continued

CONDITION	MAY PARTICIPATE?
Acute upper respiratory infection	Qualified yes
Explanation: Upper respiratory obstruction may affect pulmonary function. Athlete needs individual assessment for all but mild disease (see "Fever" listed earlier).	
Sickle cell disease	Qualified yes
Explanation: Athlete needs individual assessment. In general, if status of the illness permits, all but high-exertion, collision, or contact sports may be played. Overheating, dehydration, and chilling must be avoided.	
Sickle cell trait	Yes
Explanation: It is unlikely that individuals with sickle cell trait (AS) have an increased risk of sudden death or other medical problems during athletic participation except under the most extreme conditions of heat, humidity, and, possibly, increased altitude. These individuals, like all athletes, should be carefully conditioned, acclimatized, and hydrated to reduce any possible risk.	
Skin: Boils, herpes simplex, impetigo, scabies, molluscum contagiosum	Qualified yes
Explanation: While the patient is contagious, participation in gymnastics with mats, martial arts, wrestling, or other collision, contact, or limited contact sports is not allowed. Herpes simplex virus probably is not transmitted via mats.	
Spleen: Enlarged	Qualified yes
Explanation: Patients with acutely enlarged spleens should avoid all sports because of risk of rupture. Those with chronically enlarged spleens need individual assessment before playing collision, contact, or limited contact sports.	
Testicle: Absent or undescended	Yes
Explanation: Certain sports may require a protective cup.	

*This table is designed to be understood by medical and nonmedical personnel. In the "Explanation" section, "needs evaluation" means that a physician with appropriate knowledge and experience should assess the safety of a given sport for an athlete with the listed medical condition. Unless otherwise noted, this is because of the variability of the severity of the disease or of the risk of injury among the specific sports listed in Table 12-2, or both.

Used with permission of the American Academy of Pediatrics. American Academy of Pediatrics Committee on Sports Medicine: Medical conditions affecting sports participation. Pediatrics 94:757–760, 1994. Copyright 1994 by the American Academy of Pediatrics.

███ NEUROLOGICAL SPORTS INJURIES—RECOGNITION AND MANAGEMENT

ASSESSMENT. Neurological injuries are among the most serious that young athletes may encounter. Concussions can lead to brain dysfunction with short-term and long-term consequences. The "second impact syndrome" in which a person incurs a brain injury before having recovered from a recent previous event can result in serious brain pathology and possibly death. Health care providers need to recognize and manage concussions and help prevent second impact syndrome. Table 12-4 summarizes signs and symptoms of a concussion, and Table 12-5 summarizes the sideline neurological evaluation for head

T A B L E 12–4 ████████████████████████████████████
Recognizing a Concussion in Athletes

SYMPTOMS	SIGNS FREQUENTLY OBSERVED
Early (min to hr)	Vacant stare (befuddled facial expression)
Headache	Delayed verbal and motor responses (slower
Dizziness or vertigo	to answer questions or follow
Unawareness of surroundings	instructions)
Nausea or vomiting	Confusion/distractibility (easily distracted
Late (d to wk)	and unable to follow through with normal
Light-headedness	activities)
Persistent mild headache	Disorientation—time, place, date (walking in
Poor attention/concentration	wrong direction; unaware of time, date,
Memory dysfunction	place)
Fatigue	Slurred, incoherent speech (making
Irritability/low frustration	disjointed or incomprehensible
tolerance	statements)
Sleep disturbance	Gross incoordination (stumbling, unable to
	walk tandem/straight line)
	Emotions out of proportion to situation
	(appearing distraught, crying for no
	apparent reason)
	Memory deficits (asking same question
	repeatedly, can't remember words,
	numbers for 5 min)
	Any period of loss of consciousness
	(paralytic coma, unresponsive to stimuli)

From American Academy of Neurology Quality Standards Subcommittee: Practice parameter: The management of concussion in sports (summary statement). Neurology 48:581–585, 1997.

T A B L E 12–5

Sideline Evaluation for Assessment of Head and Neck Trauma

MENTAL STATUS TESTING

ORIENTATION	Time, place, person, activity, situation before and after the trauma
CONCENTRATION	Digits said backward: 3-1-7, 4-6-8-2, 5-3-0-7-4 Months of year said backward
MEMORY	Names of teams in prior contest Details of contest, such as plays or strategies used Recall of three words and three objects at 0 and 5 min Recent newsworthy events

EXERTIONAL PROVOCATIVE TESTS

EXERCISES*	40-yd sprint 5 push-ups, 5 sit ups, 5 knee bends

NEUROLOGICAL TESTS

PUPILS	Symmetry and reaction
COORDINATION	Finger-nose-finger Tandem walk
SENSATION	Finger-nose with eyes closed Romberg test

*Any associated symptoms are abnormal, including headache, dizziness, nausea, unsteadiness, photophobia, blurred or double vision, emotional lability, or mental status changes.
From American Academy of Neurology Quality Standards Subcommittee: Practice parameter: The management of concussion in sports (summary statement). Neurology 48:583, 1997.

and neck trauma that may be helpful in identifying neurological injuries.

MANAGEMENT. Management of the young person with a concussion includes not only referral to the emergency department, a pediatrician, or a neurologist, depending on the severity of symptoms, but also decisions about the appropriate time to return to sports participation. Table 12–6 provides the current recommendations for management of concussions in athletes. Prevention of further brain injury is the goal.

TABLE 12–6

Recommendations for Management of Concussion* in Sports

GRADE 1 CONCUSSION

Definition: Transient confusion, no loss of consciousness, and a duration of mental status abnormalities of <15 min.

Management: The athlete should be removed from sports activity, examined immediately and at 5-min intervals, and allowed to return that day to the sports activity only if postconcussive symptoms resolve within 15 min.

Any athlete who incurs a second grade 1 concussion on the same day should be removed from sports activity until asymptomatic for 1 wk.

GRADE 2 CONCUSSION

Definition: Transient confusion, no loss of consciousness, and a duration of mental status abnormalities of ≥15 min.

Management: The athlete should be removed from sports activity and examined frequently to assess the evolution of symptoms, with more extensive diagnostic evaluation if the symptoms worsen or persist for >1 wk. The athlete should return to sports activity only after asymptomatic for 1 full wk. Any athlete who incurs a grade 2 concussion subsequent to a grade 1 concussion on the same day should be removed from sports activity until asymptomatic for 2 wk.

GRADE 3 CONCUSSION

Definition: Loss of consciousness, either brief (sec) or prolonged (min or longer).

Management: The athlete should be removed from sports activity for 1 full wk without symptoms if the loss of consciousness is brief or 2 full wk without symptoms if the loss of consciousness is prolonged. If still unconscious or if abnormal neurological signs are present at the time of initial evaluation, the athlete should be transported by ambulance to the nearest hospital emergency department. An athlete who suffers a second grade 3 concussion should be removed from sports activity until asymptomatic for 1 mo. Any athlete with an abnormality on computed tomography or magnetic resonance imaging brain scan consistent with brain swelling, contusion, or other intracranial pathology should be removed from sports activities for the season and discouraged from future return to participation in contact sports.

*A concussion is defined as head-trauma-induced alteration in mental status that may or may not involve loss of consciousness. Concussions are graded in three categories. Definitions and treatment recommendations for each category are presented.

Data from Centers for Disease Control and Prevention: Sports-related recurrent brain injuries—United States. JAMA 277:1190–1191, 1997; American Academy of Neurology Quality Standards Subcommittee: Practice parameter: The management of concussion in sports (summary statement). Neurology 48:581–585, 1997.

CHAPTER 13

Sleep and Rest

▄▄▄ INTRODUCTION

Sleep and rest are influenced by health status, development, and family and cultural patterns. Many of the common sleep problems of children are learned behaviors. Less commonly, they are related to physiological problems, including ear infections, neurological disorders, hypothyroidism, colic or other pain, perinatal complications, or pinworms. They also may be related to psychological factors, including separation anxiety, depression, or other psychiatric problems. Family factors, including maternal stress or parental mismanagement of sleep routines, can be important. Finally, consider the child's sleep environment and temperament. A careful history of the sleep disorder and the family's management of it as well as a full physical examination should be done before a diagnosis is made and care for a sleep problem is planned.

▄▄▄ MANAGEMENT OF SLEEP PROBLEMS

Prevention of Sleep Problems

Development of good sleep habits from early infancy is the best way to prevent sleep problems later. Suggestions are given in Table 13-1.

Sleep Problems

Table 13-2 provides a summary of the most common sleep problems of children. Information about clinical findings, differential diagnosis, and interventions appropriate to each problem is given.

T A B L E 13–1

Suggested Strategies to Prevent Sleep Problems

Newborn	Daytime:	Respond to crying, hold the baby when fussy
		Hold the baby frequently to avoid fussy periods
	Nighttime:	Put the baby to bed while he or she is drowsy but still awake
		Feed the baby at the parent's bedtime; then let the baby awaken for feedings and feed with little stimulation, dim lights, no play
		Avoid bringing the baby into the parent's bed unless co-sleeping is the family norm
2–4 mo	Nighttime:	Move the baby to a separate bedroom unless this is not the cultural norm for the family
		Try to delay and then discontinue middle-of-the-night feedings
		No bottles in the crib
		Continue to keep middle-of-the-night feedings nonstimulating
6–12 mo	Nighttime:	Keep soft toy animal, doll, or blanket in the crib for snuggling, self-soothing
		Leave the bedroom door open and respond to fears or distress quickly and with reassurance
1 yr and older	Nighttime:	Keep bedtimes friendly and predictable occasions
		Always respond to nighttime fears or distress with reassurance and comfort
		Allow the child to take increasing responsibility for own management of body functions, including sleep
		Expect the child to remain in bed during the night

Summary of Common Pediatric Sleep Problems and Interventions

SLEEP PROBLEM	CLINICAL FINDINGS	DIFFERENTIAL	INTERVENTION
Dyssomnias			
Night waking	Needs help during the night to enter the next sleep cycle	Medical problem, pain, hunger, trained night feeder Depression	Always put the child to bed while still awake; keep day and nighttime cues very clear; do not reinforce calling out/crying behavior; try scheduled wakenings technique
Sleep refusals	Toddler/preschooler refuses to settle down to sleep when put to bed	Fears, separation anxiety, sleep needs less than parents' expectations Temperament irregular or low sensory threshold Emotional stress	Maintain consistent sleep routine and expectations; use transitional objects
Trained night feeder	Infant awakens predictably to be fed after age 4 mo	Night wakening, pain or medical problem, feeding needs	Move the child onto a 3–4 hr feeding schedule in the day; at first, feed the infant only once after the parents' bedtime; then, either eliminate that feeding or progressively decrease the volume of that feeding *Table continued on following page*

T A B L E 13–2 *Continued*

Summary of Common Pediatric Sleep Problems and Interventions

SLEEP PROBLEM	CLINICAL FINDINGS	DIFFERENTIAL	INTERVENTION
Dyssomnias			
Delayed sleep phase	Child goes to bed late and awakens late	Sleep refusal Depression	Have the child awaken progressively 15 min earlier until appropriate bedtimes and wakening times result
Advanced sleep phase	Child goes to bed early and awakens early		Progressively have the child stay up later; awakening will also occur later
Unpredictable schedule	Child goes to bed and awakens at random times	Family on erratic schedule; inconsistent parent expectations; excessive naps	Keep predictable eating, activity, and sleeping schedules for the family; maintain consistent expectation for bedtime and awakening, but allow child to stay awake in bed if not disruptive to others

Parasomnias

Nightmares	Child awakens in fear/crying; has memory of event; is interactive while upset; occurs in latter half of night; slow return to sleep	Night terrors; seizures; stress if nightmares recur frequently	Soothe and reassure the child; a nightlight or flashlight that the child can use may help if afraid of the dark
Night terrors and sleepwalking (variant)	Child awakens screaming/crying but is not interactive with the parent at the time; has no memory of event; occurs in first third of night; rapid return to sleep; sleepwalking is variant	Nightmares; seizures; physical exhaustion	Protect the child from injury if he or she is thrashing about or walking; help the child to lie down to return to sleep; protect child from stairways and other unsafe places sleepwalker might go

Medical/Psychiatric Problems

Depression	Insomnia or hypersomnia with other symptoms of depression	Other psychiatric disorder, dyssomnia or parasomnia disorder	Manage the psychiatric condition first
Obstructive sleep apnea	Snoring with apneic periods against increased respiratory efforts, restless sleep, daytime sleepiness/fatigue	Central apnea, benign snoring, seizure disorder	Refer for sleep studies and possible adenotonsillectomy

CHAPTER 14

Cognitive-Perceptual Patterns

INTRODUCTION

Children's thinking can be understood using an information-processing model. In this model, children must perceive internal or external stimuli, store that information in short-term and long-term memory, and then process the information in terms of past experiences. In feedback loops, children learn about patterns of stimuli and begin to anticipate what will come next. Cognition requires the perception of stimuli first; children with problems in this area will have problems with learning and interacting with their environment and the people around them. Children who are blind or deaf need special help to overcome the perceptual problems they face. Attention-deficit-hyperactivity disorder (ADHD) also causes children to have problems sorting the stimuli in their environment for appropriate storage and responses.

DEVELOPMENT OF CHILDREN WHO ARE BLIND OR DEAF

Because learning depends on reception of input and feedback from the environment, children with minimal vision or hearing are particularly vulnerable to developmental problems. Of course, for a given child, partial vision or hearing may allow for better performance. On the other hand, many children with vision or hearing problems have problems in other systems as well. For these children, performance may be even more delayed. Table 14-1 offers guidance for providers and parents about expected development of children with visual and auditory perceptual problems.

▓▓▓ ASSESSMENT AND MANAGEMENT OF ATTENTION-DEFICIT-HYPERACTIVITY DISORDER

Characteristics

ADHD is commonly diagnosed in children. The diagnosis is made when the characteristics from the *Diagnostic and Statistical Manual IV* are interpreted carefully. These characteristics are listed in Table 14-2.

Assessment

The primary care provider should collect a detailed history from the child and parent as well as gather data from other sources before arriving at the diagnosis and developing a plan of care. Main topics to address in the ADHD history are identified in Table 14-3.

Management

Management of children with ADHD requires ongoing cooperation from child, parents, school, and others. The condition should be considered chronic, that is, it has both physiological and psychological aspects; it affects the family; and it can be controlled but not cured with interventions. Repeated evaluations and assessment of interventions affecting the child's current status must be built into the plan.

Table 14-4 provides information about medications used to treat children with ADHD. Most authorities support a combination of behavioral and medication management strategies.

Various classroom management strategies can assist the child to learn effectively through behavioral management. Many of the suggestions in Table 14-5 are also useful for parents at home.

Figure 14-1 provides guidelines for assessment and management of the child with ADHD.

Continued on page 153

TABLE 14-1
Developmental Milestones of Blind and Deaf Infants and Children

	BLIND	DEAF
Infants (0–1 yr)	Tend to lie quietly in crib. Attachment problems possible due to decreased social cues and visual following. Decreased use of hands and bringing hands to midline, decreased prone position, decreased facial expressions. Head control normal but delayed pull to sit; creep, stand, and walk delayed about 4 mo. Creeping delayed until reaching on sound cue is achieved. Increased separation anxiety may begin by 6 mo. Increased echolalia (Ryan, 1988). Sensorimotor delays common. Delayed object permanence.	Sensorimotor stage normal. Language development: deaf children exposed early to sign language develop language similarly to hearing children exposed to spoken language (Meadow-Orlans, 1990). Deaf children exposed to both spoken and sign language learn both and progress as hearing children (Meadow, 1980). Deaf children exposed only to spoken language have language delays (Gregory & Mogford, 1981). Language output decreased around 6–9 mo.
Toddlers (12 mo–2 yr)	Decreased aggression but increased tantrums and motor behavior when frustrated. Continued delayed object permanence. Walks at 17 mo on average. Blindisms appear—rocking, swaying, head turning (Phillips & Hartley, 1988).	Sensorimotor stage normal.
Preschoolers (3–5 yr)	Decreased social skills, decreased self-help skills. "I" sense of self delayed to 4 yr (Phillips & Hartley, 1988).	May have preoperational delays (Quigley & Kretschmer, 1982). Symbolic play may be delayed if language skills are decreased.
School-age children (6–12 yr)	Reading and mobility delays. Conservation delayed to 9 years (Tobin, 1972).	May have concrete operations delays (Quigley & Kretschmer, 1982). Decreased self-concept.
Adolescents (13–19 yr)	Delays may continue, or adolescent may finally achieve developmental level with achievement in academic and social maturity areas.	Increased adjustment problems and decreased social maturity (Meadow, 1980); decreased self-concept. May have formal operations delays.

T A B L E 14–2

DSM-IV Criteria for Attention-Deficit-Hyperactivity Disorder

DOMAIN	CRITERIA
ESSENTIAL FEATURES	Symptoms occur in two or more settings (home, work, school, in public) *and* There is clear evidence of significant impairment in social, school, or work settings Symptoms have persisted for more than 6 mo Symptoms have been present before the age of 7 yr
INATTENTION TRAITS	At least *six* symptoms of inattention are present: Fails to tend to details, makes careless mistakes routinely in work and schoolwork Has difficulty sustaining attention on a task at work or at play Does not seem to listen when spoken to Fails to follow instructions or fails to complete tasks (not due to oppositional behavior or failure to understand instruction) Has difficulty organizing tasks and activities Often avoids or puts off tasks requiring sustained mental effort Often loses things necessary for performing tasks Is easily distracted by extraneous stimuli Is often forgetful in daily activities
HYPERACTIVITY/ IMPULSIVITY TRAITS	At least *six* of the following symptoms of hyperactivity/impulsivity are present: Often squirms in seat or fidgets with hands or feet Often leaves seat when remaining in seat is expected Often runs, climbs, or moves restlessly in situations when it is inappropriate Often has difficulty playing or enjoying quiet leisure activities Is often described as "on the go" or "driven" Often talks excessively Often answers before question is completed or blurts out answer Has difficulty taking turns Often interrupts or intrudes in others' activities

TABLE 14-3

ADHD History

ASSESSMENT AREA	SUGGESTED TOPICS TO EXPLORE
CHIEF COMPLAINT/HISTORY OF PRESENT PROBLEM	Major areas of concern First awareness of problem Beliefs about causation of problem Previous evaluations and results Medication history for behavioral, emotional, and/or learning problems
BIRTH HISTORY	Prenatal history, maternal health, use of medications, recreational drugs, alcohol, and tobacco during pregnancy Birth anoxia, difficult delivery Postpartum complications, birth defects Neonatal behavior—feeding, sleep, temperament problems
GENERAL HEALTH	Neurological status, vision, hearing, chronic diseases Hospitalizations, prolonged illness Frequent injuries Poisoning or lead or environmental exposures Outbursts of uncontrollable sounds/words Tics, habit spasms, uncontrollable twitches Ongoing medications
ATTENTION/HYPERACTIVITY SYMPTOMS HISTORY	Attention: paying attention, sustaining attention, listening, following through, organization, reluctant to engage in activities that need sustained attention, loses things, distracted, forgetful Activity: fidgets, leaves seat, runs/climbs when inappropriate, has difficulty with quiet games, talks excessively, has problems waiting turn, interrupts, "on the go"

DEVELOPMENTAL HISTORY	Milestones: motor, personal-social, language, cognitive
	Strengths (e.g., personality, activities, friendliness)
	Weaknesses
BEHAVIORAL HISTORY	Frequency that child complies when told to do something
	Methods used at home to improve behavior and effectiveness
	Parenting skills training
	Parental agreement about child management
	Counseling history for child and/or family
ACADEMIC HISTORY	Child's progress at each grade level
	Adjustment problems at school
	Difficulties with specific skills—reading, writing, spelling, math, concepts
	Performance problems—attention, grades, participation, excessive talking, disturbing others, fighting, abusive language, not completing work
	School assistance—tutoring, counseling, special help
Functional Health Patterns	
FEEDING	Not able to sit through a complete meal
	Messy and clumsy with utensils, dishes, and glasses
	Inadequate caloric intake can be result of symptoms and further exacerbated by medications used to treat ADHD
	Gastric distress may be a side effect of stimulant medication
SLEEPING	Difficulty falling asleep, night waking, needs less sleep than other family members
	Complains about fatigue interfering with completion of tasks
ACTIVITY	Difficulty maintaining routines for activities of daily living

Table continued on following page

T A B L E 14-3 *Continued*
ADHD History

ASSESSMENT AREA	SUGGESTED TOPICS TO EXPLORE
COGNITIVE	Level of performance is below potential for achievement Tends to miss the point of conversations and activities Often does things the hard way in absence of established routines
SELF-CONCEPT	Struggles with low self-esteem, moodiness
ROLE RELATIONSHIPS	Inadequate social and relational skills Lies, steals, plays with fire, hurts animals, is aggressive with other children, talks back to adults
COPING/STRESS TOLERANCE	Low tolerance for frustration Outbursts of temper Moody, worried, sad, quiet, destructive, fearful/fearless, self-deprecating Somatic complaints
SOCIAL/ENVIRONMENTAL HISTORY	Family stress and coping patterns Home, day care, and school environments Family social risk factors: recent moves, financial stress, parental job losses, births, deaths, divorces, remarriages, alcohol and drug use, involvement with law enforcement, weapons in the home
FAMILY HISTORY	ADHD, neurological problems, learning difficulties Mental health history of close family members, health or behavior problems in other family members
TEACHER HISTORY	Obtain information from school about child's problems, strengths, weaknesses, academic management of issues

ADHD = attention-deficit-hyperactivity disorder.

T A B L E 14-4
Medications Used to Manage ADHD Symptoms

MEDICATION	SIDE EFFECTS	MONITOR	COMMENTS
Stimulants			
Methylphenidate (Ritalin)	Anorexia, insomnia, stomachache, headache, irritability, "rebound" flattened affect, social withdrawal, crying, tics, weight loss, reduced growth rate	Height, weight, blood pressure, pulse	Do not chew or cut sustained-release tablets in half Avoid decongestants
Dextroamphetamine (Dexedrine, Dextrostat)	Anorexia, insomnia, stomachache, headache, irritability, "rebound," tics, stereopathy, weight loss, reduced growth rate	Height, weight, blood pressure, pulse	Avoid decongestants Risk of abuse
4 Mixed amphetamine salts (Adderall)	Same as dextroamphetamine		8–10 hr effect possible Tablet can be split Potential for abuse
Nonstimulants (not approved by FDA for ADHD use)			
Imipramine (Tofranil)	Constipation, fatigue, stomach upset, dry mouth, blurry vision, dizziness, tachycardia	Baseline ECG ECG and blood level with dose change Blood pressure, pulse	May affect cardiac conduction rate Increased levels with methylphenidate Use with ADHD + tics, enuresis, anxiety *Table continued on following page*

149

TABLE 14-4 Continued

Medications Used to Manage ADHD Symptoms

MEDICATION	SIDE EFFECTS	MONITOR	COMMENTS
Desipramine (Norpramin)	Tachycardia, dizziness, fatigue, stomach upset, dry mouth, blurry vision, constipation	Baseline ECG ECG and blood level with dose change Blood pressure, pulse	May affect cardiac conduction rate Increased levels with methylphenidate Use with ADHD + tics, enuresis, anxiety
Nortriptyline (Pamelor)	Dry mouth, constipation, weight gain	Baseline ECG ECG and blood level at steady state Blood pressure, pulse	Use with ADHD + tics, enuresis, anxiety
Bupropion (Wellbutrin)	Agitation, dry mouth, insomnia, headache, nausea, constipation, tremor		Lowers seizure threshold Contraindicated in patients with eating disorders or tics
Clonidine (Catapres)	Sedation, dizziness, nausea, orthostatic hypotension, clinical major depression, nightmares	Blood pressure at baseline, after dose adjustment and follow-up	Sedation decreases over time Rebound hypertension if stopped abruptly
Guanfacine (Tenex)	Sedation, dizziness, nausea, orthostatic hypotension, insomnia, agitation, headache, stomachache	Blood pressure at baseline, after dose adjustment and follow-up	

ADHD = attention-deficit-hyperactivity disorder; ECG = electrocardiogram; FDA = Food and Drug Administration.

TABLE 14-5

Suggestions for Classroom Adaptations for ADHD Children

MEMORY AND ATTENTION

Seat the child close to the teacher
Keep oral instructions brief, with repetitions
Provide written directions
"Walk" the child through assignments to be sure they are understood
Break tasks and homework into small tasks
Use visual aids
Teach active reading with underlining and active listening with note taking
Provide remedial help in small sessions
Teach subvocalization to aid memorizing

IMPULSE CONTROL

Remind the child to slow down
Teach the child to monitor quality of work before turning it in

CLASSROOM ATMOSPHERE

Provide a structured classroom with clear expectations
Use moderate, consistent discipline
Rely on positive reinforcement for good behavior

ORGANIZATIONAL SKILLS

Establish a daily checklist of tasks
List homework assignments in a special notebook with the due date and needed resources
Follow up on homework not turned in

PRODUCTIVITY PROBLEMS

Divide work sheets into sections
Reduce the amount of homework and written classwork
Cut down on the number of math problems to be completed

WRITTEN EXPRESSION

Give extra time to complete written tests and assignments
Provide help with handwriting
Allow child to dictate reports and take tests orally
Reduce the quantity of written work required
Do not reduce grades for untidy work, spelling errors, poor handwriting

SELF-ESTEEM

Reward progress
Encourage performance in areas of child's strength
Avoid humiliation
Give hand signals only the child can see as private reminders of appropriate behavior

SOCIAL RELATIONSHIPS

Provide feedback about behavior involving other children
Make sure other children do not feel the child with ADHD is doing less or allowed unacceptable behavior; change the rules for all children, if necessary

Adapted from Baren M: Managing ADHD. Contemp Pediatr 11:33, 1994.
ADHD = attention-deficit-hyperactivity disorder.

Child presents to clinic with behavioral concerns
↓
Within 1–2 clinic visits, primary care provider should
1. Take a behavioral, social, medical history (see ADHD history form, Table 14–3)
2. Perform physical assessment; hearing, vision, hemoglobin, and other labs as indicated
3. Obtain previous records: medical, school testing, teacher records
4. Send family home with behavioral data-gathering forms (e.g., Connors forms [Connors, 1969; Goyette et al., 1978]) and send forms to school
5. Review returned data
↓

ADHD Probable
Refer for mental health evaluation
↓

ADHD Not Likely
Suggest counseling, provide reassurance, monitor behavior

Mental Health Consultant's Evaluation
1. Interview child and family
2. Conduct mental status examination
3. Determine DSM-IV diagnosis
4. Recommend treatment plan for child
↓

ADHD Diagnosis
Medication indicated?
↓

ADHD Not Diagnosed
Provide referral, counseling, monitoring as indicated

Medication Indicated
1. Medication (may require physician prescription) and behavioral and classroom management plans started
   • Obtain weight and blood pressure baseline data
   • Send out behavioral reports for parent and teacher to complete

No Medication Indicated
Begin behavioral and classroom management plan and follow-up

F I G U R E 14–1
Assessment and management guidelines for the child with attention-deficit-hyperactivity disorder (ADHD).

2. Follow-up appointment in 2 weeks
   - Obtain weight and blood pressure data
   - Assess side effects and concerns; review medication effectiveness
   - Follow up with behavioral and classroom plans
   - Adjust medication doses as needed
   - Plan for completion of follow-up parent and teacher questionnaires before next visit

   ↓

Ongoing Follow-Up: 3-Month Visits
- Obtain weight and blood pressure data
- Document refills of medications
- Review follow-up questionnaires from parents and teacher
- Review child's progress following topics from the ADHD history
- Discuss child's progress with teacher as needed
- Follow up with mental health consultant as needed

F I G U R E 14–1 *Continued*

REFERENCES

American Psychiatric Association: Diagnostic and Statistical Manual of Mental Disorders. Washington, DC: American Psychiatric Association, 1994.

Connors CK: A teacher rating scale for use in drug studies with children. Am J Psychiatry 126:884–888, 1969.

Goyette C, Connors CK, Ulrich R: Normative data on Revised Connors Parent and Teacher Rating Scales. J Abnorm Child Psychol 6:221-236, 1978.

Gregory S, Mogford K: Early language development in deaf children. *In* Kyle WJ, Deuchar M (eds): Perspectives on British Sign Language and Deafness. London, Croom Helm, 1981, pp 218-237.

Meadow K: Deafness and Child Development. Berkeley, University of California Press, 1980.

Meadow-Orlans KP: Research on developmental aspects of deafness. *In* Moores DE, Meadow-Orlans KP (eds): Educational and Developmental Aspects of Deafness. Washington, DC, Gallaudet University Press, 1990, pp 283-298.

Phillips S, Hartley J: Developmental differences and interventions for blind children. Pediatr Nursing, 14:201-204, 1988.

Quigley S, Kretschmer R: The Education of Deaf Children: Issues, Theory, and Practice. Baltimore, University Park Press, 1982.

Ryan J: Hearing and speech assessment. *In* Ballard R (ed): Pediatric Care of the ICN Graduate. Philadelphia, WB Saunders, 1988, pp 111-120.

Tobin M: Conservation of substance in the blind and partially blind. Br J Educ Psychol 142:192-197, 1972.

CHAPTER 15

Self-Perception

DEFINITION AND DEVELOPMENT OF SELF-PERCEPTION

Self-perception, being both personal and subjective, includes a *description* of the self and an *evaluation* of that description. The three key components of self-perception are listed in Table 15-1.

Research from the Search Institute (1997) has identified 40 developmental assets, listed in Table 15-2, which lay a foundation for young people to grow into caring, responsible adults with a positive self-perception.

The development of self-perception parallels normal growth and development. Two stages, the emergence of self and the refining of the self, are described further in Table 15-3.

Children often compare themselves with others when developing their own self-perception. These external measures of self are listed in Table 15-4. Excessive dependence on these measures causes the child to feel insecure, inferior, and inadequate.

There are other risk factors that contribute to a low self-perception. Table 15-5 lists conditions a child may have no control over, and Table 15-6 identifies roadblocks or developmental deficits that are likely to cause a child or teenager to make negative choices or decisions that adversely affect self-perception.

TABLE 15-1

Key Components of Self-Perception

- Significance: I am loved!
- Worthiness: I am OK! I like and respect myself!
- Competence: I can do it!

40 Developmental Assets that Lay a Foundation for Positive Self-Perception

CATEGORY	ASSET NAME AND DEFINITION

EXTERNAL ASSETS

Support

1. *Family support*—Family life provides high levels of love and support.
2. *Positive family communication*—Young person and her or his parent(s) communicate positively, and young person is willing to seek advice and counsel from parent(s).
3. *Other adult relationships*—Young person receives support from three or more nonparent adults.
4. *Caring neighborhood*—Young person experiences caring neighbors.
5. *Caring school climate*—School provides a caring, encouraging environment.
6. *Parent involvement in schooling*—Parent(s) are actively involved in helping young person succeed in school.

Empowerment

7. *Community values youth*—Young person perceives that adults in the community value youth.
8. *Youth as resources*—Young people are given useful roles in the community.
9. *Service to others*—Young person serves in the community one hour or more per week.
10. *Safety*—Young person feels safe at home, at school, and in the neighborhood.

Boundaries and expectations

11. *Family boundaries*—Family has clear rules and consequences and monitors the young person's whereabouts.
12. *School boundaries*—School provides clear rules and consequences.
13. *Neighborhood boundaries*—Neighbors take responsibility for monitoring young people's behavior.
14. *Adult role models*—Parent(s) and other adults model positive, responsible behavior.
15. *Positive peer influence*—Young person's best friends model responsible behavior.
16. *High expectations*—Both parent(s) and teachers encourage the young person to do well.

Constructive use of time

17. *Creative activities*—Young person spends three or more hours per week in lessons or practice in music, theater, or other arts.
18. *Youth programs*—Young person spends three or more hours per week in sports, clubs, or organizations at school and/or in the community.
19. *Religious community*—Young person spends one or more hours per week in activities in a religious institution.
20. *Time at home*—Young person is out with friends "with nothing special to do" two or fewer nights per week.

Table continued on following page

T A B L E 15–2

40 Developmental Assets that Lay a Foundation for Positive Self-Perception *Continued*

CATEGORY	ASSET NAME AND DEFINITION

INTERNAL ASSETS

Commitment to learning

21. *Achievement motivation*—Young person is motivated to do well in school.
22. *School engagement*—Young person is actively engaged in learning.
23. *Homework*—Young person reports doing at least one hour of homework every school day.
24. *Bonding to school*—Young person cares about her or his school.
25. *Reading for pleasure*—Young person reads for pleasure three or more hours per week.

Positive values

26. *Caring*—Young person places high value on helping other people.
27. *Equality and social justice*—Young person places high value on promoting equality and reducing hunger and poverty.
28. *Integrity*—Young person acts on convictions and stands up for her or his beliefs.
29. *Honesty*—Young person tells the truth even when it is not easy.
30. *Responsibility*—Young person accepts and takes personal responsibility.
31. *Restraint*—Young person believes it is important not to be sexually active or to use alcohol or other drugs.

Social competencies

32. *Planning and decision making*—Young person knows how to plan ahead and make choices.
33. *Interpersonal competence*—Young person has empathy, sensitivity, and friendship skills.
34. *Cultural competence*—Young person has knowledge of and comfort with people of different cultural/racial/ethnic backgrounds.
35. *Resistance skills*—Young person can resist negative peer pressure and dangerous situations.
36. *Peaceful conflict resolution*—Young person seeks to resolve conflict nonviolently.

Positive identity

37. *Personal power*—Young person feels he or she has control over "things that happen to me."
38. *Self-esteem*—Young person reports having a high self-esteem.
39. *Sense of purpose*—Young person reports that "my life has a purpose."
40. *Positive view of personal future*—Young person is optimistic about her or his personal future.

T A B L E 15–3
Developmental Stages of Self-Perception

EMERGENCE OF SELF (1ST STAGE)

- Infants—learn that they are separate individuals who affect others by their behavior, view the world as responsive or unresponsive to their needs.
- Toddlers—explore their capabilities and limits and make others aware of their needs, desires, and concerns.
- Preschoolers—begin to use "I," become aware of discrepancies in abilities, discover their bodies, begin to do simple problem solving, move from seeing themselves as the center of the world.

REFINING THE SELF (2ND STAGE)

- School-age children—evaluate self on the basis of external evidence, compare themselves with others, criticize and ridicule deviations from normal.
- Early adolescents—finalize body image, focus on physical and emotional changes with peer acceptance determining self-evaluation.
- Late adolescents—refine and crystallize self-perception (physical, social, spiritual) with values, goals, and competencies guiding their future in place.

Data from Kump T: Self-esteem: Why little kids need BIG egos. Healthy Kids Oct/Nov: 53–58, 1998; Hunsberger M: Fostering self-esteem. *In* Betz CL, Hunsberger M, Wright S (eds): Family Centered Nursing Care of Children, 2nd ed. Philadelphia, WB Saunders, 1994, pp 513–526; Sieving RE, Zirbel-Donisch ST: Development and enhancement of self-esteem in children. J Pediatr Health Care 4:290–296, 1990.

T A B L E 15–4
External Measures Used to Build Self-Perception

- Physical appearance or attractiveness: How do I look?
- Intelligence: What do I know?
- Performance: How do I do?
- Importance: Who do I know?
- Financial status: What and how much do I have?
- Control: What and whom do I control?

T A B L E 15-5

Childhood Conditions That Are Risk Factors for Low Self-Perception

1. *Physical alterations, including body image:* Chronic illness (visible or not), disfiguring disabilities, sensory disabilities, obesity, anorexia
2. *Mental/emotional alterations:* School problems such as being a slow learner, semi-illiterate, an underachiever, culturally deprived, a late bloomer; having a "difficult" temperament; suffering emotional or mental illness or abuse
3. *Environmental/relational alterations:* Disrupted families and family relationships or ability to meet basic needs, unrealistic expectations or faulty thinking, lack of parent–child temperament or personality fit, social disorders, stress, past experiences of failure, rejection, criticism

STRATEGIES TO DEVELOP POSITIVE SELF-PERCEPTION

The nurse practitioner can be instrumental in helping a child develop positive self-esteem by working with both the child and family. Some specific strategies are outlined in Table 15-7.

T A B L E 15-6

Ten Roadblocks or Developmental Deficits to Building Developmental Assets *(see Table 15–2)*

1. Spending 2 hr or more a day alone at home without an adult.
2. Putting a lot of emphasis on selfish values.
3. Watching more than 2 hr of television a day.
4. Going to parties where friends will be drinking alcohol.
5. Feeling stress or pressure most or all of the time.
6. Being physically abused.
7. Being sexually abused.
8. Having a parent with alcohol or drug problem.
9. Feeling socially isolated from people who provide care, support, and understanding.
10. Having numerous close friends who often get into trouble.

T A B L E 15–7

Strategies to Help Build a Positive Self-Perception

1. Facilitate good parenting
   - Parental self-perception
   - Parental roles
   - Know your children
   - Value children
   - Be there
   - Know their friends
   - Avoid comparing
   - Let go
2. Maintain appropriate expectations of the child
   - Keep expectations age-appropriate
   - Keep expectations child-appropriate
   - Differentiate parent- vs. child-driven expectations
   - Ensure expectations are clearly stated
   - Give a positive response to failure
3. Use discipline techniques that enhance self-esteem
   - Identify limits and consequence
   - Choose acceptable behaviors
   - Foster problem solving
   - Avoid rescuing
   - Give guidance
   - Use positive manner and intent
4. Communicate positively
   - Listen
   - Watch your words
   - Praise and encourage
   - Help identify, handle, and express feelings
   - React with "I" statements
   - Be aware of self-talk
5. Provide helpful strategies for the child and adolescent
   - Support early and ongoing self-assertion
   - Find child's "island of competence"
   - Help the child compete
   - Encourage healthy connectedness
   - Promote a sense of ownership
   - Keep a close eye on the classroom
   - Offer genuine encounter moments (focused attention with time directed by child)
   - Defuse feelings of inferiority
   - Prepare for adolescence
6. Encourage developmental asset building (see Table 15–2)
   - Build relationships
   - Give consistent messages
   - Get involved in structured adult-led activities
   - Set boundaries and limits
   - Nurture a strong commitment to education
   - Provide support and care in all areas of life, not just the family
   - Cultivate positive values and concern for others

REFERENCES

Hunsberger M: Fostering self-esteem. *In* Betz CL, Hunsberger M, Wright S (eds): Family-Centered Nursing Care of Children, 2nd ed. Philadelphia, WB Saunders, 1994, 513–526.

Kump T: Self-esteem: Why little kids need BIG egos. Healthy Kids Oct/Nov: 53–58, 1998.

Search Institute: 40 Developmental Assets. Minneapolis, MN: Search Institute, 1997.

Sieving RE, Zirbel-Donish ST: Development and enhancement of self-esteem in children. J Pediatr Health Care 4:290–296, 1990.

CHAPTER 16

Role Relationships

▬ INTRODUCTION

Child abuse and divorce are two role relationship issues identified in this chapter. Information about selecting a child care or day care provider and screening criteria for international adoption also are addressed to assist nurse practitioners (NPs) in counseling families with these concerns.

▬ CHILD ABUSE

Child abuse is a significant problem that encompasses physical, emotional, and sexual abuse as well as neglect. Inflicting or allowing injury to occur are the key determinants. The NP must be vigilant in identifying families and children who are experiencing or who are at risk for maltreatment.

Table 16-1 lists behavioral signs associated with (but not diagnostic for) maltreatment that should alert the NP to further investigation.

Suspicion of physical abuse can involve a disclosure of inflicted injury or discrepancies between the history and the injury (consider the type and severity of injury together with age and developmental capabilities of the child), including behavioral or physical findings or both. Key indicators for physical abuse related to location of injury and common characteristics by type of physical abuse are listed in Tables 16-2 and 16-3. Information for approximate dating of contusion injury is listed in Table 16-4.

General indicators for neglect (willful neglect, not attributable to ignorance) and behavioral findings associated with emotional mal-

T A B L E 16-1

Behavioral Signs Associated With Child Maltreatment

Overly compliant or exhibits exaggerated fearfulness
Clingy and indiscriminate attachment
Extremes in behavior (aggressive/passive)
Apprehensive when other children cry
Wary of physical contact with adults
Frightened of parents or of going home, or both
Exhibits drastic behavioral changes in and out of parental or caregiver presence
Depressed, hypervigilant, withdrawn, apathetic, antisocial, exhibits destructive
    behavior
Suicidal (suicide attempts and/or plans) and/or engages in self-mutilation
Overprotective of parents or caregivers
Displays sleep or eating disorders

T A B L E 16-2

Physical Abuse of Children: General Considerations Related to the Location of the Injury

Typical sites of accidental injuries
    Shins, elbows, knees
Common site of intentional injuries
    Back surface of the body—neck to knees
Common type of intentional injury by location
    Head area
        Eyes—bilateral black eyes
        Earlobe—pinch and pull marks
        Cheek—slap marks, squeeze marks
        Upper lip and frenulum—lacerations or bruises
        Scalp—bare and broken hair, bruises
    Neck—choke marks
    Trunk
        Chest—bite marks, fingertip encirclement marks
        Buttocks and lower back—paddling and strap marks
    Genitals—pinch marks, penile wrapping with constrictive materials
    Extremities
        Upper arms—grab marks
        Ankles or wrists—tethering, friction burn marks
        Feet—pin or razor tattoo marks

T A B L E 16–3

Common Characteristics of Physical Abuse by Type of Injury

TYPE OF INJURY	KEY CONSIDERATIONS
Bruises—surface and soft tissue	Pattern, shape, outline Location Stages of coloring
Burns	Location Patterns, such as sharply demarcated or circumferential (e.g., sock, glove, zebra, branding, doughnut or cigarette shaped)
Bites	Pattern such as doughnut or double-horseshoe shape; adult >3 cm between canine teeth
Abrasions and lacerations	Location "C" or "U" shape typical of belt buckle mark
Central nervous system	Radiographic findings (e.g., subdural hematomas, subarachnoid hemorrhages, skull fractures), retinal hemorrhages
Shaken infant syndrome	Retinal hemorrhage, subdural hematoma, posterior rib and metaphyseal fractures
Internal organs	Liver, bowel, spleen, pancreas, kidney consistent with blunt-force trauma
Skeletal	Spiral fractures of long bones, avulsion of metaphyseal tips, multiple rib fractures in different stages of healing, subperiosteal proliferation reaction
Poisoning/ingestion of medication	Deliberate poisoning or exposure to substance abuse
Munchausen-by-proxy syndrome	Creates a fictitious illness or induces illness in child

T A B L E 16–4

General Dating of Contusion Injury

BRUISE CHARACTERISTIC	AGE OF BRUISE
Swollen, tender	0–2 d
Red/purple/blue	0–5 d
Green	5–7 d
Yellow	7–10 d
Brown	10–14 d
Clear	2–4 wk

treatment are summarized in Tables 16-5 and 16-6, respectively. Behavioral and physical findings suggestive of sexual abuse are listed in Table 16-7. Remember that most incidents of sexual maltreatment leave **no physical findings.** Statements made by any child relative to inappropriate sexual contact by another (any adult or child) must be investigated and reported.

SEPARATION AND DIVORCE

Key considerations for the NP to remember in assisting families during periods of separation or divorce center around the child's developmental stage and the need for anticipatory guidance (Tables 16-8, 16-9, and 16-10).

Text continued on page 169

T A B L E 16–5

General Indicators of Neglect: Child, Home, Supervision Factors

1. Child
     Dirty, malnourished, poor hygiene, inadequately dressed for weather
     Inadequate medical and dental care (has multiple caries)
     Always sleepy (chronic fatigue) or hungry
2. Home
     Fire hazards or other unsafe conditions
     No heating or plumbing
     Nutritional quality of the food inadequate
     Meals not prepared; food spoiled in refrigerator or cupboards
3. Supervision
     Child has a history of repeated physical injuries or ingestion of harmful
       substances with evidence of poor supervision by adult caretaker
     Child cared for by another child
     Child left alone in the home, car, or anywhere without supervision (typically
       defined as a child under age of 12 yr who is left unsupervised during the
       daytime or child under age 16–18 yr, left unsupervised by an adult at
       night)

T A B L E 16-6

Behavioral Findings Associated With Emotional Maltreatment

BEHAVIORAL FINDINGS SUGGESTIVE OF EMOTIONAL ABUSE

1. Behavioral indicators seen in children

   Withdrawn, depressed, apathetic

   Act out or have behavioral problems

   Overly rigid in conforming to instructions or attention to details as if fearful of doing something wrong

   Somatic signs of emotional distress (e.g., repetitive rhythmical movements, enuresis, encopresis)

   Talk about or report negative comments made by parent about themselves
2. Behavioral indicators seen in parents or caregivers

   Unrealistic demands or impossible expectations placed on child in terms of child's developmental capacity

   Child used to satisfy parents' ego needs or as a battleground for marital conflicts

   Child referred to as "it" or treated as an object

BEHAVIORAL FINDINGS SUGGESTIVE OF EMOTIONAL DEPRIVATION

On presentation, these children can have the following characteristics:

  Be developmentally delayed for age with no organic reason

  Appear frail or refuse to eat adequate amounts of food

  Display any of the following behaviors:

    Antisocial behavior, delinquency, unresponsiveness, sadness, and/or withdrawal

  Exhibit exaggerated fears

  Crave attention and affection from other adults, such as teachers or neighbors

T A B L E 16-7

Sexual Maltreatment: Associated Findings

BEHAVIORAL FINDINGS*

Loss of bowel and bladder control

Regressive behaviors such as newly manifested clinging and irritability in young children, thumb sucking, renewed need for a security object

Night terrors, inability to sleep alone

Overeating or lack of appetite; compulsive behaviors or unusual fears and phobias

Change in school performance, loss of concentration or easy distractibility

Sexualized behavior or play inappropriate for developmental level

Depression or inactivity, poor peer relationships, poor self-esteem, acting out, excessive anger

Runaway, suicide attempts, prostitution or promiscuity, substance abuse, teenage pregnancy, psychosomatic gynecological and gastrointestinal complaints

MEDICAL INDICATORS—NONSPECIFIC

Pain on urination; vaginal or penile discharge; vaginal, rectal, or penile bleeding; enuresis (bed wetting after having been dry at night) and encopresis

Urethral or lymph gland inflammation, genital or perianal rashes, labial adhesions

Pain in anal, gastrointestinal, pelvic, and urinary areas

Genital injuries or signs (e.g., bruising, scratches, bites, grasp marks, swelling of the genitalia) unexplained or inconsistent with history

MEDICAL INDICATORS—SPECIFIC

Blunt-force trauma (lacerations, bruising, abrasions, tears) to the genital or rectal areas, or both, inconsistent with the history, or these same findings with a history of sexual contact or penetration

Commonly encountered sexually transmitted diseases (by probability of sexual abuse in infants and prepubertal children from certain to uncertain):

1. Certain—gonorrhea (by culture) and syphilis if not perinatally acquired
2. Probable—chlamydia (culture is only reliable diagnostic method), condyloma acuminatum (if not perinatally acquired), *Trichomonas vaginalis,* herpes type 2
3. Possible—herpes type 1 (in the genital area)
4. Uncertain—bacterial vaginosis

Pregnancy and semen are certain indicators in young children

---

* Behavioral indicators are not diagnostic but indicate a need for careful assessment.

TABLE 16-8

Child-Related Assessment Factors in Divorce

DEVELOPMENTAL STAGE OF CHILDREN

Age and developmental stage of children greatly affect their response to separation and divorce of parents

Common reactions of children to divorce by age group:

2–5 yr: Regression, irritability, sleep disturbances, aggression

6–8 yr: Open grieving and feelings of rejection or being replaced; whiny, immature behavior, sadness, fearfulness

9–12 yr: Fear and intense anger at one or both parents

≥13 yr: Worried about own future, depressed and/or acting-out behaviors (e.g., truancy, sexual activity, alcohol or drug use, suicide attempts)

COMMON ISSUES FOR CHILDREN OF DIVORCING PARENTS

Continued tension, conflict, and fighting between parents

Litigation disputes over custody and visitation arrangements

Abandonment by one parent or sporadic visitation (decreased availability) vs. denial of visitation

Diminished parenting resulting from such factors as availability issues or emotional inaccessibility, distress, or instability

Limited social support system outside nuclear family

Feelings of loneliness or emotional abandonment, or both

T A B L E 16-9

Key Anticipatory Guidance Issues for Families Experiencing Divorce

Advise parents to prepare the child for the impending breakup.
- If possible, prepare the child for the impending breakup of the family and departure of a parent from the home. Children who are told of the impending divorce before the departure of a parent handle the situation in a calmer manner than those who are given no preparation and wake up to find the parent gone.
- Discussions about the impending divorce should be an ongoing supportive process for the child.

Explain the need for parents to discuss with their children the following key issues about the separation and decision to divorce.
- Assure children that they will continue to see the departing parent if this is true.
- Explain what divorce means in language that the child can understand, what the family structure will be like afterward, and what imminent changes will occur in the living arrangements and daily routines.
- Reassure children that they will be cared for and are not being abandoned by either parent unless a parent has disappeared or indicates noninvolvement.
- Explain the visitation arrangements as soon as established.
- Offer an explanation of the reasons for the divorce appropriate to age and level of understanding of the child. Young children can simply be told that their parents are unhappy and that the purpose of the divorce is to end the unhappiness and conflict between their parents.

- Reassure children that they did not cause the divorce, they can do nothing to correct their parents' unhappiness in the marriage, and the divorce is the parents' decision.
- Tell children that they are not expected to take sides against one parent or the other. They should love both parents, and feelings of sadness, anger, and disappointment are normal.

Suggest self-help measures.
- Attendance at divorce recovery workshops or classes about families in transition as well as participation in support groups for children can be helpful.
- Working with school counselors, religious groups, or community and government agencies is another option that can be explored.

Discuss indications for referrals for mental health counseling.
- Professional counseling can be an essential component of the recovery process. The type of referral depends on the nature of the problem, the severity of symptoms, and the continuance of symptoms or problems without signs of improvement.
- Referrals can include individual or family counseling with mental health practitioners.

T A B L E 16-10

Factors Affecting a Child's Ability to Achieve Healthy Adjustment to Divorce in Their Families

The opportunity for continued participation of the noncustodial or visiting parent in the child's life on a regular basis

The ability of the custodial parent to handle and successfully parent the child

The ability of parents to separate their own feelings of anger and conflict and resolve their own hostility toward the other parent so that the child's need for a relationship with both parents is met

The child does not become involved in parental conflict and does not feel rejected

The availability of a social support network

The ability of parents to meet the child's developmental needs and to help the child master the developmental tasks before him or her

The child's overall personality and personal assets as well as deficits

CHILD CARE

The NP often is called on to advise parents about selecting a suitable child care provider. Counseling parents to use a four-step approach when selecting this individual or setting will assist them in providing an environment that is safe and meets their child's unique needs. Table 16-11 summarizes these steps.

T A B L E 16-11

Guidelines for Selecting a Child-Care Provider: A Four-Step Approach

STEP 1: INTERVIEW POTENTIAL CHILD-CARE PROVIDERS AND OBSERVE THE PROGRAM OR SETTING

Ask questions about

1. Cost—cost calculation per hour, daily, weekly, monthly; any late fees; policy about fee structure and rules (e.g., if the child is absent)
2. Enrollment—number of children enrolled in the program, the maximum daily capacity of setting
3. Child factors—age of the children served in the setting/program
4. Daily activities or program plan—structured vs. unstructured activities
5. Accreditation and licensing regulations related to the provider or setting; review copy of any license or certificate

Table continued on following page

T A B L E 16–11

Guidelines for Selecting a Child-Care Provider:
A Four-Step Approach Continued

6. Caretaker issues—credentials and/or experience (e.g., academic degrees, course, cardiopulmonary resuscitation certification)
7. Policies—open visiting, illness in the child, emergency care, nutrition and feeding policies
8. Preventable illness measures—immunization requirements for child and staff

Carefully observe the environment

1. Look at provider–child interactions—check for evidence of nurturing, responsive, comforting interactions
2. Look at safety issues of the physical environment—the play areas, toileting and diaper changing areas, outdoor environment, napping and eating areas
3. Assess the quality of the learning materials and/or toys (from an educational and safety perspective)

STEP 2: CHECK REFERENCES

1. Talk to parents with children enrolled in the program or being cared for by the provider; ask about their experiences relative to how the providers handled the care (discipline) and whether they were nurturing and responsive to parents as well as the child; ask about reliability and consistency of the providers
2. Talk to local child-care resource and referral program or licensing office; Child Care Aware (800) 424-2246 provides information about the nearest child-care resource and referral programs

STEP 3: MAKE A DECISION BASED ON SPECIFIC CRITERIA

1. The child will be happy with this care provider and have a safe, nurturing, and developmentally appropriate environment
2. If the child has special needs, these will be met
3. The values of the provider and parents are compatible
4. The child care is affordable

STEP 4: BE AN INVOLVED PARENT

1. Regularly talk to the provider about how the child is doing
2. Talk to the child daily about activities and experiences at the facility
3. If possible, visit the setting unannounced and observe at various times of the day
4. Communicate with other parents, and become involved in child-care events as much as possible

From US Department of Health and Human Services Administration for Children and Families. March 1999. (http://www.acf.dhhs.gov/programs/ccb/faq/4steps.htm)

TABLE 16–12

Recommended Screening Tests for Children Adopted From Foreign Countries

Complete blood count and differential, platelet count, and indices
Hemoglobin electrophoresis and G6PD screening
Hepatitis B panel, HIV, and RPR
Urinalysis, tuberculosis skin test, lead level, and stool for ova and parasites
If a young infant, standard newborn screening
Thyroid function test (if not done as part of newborn screen)
Developmental, dental, hearing, and vision screening (Barnett & Miller, 1996)

G6PD = glucose-6-phosphate deficiency; HIV = human immunodeficiency virus; RPR = rapid plasma reagin.

ADOPTION

The number of international adoptions has dramatically increased over the past 10 years. Recommended screening tests for these children are identified in Table 16–12.

REFERENCES

Administration for Children and Families, U.S. Department of Health and Human Services, March 1999: http://www.acf.dhhs.gov/programs/ccb/faq/4steps.htm.

Barnett ED, Miller LC: International adoption. The pediatrician's role. Contemp Pediatr 13(8):29–46, 1996.

CHAPTER 17

Sexuality

Achieving a sense of one's sexuality is a part of normal growth and development. At each stage of childhood, physical and psychosocial processes related to sexual function, self-concept, roles, and relationships can be identified (Table 17-1). Many parents may be surprised or distressed by their child's expressions of sexuality and unsure about how to best respond. Children, especially adolescents, may feel awkward, insecure, and embarrassed about feelings and changes related to sexuality. The nurse practitioner (NP) can offer reassurance, provide accurate developmental information, and help establish good communication between parents and children in order to facilitate healthy sexual development.

As children enter adolescence, sexual development accelerates and issues of sexual identity, sexual activity, reproduction, and sexually transmitted diseases arise. Accurate assessment of the adolescent's evolving sexuality can help the NP identify healthy behaviors that can be reinforced, as well as potential or actual problems, so that early intervention can occur. Questioning of adolescents must be respectful, supportive, and nonjudgmental. Table 17-2 outlines areas of inquiry for a sexual and reproductive history in adolescents.

Decisions about contraceptive use among adolescents are based on both psychosocial and physical factors. For any contraceptive to be used successfully, adolescents must:

- Be able to plan for the future; to prepare to be sexually active; to acknowledge that they are sexually active
- Be willing to acquire contraceptives publicly; to seek advice, services, and products from health-care providers and pharmacies.

TABLE 17-1

Sexual Function, Self-Concept, and Relationships During Childhood Through Young Adulthood

	SEXUAL FUNCTION	SEXUAL SELF-CONCEPT	SEXUAL ROLE/RELATIONSHIP
Infancy	Orgasmic potential present Erectile function present	Gender identity reinforced Association of sexuality with "good/bad" Distinction between self and others	
Toddler	Genital pleasuring and exploration Sensual activity (e.g., hugging, stroking)	Core gender identity solidified by age 3 years	Sex role differences learned Discrimination between male and female role models Sexual vocabulary learned
Preschool	Sex play—exploration of own body and those of playmates		Sex roles learned Parental attachment and identification
School age	Self-pleasuring (masturbation)	Curiosity about sex Sexual fears and fantasies Interest in aspects of sexual development Self-awareness as sexual being	Same-sex friends Off-color humor related to sexuality

Table continued on following page

TABLE 17-1

Sexual Function, Self-Concept, and Relationships During Childhood Through Young Adulthood *Continued*

	SEXUAL FUNCTION	SEXUAL SELF-CONCEPT	SEXUAL ROLE/RELATIONSHIP
Adolescence, prepubertal	Menarche (female) Seminal emissions (male)	Concerns about body image	Same-sex friends Sexual experiences as part of friendship
Adolescence, early	Awkwardness in first sexual encounter Masturbation, petting May or may not be sexually active	Anxiety over inadequacy, lack of partner, virginity	Appropriate sex friendships Dating
Adolescence, late	May or may not be sexually active	Responsibility for sexual activity	Intimacy in relationships learned
Young adult	Experimentation with sexual positions, expressions Exploration of techniques	Responsibility for sexual health (e.g., contraception, sexually transmitted disease prevention) Development of adult sexual value system, tolerance for others	Giving and receiving pleasure learned Long-term commitment to relationship developed

T A B L E   17–2

Adolescent Sexual and Reproductive History: Areas to Assess

FOCUS AREA OF ASSESSMENT	CONTENT
Background information	• Age • Gender • History of risky behaviors • Relationship patterns in family and with parents during childhood and adolescence
Physical development Self-concept	• Pubertal changes • Body image • Emotions and feelings about body changes and sexual behaviors
Sexual activity and responsibility	• Masturbation • Petting and necking • Number of partners • Contraception • Abstinence • Heterosexual/homosexual relations • Nature of intimate relationships
Reproduction	• Contraception • Pregnancy • Abortion
Sexual exploitation and abuse	• Sexually-transmitted diseases • Rape • Incest • Abuse • Prostitution

T A B L E 17–3

Choosing a Combined Oral Contraceptive with Less than 50 Micrograms of Estrogen
Start by determining if the woman can safely use estrogen

STEP 1	STEP 2
Is this person a good candidate for a pill with estrogen?	YES, she can use an estrogen; if oral contraceptive is prescribed, use lowest dose of estrogen that is effective
In general, avoid prescribing a pill with estrogen to women with:	NO, it would be best if she did not use an estrogen. Therefore, you can consider:

• Current or a history of circulatory diseases due to blood clots (including heart attack, stroke, or blood clots in deep veins) or cardiovascular disease due to diabetes.	• Progestin-only pills, such as
	  • Micronor (0.35 mg norethindrone daily)
	    NOR QD (0.35 mg nonrethindrone daily)
	  • Ovrette (0.075 mg nogestrel daily)

• Structural heart disease with complications such as atrial fibrillation or subacute bacterial endocarditis.	• Norplant (5-year levonorgestrel implants) • Depo-Provera (150 mg medroxyprogesterone acetate injection every 3 months)
• Blood pressure of 160/100 or greater.	• Intrauterine device
• Age of 35 or more who are smokers.	• Copper T 380-A
• Breast cancer or history thereof (exceptions may be made if no evidence of disease in past 5 years).	• Levonorgestrel IUD • Progestasert system
• Active hepatic disease including symptomatic viral hepatitis, severe or mild cirrhosis, or benign or malignant liver tumors.	

- Past history of jaundice (cholestasis) related to oral contraceptives.
- Migraine headaches with neurological impairment such as blurred or lost vision, seeing flashing lights or zigzag lines, trouble speaking or moving.
- Diabetes and damaged vision (retinopathy), kidneys (nephropathy) or nervous system (neuropathy), or women who have had diabetes for 20 years or longer.
- Plan to undergo major surgery or any leg surgery requiring immobilization for several days or more. Estrogen-containing pills should be discontinued 4 weeks before major surgery.

- Condoms (male or female)
- Diaphragm, cervical cap, Reality female condom
- Foam, VCF film, suppository
- Fertility awareness
- Male or female sterilization

Breastfeeding women, in general, should avoid estrogen until they start weaning the baby from breastfeeding.

Exceptions may be made in specific cases and occasionally pills may be prescribed for women in the above categories, provided that the specialized (individualized) grounds are well documented in the record.

VCF = vaginal contraceptive film.
From Hatcher RA: Contraceptive Technology. New York, Ardent Media, 1998.

177

An algorithm for selecting oral contraceptives is given in Table 17-3. If an oral contraceptive is prescribed, the lowest dosage of estrogen that is effective should be used.

REFERENCE

Hatcher RA: Contraceptive Technology. New York, Ardent Media, 1998.

CHAPTER 18

Coping and Stress Tolerance

All people, including children, use a variety of strategies to cope with the many stressors in their lives. The kinds of strategies used increase in complexity as children progress developmentally, as they experience successful outcomes, and as they encounter more severe stressors. Parents have a significant role as mediators of the environment for children, helping them cope on a daily basis. When stressors exceed normal coping responses, children develop psychological problems that require intervention, just as with physiological or developmental problems.

▬▬ POSITIVE PARENTING TO SUPPORT COPING

Positive parenting strategies are outlined in Table 18-1. These suggestions can help parents serve as teachers and mediators and not as additional sources of stress for children.

▬▬ DEPRESSION

ASSESSMENT. There are three categories of depression that may be assigned regardless of age (American Psychiatric Association, 1994):

- A *major depressive episode* is defined as the presence of a depressed or irritable mood and/or a markedly diminished interest and pleasure in almost all of the usual activities for a period of at least 2 weeks.

T A B L E 18–1

Positive Parenting Strategies

ATTENDING TO THE CHILD INDIVIDUALLY

Allow the child to make reasonable choices

Respond to child's bids for attention with eye contact, smiles, and/or physical contact

Comment on child's appropriate/desirable behavior frequently and positively throughout the day

Provide guaranteed special time daily: no interruptions, no directions, no interrogations

Avoid secondary gains for the child's minor transgressions by having no discussion, physical contact, perhaps even eye contact with the child; be neutral and simply state the preferred behavior.

LISTEN ACTIVELY

Paraphrase or describe what child is saying

Reflect the child's feelings

Share the child's affect by matching the child's body posture and tone of voice

Avoid giving commands, judging, or editorializing

Follow the child's lead in the interaction

CONVEY POSITIVE REGARD

Communicate positive feelings (e.g., love) directly

Give directions positively, firmly, specifically

Provide notice before requiring child to change activities

Label the behavior, not the child

Praise competency and compliance; say thank you

Apologize when appropriate

Avoid shaming or belittling the child

Strive for consistency

- A *dysthymic disorder* is characterized by a depressed or irritable mood more often than not, extending over a year-long period of time with symptom relief for no more than 2 months.
- *Adjustment disorder with depressed mood* typically occurs within 3 months after a major life stressor and is relatively mild and brief.

CLINICAL FINDINGS. Any disturbance in mood that is attended by functional impairment should be assessed. Talking directly with the child or adolescent is essential, as it is thought that half of depression cases are missed when parents alone are interviewed.

The interview should include discussion of

- Recent life events and losses
- Family history of depression or other psychiatric disorders

- Family dysfunction
- Changes in school performance
- Risk-taking behavior, including sexual activity and substance use
- Deteriorating relationships with family
- Changes in peer relations, especially social withdrawal

Common clinical findings of depression are listed in Table 18-2.

Suicide needs to be considered for any school-age child or adolescent who is depressed. Key warning signs of suicide in children are listed in Table 18-3.

MANAGEMENT OF DEPRESSION AND SUICIDE. Acute suicidal intent requires immediate psychiatric evaluation. Establishment of a safe

T A B L E 18–2

Clinical Findings of Depression in Infants and Children

AGE	SYMPTOMS
Infants and preschoolers	• Anorexia with a lack of expected weight gain • Weight loss or failure to thrive • Sleep problems • Apathy and social withdrawal • Developmental delays
Both school-age children and adolescents	• Depressed mood: sad, blue, down, angry, bored • Loss of interest and pleasure in usual activities • Change in appetite/weight (loss or gain) • Insomnia or hypersomnia • Low energy/fatigue • Difficulty concentrating; indecision • Feelings of worthlessness and/or inappropriate or excessive guilt • Recurrent thoughts of death and/or suicidal ideation
School-age children: additional symptoms	***Externalizing symptoms*** • Hyperactivity or difficulty handling aggression • School phobia or school problems ***Internalizing symptoms*** • Anxiety • Irritability • Social withdrawal • Somatic complaints (gastrointestinal, headaches, chest pain) • Eating or sleep disturbances • Enuresis or encopresis
Adolescents: additional symptoms	• Impulsivity • Hopelessness • Substance abuse

T A B L E 18-3

Warning Signs for Suicide

AREA OF FUNCTIONING	SIGNS*
Change in behavior	Accident prone
	Drug and alcohol abuse
	Physical violence toward self, others, or animals
	Loss of appetite
	Sudden alienation from family, friends, coworkers
	Worsening performance at work/school
	Putting personal affairs in order
	Loss of interest in personal appearance
	Disposal of possessions
	Writing letters, notes, or poems with suicidal content
	Taking unnecessary risks
	Buying a gun
Changes in mood	Expressions of hopelessness or impending doom
	Explosive rage
	Dramatic swings in affect
	Crying spells
	Sleep disorders
	Talk about suicide
Changes in thinking	Preoccupation with death
	Difficulty concentrating
	Irrational speech
	Hearing voices, seeing visions
	Sudden interest (or loss of interest) in religion
Major life changes	Death of a family member or friend (especially by suicide)
	Separation or divorce
	Public humiliation or failure
	Serious illness or trauma
	Loss of financial security

* These signs must be interpreted in context. Many of them are common outside the realm of presuicidal behavior.

From Oregon Health Division: Suicidal thoughts, suicidal deaths. CD Summary 46:24, 2, 1997.

environment is also important. Lethal medications and firearms need to be removed from the environment. Community resources such as hotlines can be used. A commitment to a no-suicide agreement by which the adolescent agrees to refrain from harming himself or herself should be elicited and the caretaker or care provider notified if suicidal ideation returns.

All depressive episodes in children require intervention by a mental health specialist. Therapies typically include cognitive behavior strategies in an individual or group format. Family therapy may be indicated. Pharmacological approaches including selective serotonin reuptake inhibitors are being used more commonly with children.

FEARS AND PHOBIAS

Fear is the occurrence of various avoidance responses to particular stimuli, a state of apprehension, or a response to a threatening situation. Fears are developmentally normal. A *phobia* is a persistent, extreme, and irrational fear that interferes with functioning. The onset of fears occurs during the transition to toddlerhood. Phobias are determined by multiple factors, with genetic influences, temperament, parental mental health problems, and individual conditioning histories converging in the development of specific phobias.

MANAGEMENT. Most fears are short-lived, not serious, and do not predict adult mental health problems. Parents absolutely must be cautioned against using fears as a form of behavioral control (e.g., threats of abandonment with toddlers) or as a strategy for discipline (e.g., leaving a preschooler alone in a dark room). The child should be referred for treatment if the fear or phobia affects the child's functioning, developmental progress, learning experiences, and level of comfort. Treatment strategies for phobias include systematic desensitization, contingency management, cognitive-behavioral procedures, and family interventions.

ANXIETIES

Anxiety is distinguished from fear on the basis of its diffuse apprehension in response to less specific stimuli. Anxiety that persists at high levels and is reflected in maladaptive behavior warrants diagnosis and treatment. Children with anxiety disorders tend to have multiple problems, are impaired in important areas of social functioning, and live with parents who have symptoms of anxiety or mood disorders.

A temperamental disposition for negative emotionality may be a predisposing factor. Youngsters with anxiety disorders are at high risk for subsequent anxiety disorders, comorbid anxiety or mood disorders, and adolescent substance use disorder. Anxiety disorders show distinct clustering in families.

Table 18-4 outlines several types of anxiety disorders, clinical findings, etiologies, and management strategies.

T A B L E 18–4

Anxiety Disorders

DISORDER AND DEFINITION	CLINICAL FINDINGS	ETIOLOGY	MANAGEMENT	COMMENTS
Separation anxiety: Excessive anxiety on separation from major attachment figures, home, or familiar surroundings.	• Developmentally inappropriate or excessive anxiety about separations. • Unrealistic worry about harm to self or attachment figures or about abandonment during separations. • Reluctance to sleep alone or away from home. • Persistently avoids being alone. • Nightmares about separation. • Physical complaints/ signs of distress in anticipation of separation. • Social withdrawal during separations.	Most common at ages 5–16 yr. Poor attachment relationship or problem in response to life events that threaten safety and/or primary relationships.	Family-system or relationship-based problem. Both symptoms and source of problem must be addressed. Refer to child therapist for early intervention. Antidepressants and benzodiazepines seem to have benefits.	Precursor to agoraphobia or panic disorder in adolescence or adulthood.

| Generalized anxiety disorder: Excessive anxiety or worry, not focused on a specific object or situation, or the result of a recent stressor. Generalized anxiety about a number of events or activities. A "worrier." | • Worry about future events.
• Preoccupation with past behavior.
• Overconcern about competence.
• Marked self-consciousness.
• Somatic complaints without physical basis.
• Need for reassurance.
• Restlessness, fatigue, difficulty concentrating, irritability, tension, disturbed sleep. | Most common at ages 9–18 yr. Familial association. | Refer to child therapist for treatment of symptoms through relaxation techniques or cognitive-behavioral therapy. Source of anxiety must be pursued through individual or family counseling. Younger children benefit from a combination of cognitive behavioral strategies and family intervention. Pharmacological intervention may be warranted, especially with comorbid social phobia or separation anxiety disorder. | Comorbidity with other anxiety disorders and/or mood disorder is common. |

Table continued on following page

TABLE 18-4 Continued

Anxiety Disorders

DISORDER AND DEFINITION	CLINICAL FINDINGS	ETIOLOGY	MANAGEMENT	COMMENTS
Obsessive-compulsive disorder: Obsessions are recurrent thoughts and/or images that are disturbing to the child and are difficult to dislodge. Compulsions are repetitive behaviors or mental acts that the child feels driven to perform to prevent harm or remove contaminants.	• Obsessive thoughts and compulsive behaviors. • No recognition by the child that the obsessions and/or compulsions are excessive or unreasonable. • No pleasure is derived from ritualistic activity. • The obsessions and compulsions are time consuming or significantly interfere with the child's or adolescent's normal routine, academic performance, and social functioning. • Washing, checking, and ordering rituals are more common in children.	Most common in preadolescents and adolescents but seen as early as age 2 yr. Serotonin and abnormalities in the basal ganglia and functionally related cortical structures are etiological factors.	Cognitive behavioral psychotherapy, alone or in combination with pharmacotherapy, is an effective treatment for obsessive-compulsive disorder (OCD) in children and adolescents. Anxiety management training and OCD-specific family interventions play an adjunctive role, especially to prevent the avoidant behavior that is a complication of OCD. Most, but not all, patients with OCD respond to antidepressant agents with prominent serotinin uptake blocking properties.	Very chronic, with high rates of comorbidity, typically with some other anxiety disorder, major depression, or substance use disorder.

REFERENCES

American Psychiatric Association: Diagnostic and Statistical Manual of Mental Disorders. Washington, DC: American Psychiatric Association, 1994.

Approaches to Disease Management

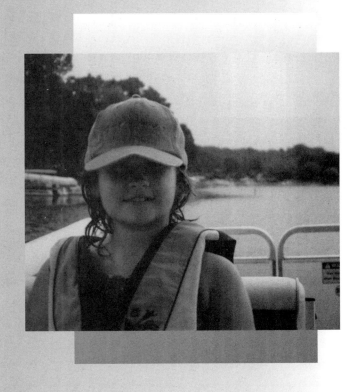

CHAPTER 19

Infectious Diseases

INTRODUCTION

Infections occur in all children at one time or another, with viruses being the leading cause of most pediatric infections. The nurse practitioner needs to quickly differentiate the insignificant illness from the more serious condition. This chapter focuses on common infectious diseases and the prevention of communicable diseases through immunizations.

THE INFECTIOUS DISEASE HISTORY

The diagnosis of a common infectious disease in pediatric patients often is based solely on history and clinical findings. Table 19-1 lists important areas to review in the history when considering the possibility of an infectious disease.

RECOMMENDED AND OTHER SELECTED IMMUNIZATIONS FOR CHILDREN

Immunization is the single best technique to halt the spread of vaccine-preventable infectious diseases. Remember that informed consent is critical when discussing the benefits and risks of vaccination. The recommended childhood immunization schedules for infants and children and for those not vaccinated in the first year of life are given in Tables 19-2 and 19-3, respectively.

If a recommended vaccination was not obtained on time, the child

T A B L E 19–1

Key Information to Obtain When Considering a Diagnosis of Infectious Disease

Evolution of the symptoms: order and timing of their presentation
Epidemiology: family, day care, school, or neighborhood contacts
Recent and previous travel
Recent medical intervention or instrumentation: dental, gastrointestinal, genitourinary, vaccinations, transfusions
Unusual occurrences, including loss of consciousness or trauma
Possible drug use
Contact with animals or animal byproducts such as hides, waste, or blood
Unusual dietary practices: ingestion of unpasteurized milk or raw meat
Pre-existing illness that may compromise the child
Congenital anomalies that increase the likelihood of illness
History of pica
Medication history: previous and current medications used (over-the-counter and prescription medications)
Genetic background of family
Hereditary diseases
Cultural practices of family or community

should be immunized as soon as possible. Do not repeat the entire series again; just continue normally from that point.

Other immunizations that may be given to selected groups of children are discussed in Table 19-4. The immunization schedule for hepatitis A is presented in Table 19-5. See Table 19-6 for guidelines for tetanus prophylaxis in wound management.

COMMON VIRAL DISEASES

Table 19-7 summarizes the assessment and management of coxsackie and parvovirus B19 (erythema infectiosum) infections. Most children with uncomplicated coxsackie and parvovirus B19 infections do not need diagnostic testing. Viral cultures and/or serologic testing can be obtained if needed to confirm the diagnosis. Important features of hepatitis A, B, and C and their management are outlined in Table 19-8, and laboratory markers for hepatitis B are identified in Table 19-9.

The human herpes viruses are double-stranded DNA viruses. Herpes simplex virus (HSV) is a widely disseminated infectious agent with two antigenic types. HSV-1 is associated chiefly with nongenital infections of the mouth, lips, eyes, and central nervous system (but

Recommended Childhood Immunization Schedule*

VACCINE	SPECIAL CONSIDERATIONS	AGES AND DOSES
Hepatitis B (HepB)	If HBsAg-negative mother	First dose by age 2 mo, second at least 1 mo later, third at least 4 mo after first dose and 2 mo after second dose but not before 6 mo of age
	If HBsAg-positive mother	First dose HepB vaccine and 0.5 ml HBIG within 12 hr of birth (separate sites), second dose at 1–2 mo of age, third at 6 mo of age
	If mother's HBsAg status is unknown	HepB within 12 hr of birth; have mother's blood drawn at delivery and, if HBsAg positive, give HBIG as soon as possible (no later than 1 wk of age)
Diphtheria, tetanus, pertussis (DTaP)	If child was never immunized	Begin series of three immediately
		Doses at 2, 4, and 6 mo of age; fourth dose at 15–18 mo of age but may be given as early as 12 mo of age if at least 6 mo since third dose and child unlikely to return; fifth dose at 4–6 yr of age
Tetanus, diphtheria (Td)	Booster doses	Recommended at 11–12 yr of age if ≥5 yr since last dose of DTaP, DTP, or DT
	Routine boostering	Recommended every 10 yr
Haemophilus influenzae type b (HIB)	Dosing depends on specific vaccine used and age at first vaccination	PRP-OMP (PedvaxHIB or Comvax [Merck]) given at 2 and 4 mo of age and third dose between 12 and 15 mo of age. HbOc or PRP-T given at 2, 4, and 6 mo with booster dose (fourth) at 12–15 mo of age
	For infants vaccinated after 7 mo of age, consult Centers for Disease Control and Prevention (CDC) or American Academy of Pediatrics (AAP) guidelines	

Table continued on following page

Recommended Childhood Immunization Schedule* Continued

VACCINE	SPECIAL CONSIDERATIONS	AGES AND DOSES
DTaP/HIB combinations	Do not use in infants 2, 4, or 6 mo of age unless FDA approved	
Inactivated poliovirus (IPV)	Recommended for routine childhood vaccination	Doses at 2, 4, and 6–18 mo of age and again at 4–6 yr
Oral poliovirus (OPV)	Recommended only under specified circumstances	Consult CDC and/or AAP guidelines
Measles, mumps, rubella		First dose between 12 and 15 mo of age; second dose at 4–6 yr; second dose may be given anytime if >4 wk elapsed since received first dose and both doses started ≥12 mo of age
Varicella	Give to children not immunized or having no reliable history of chickenpox	First dose on or after first birthday; if ≥13 yr of age, give two doses at least 4 wk apart
Hepatitis A	Recommended in certain states	Consult CDC references
Conjugate pneumococcus†		

DT = diphtheria and tetanus; DTaP = diphtheria, tetanus, and acellular pertussis; DTP = diphtheria, tetanus, and pertussis; FDA = Food and Drug Administration; HBIG = hepatitis B immune globulin; HbOC = HibTITER; HBsAg = hepatitis B surface antigen; PRP-OMP = Pedvax HIB; PRP-T = Act HIB or Omni HIB.

* Recommendations for January to December 2000 approved by the Advisory Committee on Immunization Practices (ACIP), the American Academy of Pediatrics (AAP), and the American Academy of Family Physicians (AAFP).

†Conjugate pneumococcal vaccine is expected to be added to the recommended routine childhood immunization schedule by the year 2001 or sooner, with a 2, 4, and 6 mo primary series and a booster at 12 mo to 15 mo.

T A B L E 19-3

Recommended Schedule for Children Not Vaccinated in the First Year of Life

TIME	IMMUNIZATION
CHILDREN <7 YEARS OLD	
First visit	HepB, DTaP, IPV, MMR (if >12 mo of age), HIB (15–59 mo of age), Mantoux
1 mo later	HepB, DTaP, varicella (if >12 mo of age)
2 mo later	DTaP, IPV, HIB (if first dose was given at <15 mo of age)
8 mo or later	DTaP, HepB, IPV
4–6 yr	DTaP, IPV, MMR
11–12 yr	MMR (if not given at entry to kindergarten), Td can be given if 5 yr since previous dose (then repeat Td every 10 yr)
CHILDREN >7 YEARS OLD	
First visit	HepB, Td, IPV, MMR
2 mo later	HepB, Td, IPV, varicella
8–14 mo later	HepB, IPV, Td
5 yr later	Td (then repeat Td every 10 yr)
11–12 yr	MMR

DTaP = diphtheria, tetanus, and acellular pertussis; HepB = hepatitis B; HIB = *Haemophilus influenzae* type B; IPV = inactivated polio vaccine; MMR = measles, mumps, rubella; Td = tetanus and diphtheria toxoid.

can be found in the genital tract); HSV-2 is most commonly associated with genital and neonatal infection. Varicella (human herpesvirus 3), Epstein-Barr virus (herpesvirus 4), and roseola infantum (herpesvirus 6) are three other human herpesvirus infections that cause illnesses typically seen in children (Table 19–10).

The influenza (types A and B) and parainfluenza infections are very contagious diseases. Table 19–11 outlines their assessment and management.

BACTERIAL INFECTIONS

Group A β-hemolytic *Streptococcus* (GABHS) is a common bacterial organism responsible for a variety of infections. GABHS pharyngitis is discussed in Chapter 27. Other clinical entities associated with GABHS infections are summarized in Table 19–12.

TABLE 19-4

Other Vaccines and Agents Available for Use to Prevent Communicable Diseases in Selected Children

VACCINE/AGENT	INDICATIONS	SCHEDULE/COMMENTS
Bacille Calmette-Guérin (BCG)	Prevent the spread of tuberculosis (TB) in developing countries with a high prevalence of TB; in United States, only for uninfected children at unavoidable exposure who cannot be protected by other methods of prevention (e.g., living with persons who are ineffectually or not treated or who have drug-resistant forms)	Birth to 2 mo old
Hepatitis A (Havrix and Vaqta)*	Children in communities with high case rates; Native Alaskans and Native Americans and day care centers with high rates of hepatitis A; homosexual and bisexual males; severe illness (e.g., chronic liver disease); illicit or intravenous drug users; healthy persons over 2 yr of age at nurse practitioner's discretion (e.g., child care staff and attendees and hemophiliacs)	≥2 yr old (see Table 19-5)
Influenza (use split cell 6 mo to 13 yr; whole cell >13 yr)	Chronic pulmonary disease (mild to severe asthma, bronchopulmonary dysplasia, cystic fibrosis) or significant heart disease, immunosuppressed (off chemotherapy 3–4 wk if possible), hemoglobinopathies (sickle cell anemia), diabetes mellitus, chronic renal disease, severe metabolic illness, symptomatic human immunodeficiency virus (HIV), rheumatoid arthritis, Kawasaki's disease, household contacts of high-risk patients; those receiving long-term aspirin therapy	Start in September, continue through mid November to December; two doses if <9 yr old or first time; give one dose subsequent times; dosage varies by age; skin test if severe egg allergy is present

Meningococcus	Functional or anatomical asplenia, terminal complement component deficiencies, adjunct to chemoprophylaxis, all military recruits, travelers to epidemic or hyperendemic areas	≥2 yr old unless epidemic; single dose; revaccinate after 2–3 yr if first immunized <4 yr old
Pneumococcus (23-valent polysaccharide)	Sickle cell disease; functional or anatomical asplenia; nephrotic syndrome or chronic renal failure; immunosuppression (e.g., organ transplantation or HIV infections); cerebrospinal fluid leaks; chronic pulmonary, cardiac, and liver disease; living in environments with high risk of invasive pneumococcal disease (e.g., Alaskan Natives and certain Native American groups)	≥2 yr; single dose; see AAP (2000) for revaccination guidelines
Synagis-Palivizumab (monoclonal antibody)	Prevention of lower respiratory tract infections due to respiratory syncytial virus. Given only to high-risk patients: infants with bronchopulmonary dysplasia, history of prematurity (≤35 wk)	Monthly intramuscular injections during respiratory syncytial virus season, start just before season; 15 mg/kg

* Hepatitis A vaccine is a required childhood vaccine in some states.

T A B L E 19-5
Hepatitis A Vaccination Schedule (AAP, 1997)

AGE	VACCINE	ANTIGEN	DOSAGE	#DOSE	SCHEDULE
2–18 yr	Havrix	720 EL.U	0.5 ml	2	Initial and 6–12 mo later
	Vaqta	25 U	0.5 ml	2	Initial and 6–18 mo later
19 yr	Havrix	1440 EL.U	1.0 ml	2	Initial and 6–12 mo later
	Vaqta	50 U	1.0 ml	2	Initial and 6–18 mo later

T A B L E 19–6

Tetanus Prophylaxis in Wound Management

PREVIOUS TETANUS IMMUNIZATION	CLEAN MINOR WOUND	DIRTY WOUND
Uncertain or <3 doses	Td only*	Td* and TIG within 3 d
3 doses	Td (fourth dose)*	Td (fourth dose)*
>3 doses	Td* if last dose >10 yr ago	Td* if last dose >5 yr ago

Td = tetanus and diphtheria toxoid; TIG = tetanus immunoglobulin.

*In children older than 7 years, use Td for vaccination. In children younger than 7 years of age, use diphtheria, tetanus, and pertussis (DTaP), and acellular pertussis (DTaP), or diphtheria and tetanus (DT) if pertussis is contraindicated.

T A B L E 19-7
Assessment and Management of Coxsackie and Parvovirus B19, and Human Immunodeficiency Virus Infections

VIRUS	TRANSMISSION	INCUBATION PERIOD	CLINICAL FINDINGS	MANAGEMENT
Coxsackie Type A	Fecal-oral	3–6 d	Varied: nonspecific fever with myalgia and malaise; herpangina, high fever; sore throat; dysphagia; positive viral cultures; decreased appetite; vesicles/ulcers on uvula, pharynx, soft palate; hand-foot-mouth with vesicles on buccal mucosa and maculopapular rash on hands and feet; mild upper respiratory infection to pneumonia; aseptic meningitis	Treat symptoms; fluids; rest; lasts 6–7 d
Type B			Similar to type A infections but no herpangina; also causes orchitis, congenital/neonatal infections, myocarditis	Treat symptoms
Parvovirus B19	Respiratory secretions; blood	4–14 d	Typical late winter/early spring; up to 30% have low grade fever and malaise before rash appears; "slapped cheek" rash on face with circumoral pallor; next a lacy maculopapular rash on arms, face, thighs, buttocks (can last for months); complications include arthritis, hemolytic anemias, aplastic crisis, pneumonia; fetal death, fetal hydrops, and anemia at birth if initial infection during first two trimesters of gestation	Treat symptoms and complications if occur; child in rash stage can go to school

T A B L E 19–8
Hepatitides A, B, and C

HEPATITIS	TRANSMISSION	INCUBATION	CLINICAL FINDINGS	MANAGEMENT
A	Fecal-oral, person to person; water-based, highly contagious	1–3 wk	Preicteric phase: acute febrile illness, anorexia, nausea, vomiting, dull right upper quadrant pain Jaundice phase: urine dark, stools clay colored; diarrhea in young children, constipation in older children; sick appearing; lasts few days to few mo. Self-limiting illness; low mortality	Supportive treatment; use of gamma globulin within the incubation period, up to 6 d before onset of symptoms; prevention with hepatitis A vaccination
B	Blood exposure, sexual contact, perinatally acquired	45–160 d	Varies from asymptomatic sero-conversion to fulminating severe liver disease; acute infection presents with icteric skin, sclera, mucous membranes, enlarged and tender liver; can go on to chronic illness; may have hepatocellular carcinoma as adult	Interferon used for chronic disease; prevention with hepatitis B vaccination
C	Blood transfusion, intravenous drugs, small percentage due to sexual exposure	1–5 mo	Onset of symptoms insidious; flu-like syndrome with jaundice in 25% of cases; may have hepatocellular carcinoma as adult	Interferon for chronic disease

201

TABLE 19-9

Laboratory Markers for Infection With Hepatitis B Virus: The Stages of Infection and When They Are Generally Present

TEST	PREICTERIC	ICTERIC	CONVALESCENT	CARRIAGE
HBsAg	+ + + +	+ +	+	+ +
Anti-HBs		+ or −	+ +	−
IgM anti-HBc		+ +	+ + +	
Anti-HBc		+ or −	+ + +	+ or −
Anti-HBe		+ + +	+ +	+ or −
Bilirubin	+ + + +	+ +		+ or −
Transaminase	+ + +	+ or −	+ +	+ or −

+ indicates laboratory values will be present; on a scale of 1 to 4, 4+ indicates very high levels; − indicates this laboratory marker is not present. HBc = hepatitis B core; HBe = hepatitis B envelope; HBs = hepatitis B surface; HBsAg = hepatitis B surface antigen.

Adapted from Behrman RE, Kleigman R, Nelson WE (eds): Nelson Textbook of Pediatrics, 14th ed. Philadelphia, WB Saunders, 1992.

Human Herpes Virus Infections: Herpes Simplex Virus (HSV), Epstein-Barr Virus, Varicella, and Roseola Infantum

TYPE	TRANSMISSION	INCUBATION PERIOD	CLINICAL FINDINGS	MANAGEMENT
HSV-1	Stool, urine, skin lesions, saliva, respiratory secretions; transplacental	Unknown, probably <1 wk	Primary infection: children 1–2 yr of age. Varied presentation: gingivostomatitis with temperature 103 to 105°F; painful red ulcers on mucous membranes, gums, and oropharynx last up to 2 wk; pharyngitis; neonatal herpetic infection; traumatic herpetic infections (e.g., thumb, if thumb sucker); meningoencephalitis or mild/silent infection. Recurrent infection: body does not eradicate HSV; herpes labialis most common site of recurrence	Supportive for gingivostomatitis with referral to specialists for serious infections; pharmacotherapy: acyclovir; (see Chapter 29)
HSV-2	Transplacental, sexual contact		Primary infection: maculopapular to vesicular, pustular, ulcerative lesions over genitals; pain and lymphadenopathy; may have urinary retention; meningitis possible complication. Recurrent: less severe localized disease	Supportive treatment: use acyclovir; refer to specialist for severe infections; educate teenagers to not have sex when active lesions are present
Epstein-Barr	Pharyngeal secretions and fomites	2–8 wk	Causes infectious mononucleosis: enlargement of regional lymph nodes, tonsils, spleen, and liver; moderate to high fever (1–2 days) and sore throat; rash that is maculopapular, urticarial, or scarlatiniform, hemorrhagic, or nodular; bilateral periorbital edema in 30% of cases; abnormal liver enzymes	Mono spot or serum heterophile positive (90% cases) by 2 wk after onset; symptomatic treatment; corticosteroids for severe tonsillar swelling

Table continued on following page

Human Herpes Virus Infections: Herpes Simplex Virus (HSV), Epstein-Barr Virus, Varicella, and Roseola Infantum *Continued*

TYPE	TRANSMISSION	INCUBATION PERIOD	CLINICAL FINDINGS	MANAGEMENT
Varicella	Airborne, direct contact, droplet	10–21 d	Typically seen in late autumn, winter, and spring. Prodrome: low-grade fever, headache, listlessness, abdominal pain, URI. Rash: begins on trunk; crops of lesions; lesions from maculopapular to vesicle stage, then crust; scabs last 5–20 d; lesions can develop on mucous membranes. Secondary complications: pyodermas, pneumonia, CNS problems, Reye syndrome, ITP	Symptomatic treatment; VZIG to prevent or modify if given shortly after exposure. Acyclovir within 24 hr of exposure. Prevention: vaccine
Roseola infantum	Unknown	Probably 7–17 d	Child 3 mo to 3 yr old; fever to 105°F for 3–5 d; child does not look ill, then diffuse, discrete, pinkish, maculopapular rash that fades on pressure; rash lasts 3–5 d; febrile convulsion is a possible complication	Treat symptoms

CNS = central nervous system; ITP = idiopathic thrombocytopenic purpura; URI = upper respiratory infection; VZIG = varicella zoster immune globulin.

T A B L E 19–11

Influenza and Parainfluenza Infections

TYPE	TRANSMISSION	INCUBATION PERIOD	CLINICAL FINDINGS	MANAGEMENT
Influenza	Droplet, direct contact, nasopharyngeal secretions	1–3 d	Looks sick; has hacking cough, fever 102–106°F, headache, sore throat, pain in back and extremities; in young children, vomiting and diarrhea; infants can get septic; pneumonia and anoxia are possible complications	Treatment is supportive; amantadine (5 mg/kg/d or 150 mg/d in one or two divided doses ≤40 kg; if >40 kg, 200 mg/d) as soon as possible for 2–5 d; bedrest. Prevention: influenza vaccine
Parainfluenza	Direct contact with nasopharyngeal secretions, fomites	2–6 d	Types 1 and 2 cause infection in 2–6 yr olds and reinfections at any age. Type 3 causes LRI in infants <12 mo. Type 4 infections are mild. 80% of cases have signs and symptoms of URI; fever in 20% of cases; discrete maculopapular rash of short duration; complications include otitis media, pneumonia	Symptomatic treatment; cefuroxime if secondary bacterial infection

LRI = lower respiratory infection; URI = upper respiratory infection.

205

T A B L E 19-12

Group A β-Hemolytic Streptococcal Infections: Clinical Findings and Treatment

INFECTION	CLINICAL FINDINGS
Scarlet fever	Abrupt onset of sore throat, vomiting, headache, chills, malaise; fever to 103°F; tonsils erythematous, swollen, usually covered in exudate; pharynx inflamed, can have exudate; palate and uvula erythematous, reddened with petechiae; tongue coated and red with desquamates (strawberry tongue). Rash appears within 12–24 h; is red, finely papular, coarse (sandpaper) with Pastia's lines; begins in the axilla, groin, neck; spreads centripetally, blanches on pressure, face usually spared; circumoral pallor, cheeks flushed. Rash, sore throat, and constitutional symptoms resolve in about 7 days; rash begins to desquamate, leaving fine branny flakes on the skin (this takes about 3 wk)
Skin infections	Lesions are honey-colored scab on an erythematous base; small transient vesicular lesion can precede the scab lesion (impetigo); deep soft tissue infection can follow; localized lymphadenopathy is common. Areas of eczema often develop the typical impetiginous lesions. Erysipelas (acute cellulitis and lymphadenitis) characterized by red and indurated skin, beginning with a small lesion, spreading marginally with firm, raised, and tender borders. Fever, chills, vomiting, irritability, and other constitutional symptoms are present
Bacteremia	Follows pharyngitis, tonsillitis, and localized skin infection. Some children have no obvious source of infection
Vaginitis	Severe vaginitis in prepubertal females. Vulvar erythema, serous discharge, and pain

REFERENCES

Advisory Committee on Immunization Practices (ACIP): Prevention of hepatitis A through active or passive immunization: Recommendations of the Advisory Committee on Immunization Practices. MMWR 48(RR12):1–37.

American Academy of Pediatrics (AAP): 2000 Red Book: Report of the Committee on Infectious Diseases, 25th ed. Elk Grove Village, IL: American Academy of Pediatrics, 2000.

CHAPTER **20**

Atopic Disorders and Rheumatic Diseases

INTRODUCTION

Asthma, allergic rhinitis, and atopic dermatitis are three atopic or allergic conditions commonly seen in children. The development of these conditions involves three main features: individual susceptibility, exposure to an offending allergen, and the emergence of an immunological response that results in a cascade of biochemical reactions, with inflammation being a significant component. Assessment for each of these key factors is an important part of the history taking.

ASTHMA

Coughing (especially nighttime or with exercise or exertion) and wheezing are characteristic of asthma. The National Heart, Lung, and Blood (NHLB) Institute guidelines (1997) for the management of asthma serve as standards for the treatment of childhood asthma. Individualization of care is important, however, and is based on the child's response to treatment. Determining the classification of asthma severity in children (Table 20-1) allows the nurse practitioner to identify an appropriate pharmacological management plan. Remember that the degree of airway hyperresponsiveness is usually related to the severity of asthma. Children less than 5 years of age experience greater airway hyperresponsiveness than do older children.

Early asthmatic response (EAR) phase is characterized by activation of mast cells and their mediators; bronchospasm is the key feature. It starts within 20 to 30 minutes of mast cell activation and resolves within approximately 1 hour if the individual is removed from the

TABLE 20-1
Classification of Asthma Severity in Children: Clinical Features Before Treatment

CLASSIFICATION & STEP	SYMPTOMS*	NIGHTTIME SYMPTOMS	LUNG FUNCTION
Step 1: Mild intermittent	Symptoms ≤2 times per wk Asymptomatic and normal PEF between exacerbations Exacerbations brief (few hr or d); varying intensity	≤2 times per mo	FEV_1 or PEF ≥80% predicted PEF variability <20%
Step 2: Mild persistent	Symptoms >2 times per wk but <1 time per d Exacerbations may affect activity	>2 times per mo	FEV_1 or PEF ≥80% predicted PEF variability 20–30%
Step 3: Moderate persistent	Daily symptoms Daily use of inhaled short-acting β_2-agonist Exacerbations affect activity ≥2 times per week; may last days	>1 time per wk	FEV_1 or PEF >60%; ≤80% predicted PEF variability >30%
Step 4: Severe persistent	Continual symptoms Limited physical activity Frequent exacerbations	Frequent	FEV_1 or PEF ≤60% predicted PEF variability >30%

* Having at least one symptom in a particular step places the child in that particular classification.

FEV_1 = forced expiratory volume in 1 second; PEF = peak expiratory flow.

Adapted from Highlights of the Expert Panel Report 2: Guidelines for the Diagnosis and Management of Asthma (National Heart, Lung, and Blood Institute [NHLBI] Publication No. 97-4051A). Bethesda, MD, National Institutes of Health, 1997.

offending allergen. Late phase asthmatic response is a prolonged inflammatory state, usually follows the EAR within a few hours, often is associated with respiratory symptoms more severe than the EAR presentation, and can last from hours to days (May, 1998). Exercise-induced bronchospasm describes the phenomenon of airway narrowing during or minutes after the onset of vigorous activity.

Tables 20-2 and 20-3 outline the stepwise approach for managing asthma during childhood; Tables 20-4 and 20-5 describe the use of long-term control and quick relief medications.

Because corticosteroids are an essential factor in successful control of asthmatic symptoms, various commonly prescribed inhaled corticosteroid agents are compared in Table 20-6 as to their dosing and frequency of use.

Peak flow rate is an important management tool used to monitor asthma control (Table 20-7). A sample peak flow nomogram is presented in Figure 20-1, and Table 20-8 lists predicted average peak expiratory flows for normal children and adolescents. Instructions about the proper use of metered-dose inhalers and dry-powdered inhalers are provided in Table 20-9. Children and their families need to be educated about the correct technique to use these devices.

The initial pharmacological treatment for *acute asthma exacerbations* is

- Inhaled short-acting β_2-agonists 2 to 4 puffs every 20 minutes for three treatments via metered-dose inhaler with or without a spacer

or

- Single nebulizer treatment (0.05 mg/kg; minimum 1.25 mg, maximum 2.5 mg of 0.5% solution of albuterol in 2 to 3 ml of normal saline).

If the initial treatment results in a good response (peak expiratory flow rate >80% of patient's best), continue the inhaled short-acting β_2-agonist every 3 to 4 hours for 24 to 48 hours. If a child has been on corticosteroids, the dose should be doubled for 7 to 10 days.

An *incomplete response* (peak expiratory flow rate between 50% and 80% of personal best and/or symptoms recur within 4 hours of therapy) is treated by continuing β_2-agonists and adding an oral corticosteroid. The β_2-agonist can be given via nebulizer.

▨ ALLERGIC RHINITIS

Allergic rhinitis can be a seasonal, perennial, or acute allergic reaction. Key features are summarized in Table 20-10.

Text continued on page 225

TABLE 20-2

Stepwise Approach* for Managing Asthma in Infants and Children 5 Years of Age and Younger for Long-Term Control and Quick Relief

LONG-TERM CONTROL	QUICK RELIEF
STEP 1: MILD INTERMITTENT ASTHMA	• For symptoms <2 times per wk, use bronchodilators; frequency of medications depends on severity of exacerbation
No daily medications	Use one of the following:
	Inhaled short-acting β_2-agonist by way of nebulizer or face mask and spacer/holding chamber
	or
	Oral β_2-agonist
	• With viral respiratory infections use bronchodilator q 4-6 hr up to 24 hr (longer use, consult with asthma specialist); repeat no more than every 6 wk without further review
	• Consider systemic corticosteroids if severe exacerbation or previous history of severe exacerbations
	• Use of short-acting bronchodilators >3 or 4 times in 1 d or daily use indicates need for additional therapy
STEP 2: MILD PERSISTENT ASTHMA*	Bronchodilators as needed for control of symptoms (see Step 1 recommendations)
Daily anti-inflammatory medications	
Use either of the following:	
Cromolyn (nebulizer preferred or MDI) or nedocromil (MDI) 3 or 4 times per d	
Usually try these drugs first in infants and young children	
or	
Low-dose inhaled corticosteroid via spacer/holding chamber and face mask	

STEP 3: MODERATE PERSISTENT ASTHMA*

Daily anti-inflammatory medications
Use either of the following:
  Medium-dose inhaled corticosteroid by way of spacer/holding
  chamber and face mask

  or

  Once symptoms controlled
  Medium-dose inhaled corticosteroid and nedocromil

  or

  Medium-dose inhaled corticosteroid by way of spacer/holding
  chamber and face mask

Bronchodilator as needed for symptoms up to 3 times a day (see
Step 1 recommendations)

STEP 4: SEVERE PERSISTENT ASTHMA*

Daily anti-inflammatory medications
Use either of the following:
  High-dose inhaled corticosteroid via spacer/holding chamber
  and face mask

  If needed, add systemic corticosteroids at 2 mg/kg per day,
  reducing to lowest daily or alternate-day dose that will
  stabilize symptoms

Bronchodilator as needed for symptoms up to 3 times a day (see
Step 1 recommendations)

* NHLBI Guidelines recommend consultation with an asthma specialist for infants and young children (≤5 years old) in step 3 and 4 classifications; a step 2
classification merits consideration of a consultation.

MDI = metered-dose inhaler.

Adapted from Highlights of the Expert Panel Report 2: Guidelines for the Diagnosis and Management of Asthma (National Heart, Lung, and Blood Institute
[NHLBI] Publication No. 97-4051A). Bethesda, MD, National Institutes of Health, 1997.

TABLE 20-3

Stepwise Approach for Managing Asthma in Children Older Than 5 Years of Age for Long-Term Control and Quick Relief

LONG-TERM CONTROL	QUICK RELIEF
STEP 1: MILD INTERMITTENT ASTHMA	
No daily medications	Short-acting bronchodilator for symptom control Inhaled short-acting β₂-agonist is preferred Intensity of treatment depends on severity of exacerbation Use of short-acting inhaled β₂-agonists >2 times per week indicates need to consider long-term control therapy
STEP 2: MILD PERSISTENT ASTHMA	
Daily medication: Anti-inflammatory medications Low-dose inhaled corticosteroid or cromolyn or nedocromil is the *preferred treatment*. Usually begin with trial of cromolyn or nedocromil in children Sustained-release theophylline is an alternate but not preferred therapy in pediatrics. Used only with older children. Zafirlukast or zileuton may be considered for children 12 years of age or older.	Short-acting bronchodilators: Prefer inhaled β₂-agonist for relief of symptoms Intensity of therapy depends on severity of exacerbation Daily or increasing use of a short-acting bronchodilator indicates need for additional long-term control therapy

STEP 3: MODERATE PERSISTENT ASTHMA

Daily medication

Either

Anti-inflammatory: inhaled medium-dose corticosteroid is the *preferred treatment*

or

Inhaled low-medium dose corticosteroid and a long-acting bronchodilator, especially for nighttime symptoms: either a long-acting inhaled β_2-agonist (for children 12 years or older), which *is preferred*, or sustained-release theophylline, or long-acting β_2-agonist tablets

If needed:

Anti-inflammatory: inhaled corticosteroid (medium-high dose) *and*

Long-acting bronchodilator, especially for nighttime symptoms: either a long-acting inhaled β_2-agonist (for children 12 years of age or older), which *is preferred*, or sustained-release theophylline, or long-acting β_2-agonist tablets

Short-acting bronchodilators:
Prefer inhaled β_2-agonist for relief of symptoms
Intensity of therapy depends on severity of exacerbation
Daily or increasing use of short-acting bronchodilator indicates
  need for additional long-term therapy

Table continued on following page

213

TABLE 20-3

Stepwise Approach for Managing Asthma in Children Older Than 5 Years of Age for Long-Term Control and Quick Relief
Continued

LONG-TERM CONTROL	QUICK RELIEF
STEP 4: SEVERE PERSISTENT ASTHMA	Short-acting inhaled bronchodilator as needed for symptoms
Daily medications	Intensity of treatment depends on severity of exacerbation
Anti-inflammatory: inhaled high-dose corticosteroid *is preferred*	Daily or increasing use of short-acting bronchodilator indicates need for additional long-term control therapy
and	
Long-acting bronchodilator: either a long-acting inhaled β$_2$-agonist for children 12 years of age or older, sustained-release theophylline, or long-acting β$_2$-agonist tablets	
and	
Corticosteroid tablets or syrup long term (2 mg/kg per d, generally not to exceed 60 mg per d) reducing to lowest daily dose or alternate day dose that stabilizes symptoms	

Adapted from Highlights of the Expert Panel Report 2: Guidelines for the Diagnosis and Management of Asthma (National Heart, Lung, and Blood Institute [NHLBI] Publication No. 97-4051A). Bethesda, MD, National Institutes of Health, 1997.

TABLE 20-4

Long-Term Control Medications for the Treatment of Asthma

MEDICATION	DOSAGE FORM	ADULT DOSE	CHILD DOSE	COMMENTS
SYSTEMIC CORTICOSTEROIDS				
Methylprednisolone	2, 4, 8, 16, 32 mg tablets	7.5–60 mg daily in a single dose or every other day as needed for control	0.25–2 mg/kg daily in single dose or every other day as needed for control	For long-term treatment of severe persistent asthma, administer single dose in morning either daily or on alternate days (alternate-day therapy may produce less adrenal suppression). If daily doses are required, one study suggests improved efficacy and no increase in adrenal suppression when administered at 3:00 PM.
Prednisolone	5 mg tabs, 5 mg/5 ml, 15 mg/5 ml	Short-course "burst": 40–60 mg/d as single or 2 divided doses for 3–10 d	Short course "burst": 1–2 mg/kg/d, maximum 60 mg/d for 3–10 d	Short courses or "bursts" are effective for establishing control when initiating therapy or during a period of gradual deterioration.
Prednisone	1, 2.5, 5, 10, 20, 25 mg tablets; 5 mg/ml, 5 mg/5 ml			The bursts should be continued until patient achieves 80% PEF personal best or symptoms resolve. This usually requires 3–10 d but may require longer. There is no evidence that tapering the dose following improvement prevents relapse.
Table continued on following page

215

TABLE 20-4

Long-Term Control Medications for the Treatment of Asthma *Continued*

MEDICATION	DOSAGE FORM	ADULT DOSE	CHILD DOSE	COMMENTS
CROMOLYN AND NEDOCROMIL				
Cromolyn	MDI 1 mg/puff	2–4 puffs tid–qid	1–2 puffs tid–qid	One dose before exercise or allergen exposure provides effective prophylaxis for 1–2 hr.
	Nebulizer solution 20 mg/ampule	1 ampule tid–qid	1 ampule tid–qid	
Nedocromil	MDI 1.75 mg/puff	2–4 puffs bid–qid	1–2 puffs bid–qid	See cromolyn above.
LONG-ACTING β_2-AGONISTS				
Salmeterol	**Inhaled**			
	MDI 21 μg/puff, 60 or 120 puffs	2 puffs q12h	1–2 puffs q12h	May use one dose nightly for symptoms.
	DPI 50 μg/blister	1 blister q12h	1 blister q12h	Do not use as a rescue inhaler for symptom relief or for exacerbations.
Sustained-release albuterol	**Tablet**			
	4 mg tablet	4 mg q12h	0.3–0.6 mg/kg/d, not to exceed 8 mg/d	

METHYLXANTHINES

Theophylline (numerous manufacturers)	Liquids Sustained-release tablets and capsules	Starting dose 10 mg/kg per d up to 300 mg maximum; usual maximum 800 mg/d	Starting dose 10 mg/kg per d: usual maximum: <1 yr: 0.2 (age in wk) + 5 = mg/kg per d ≥1 yr of age: 16 mg/kg per d	Routine serum theophylline level monitoring is required; not commonly used with pediatric patients.

LEUKOTRIENE MODIFIERS

Montelukast	5 mg chewable tablet 10 mg tablet	10 mg tablet daily in evening (≥15 years of age or older)	5 mg chewable tablet daily in evening (6–14 years of age)	Approved for use in children 6 years of age or older.
Zafirlukast	20 mg tablet	40 mg daily (1 tablet bid)		Take zafirlukast at least 1 hr before or 2 hr after meals.
Zileuton	300 mg tablet 600 mg tablet	2400 mg daily (two 300 mg tablets or one 600 mg tablet qid)		Monitor hepatic enzymes (ALT).

DPI = dry-powdered inhaler; MDI = metered-dose inhaler; PEF = peak expiratory flow.

Adapted from Highlights of the Expert Panel Report 2: Guidelines for the Diagnosis and Management of Asthma (National Heart, Lung, and Blood Institute [NHLBI] Publication No. 97-4051A). Bethesda, MD, National Institutes of Health, 1997.

TABLE 20-5

Quick-Relief Medications for the Treatment of Asthma

MEDICATION	DOSAGE FORM	ADULT DOSE	CHILD DOSE	COMMENTS
SHORT-ACTING INHALED BETA₂-AGONISTS				
	MDIs			
Albuterol	90 μg/puff, 200 puffs	2 puffs 5 min before exercise	1–2 puffs 5 min prior to exercise	An increasing use or lack of expected effect indicates diminished control of asthma.
Albuterol HFA	90 μg/puff, 200 puffs	2 puffs tid–qid	2 puffs tid–qid	Not generally recommended for long-term treatment. Regular use on a daily basis indicates the need for additional long-term control therapy.
Bitolterol	370 μg/puff, 300 puffs			Differences in potency exist so that all products are essentially equipotent on a per puff basis.
Pirbuterol	200 μg/puff, 400 puffs			May double usual dose for mild exacerbations.
Terbutaline	200 μg/puff, 300 puffs			Nonselective agents (i.e., epinephrine, isoproterenol, metaproterenol) are not recommended because of their potential for excessive cardiac stimulation, especially at high doses.
	DPIs			
Albuterol Rotahaler	200 μg/capsule	1–2 capsules q4–6h as needed and before exercise	1 capsule q4–6h as needed and before exercise	

Albuterol	**Nebulizer solution** 5 mg/ml (0.5%)	1.25–5 mg (0.25–1 ml) in 2–3 ml of saline q4–8h	0.05 mg/kg (min 1.25 mg, max 2.5 mg) in 2–3 ml of saline q4–6h	May mix with cromolyn or ipratropium nebulizer solutions; may double dose for mild exacerbations.
Bitolterol	2 mg/ml (0.2%)	0.5–3.5 mg (0.25–1 ml) in 2–3 ml of saline q4–8h	Not established	May not mix with other nebulizer solutions.
ANTICHOLINERGICS				
Ipratropium	**MDIs** 18 µg/puff, 200 puffs	2–3 puffs q6h	1–2 puffs q6h	Evidence is lacking for producing added benefit to β_2-agonists in long-term asthma therapy.
	Nebulizer solution 0.25 mg/ml (0.025%)	0.25–0.5 mg q6h	0.25 mg q6h	

Table continued on following page

TABLE 20-5

Quick-Relief Medications for the Treatment of Asthma *Continued*

MEDICATION	DOSAGE FORM	ADULT DOSE	CHILD DOSE	COMMENTS
SYSTEMIC CORTICOSTEROIDS				
Methylprednisolone	2, 4, 8, 16, 32 mg tablets	Short course "burst": 40–60 mg per d as single or 2 divided doses for 3–10 d	Short course "burst": 1–2 mg/ kg/d, maximum 60 mg/d, for 3–10 d	Short courses or "bursts" are effective for establishing control when initiating therapy or during a period of gradual deterioration.
Prednisolone	5 mg tabs, 5 mg/5 ml, 15 mg/5 ml			The burst should be continued until patient achieves 80% PEF personal best or symptoms resolve; this usually requires 3–10 d but may require longer; there is no evidence that tapering the dose following improvement prevents relapse.
Prednisone	1, 2.5, 5, 10, 20, 25 mg tablets: 5 mg/ ml, 5 mg/5 ml			

DPIs = dry-powdered inhalers; MDIs = metered-dose inhalers; PEF = peak expiratory flow.

From the Highlights of the Expert Panel Report 2: Guidelines for the Diagnosis and Management of Asthma. NHLBI Publication No. 97-4051A, Bethesda, MD, National Institutes of Health, 1997.

TABLE 20-6

Daily Doses of Inhaled Corticosteroids (Long-Term Control Medications) for Children: Comparison of Agents and Frequency of Delivery

DRUG	LOW DOSE	MEDIUM DOSE	HIGH DOSE	FREQUENCY
Beclomethasone dipropionate	84–336 µg	336–672 µg	>672 µg	
42 µg/puff	2–8 puffs	8–16 puffs	>16 puffs	Divided doses 2 or 3–4 times per d
84 µg/puff (double strength)	1–4 puffs	4–8 puffs	>8 puffs	Divided doses twice a day
Budesonide Turbuhaler	100–200 µg	200–400 µg	>400 µg	
200 µg/dose		1–2 inhalations	>2 inhalations	Once or twice daily (divided doses)
Flunisolide	500–750 µg	1000–1250 µg	>1250 µg	
250 µg/puff	2–3 puffs	4–5 puffs	>5 puffs	Divided doses twice daily
Fluticasone	88–176 µg	176–440 µg	>440 µg	
MDI: 44 µg/puff	2–4 puffs	4–10 puffs		Divided doses twice daily
110 µg/puff		2–4 puffs	>4 puffs	
220 µg/puff			>2 puffs	
Triamcinolone acetonide	400–800 µg	800–1200 µg	>1200 µg	
100 µg/puff	4–8 puffs	8–12 puffs	>12 puffs	Divided doses 3–4 times daily

From Highlights of the Expert Panel Report 2: Guidelines for the Diagnosis and Management of Asthma (National Heart, Lung, and Blood Institute [NHLBI] Publication No. 97-4051A). Bethesda, MD, National Institutes of Health, 1997, and from information in Taketomo CK, Hodding JH, Kraus DM: Pediatric Dosage Handbook, 5th ed. Hudson, OH: Lexi-Comp, Inc., 1998.

T A B L E 20–7

Use of the Peak Flow Meter and Its Interpretation

STEPS TO FOLLOW IN USING A PEAK FLOW METER

1. Have child stand up.
2. Make sure that indicator is at the base of the numbered scale.
3. Ask child to take a deep breath.
4. Have the child place the peak flow meter in the mouth with the lips sealing the mouthpiece.
5. Tell the child to blow out as hard and fast as possible.
6. Record the rate.
7. Repeat steps 2 through 6 two more times.
8. Record the highest of the three values.

PEAK EXPIRATORY FLOW RATE (PEFR)

The maximum flow rate that is produced during forced expiration with fully inflated lungs.

PERSONAL BEST VALUE

The highest value that an individual achieves in measuring PEFR is known as one's "personal best" value or rate. The personal best value is the most accurate gauge to use to interpret changes in peak flow measurements, as the child's own scores are used as the standard for comparison.

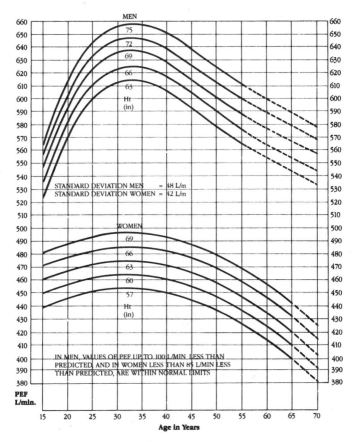

F I G U R E 20–1

Sample peak expiratory flow rate nomogram. (From National Heart, Lung, and Blood Institute [1994]. *Executive summary: Guidelines for the diagnosis and management of asthma* [Publication No. 94–3042A]. Bethesda, MD: National Institutes of Health.) (Figure on this page, Adapted from Nunn, A.J., Gregg, J. [1989]. BMJ, 298, 1068–1070. Figure on next page, Adapted from Godfrey, S., et al. [1970]. Br. J. Dis. Chest., 64, 15–24.)

Illustration continued on following page

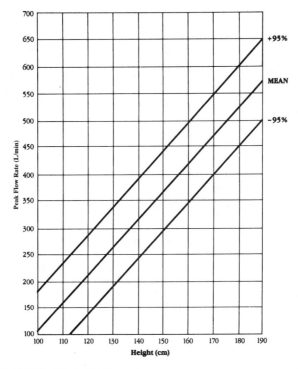

F I G U R E 20-1 *Continued*

T A B L E 20–8

Predicted Average Peak Expiratory Flow for Normal Children and Adolescents

HEIGHT (in)	MALES AND FEMALES (L/min)
43	147
44	160
45	173
46	187
47	200
48	214
49	227
50	240
51	254
52	267
53	280
54	293
55	307
56	320
57	334
58	347
59	360
60	373
61	387
62	400
63	413
64	427
65	440
66	454
67	467

Note: It is recommended that peak expiratory flow rate (PEFR) objectives for therapy be based on each individual's "personal best," which is established after a period of PEF rate monitoring while the individual is under effective treatment.

From National Heart, Lung, and Blood Institute: Executive Summary: Guidelines for the Diagnosis and Management of Asthma (Publication No. 94-3042A). Bethesda, MD, National Institutes of Health, 1994. Adapted from Polger G, Promedhar V: Pulmonary Function Testing in Children: Techniques and Standards. Philadelphia, WB Saunders, 1971.

The use of intranasal corticosteroid preparations is important in the management of problematic allergic rhinitis. Table 20–11 provides dosage information about commonly used products.

Text continued on page 232

T A B L E 20-9

How To Use a Metered-Dose Inhaler and Dry-Powdered Inhaler

METERED-DOSE INHALER

CHILDREN <5 YEARS

1. The use of a mask chamber, such as the InspirEase, with an MDI allows the delivery of inhaled medications even in an uncooperative child.
2. The child should be placed in the parent's lap and the mask placed around the child's mouth.
3. Press down on the MDI while firmly holding the mask around the child's mouth. The child will eventually take a deep breath and inhale the medication.

CHILDREN ≥5 YEARS

1. Remove the cap and hold the MDI upright.
2. Shake the MDI.
3. Tilt head back slightly and breathe out.
4. Position the inhaler in one of the following ways:
   a. If a spacer is used, put the spacer in the mouth and seal with the lips.
   b. If a spacer is not used, the most effective method of delivery is to open the mouth and hold the inhaler 1–2 inches away.
   c. If a spacer is not used and the child cannot coordinate the method outlined in b, have the child put the inhaler in his or her mouth and seal with the lips.
   d. If a breath-activated β_2-agonist MDI is used, place inhaler in mouth.
5. Press down on the MDI to release the medication, while slowly taking a deep breath (3–5 sec) through mouth.
6. Hold breath for 10 sec.
7. Wait for at least 1 min between inhalations.

DRY-POWDERED INHALER

1. Exhale and then close mouth tightly around the mouthpiece.
2. Rapidly inhale.
3. Hold breath for 10 seconds (slow count to 10) and exhale (not into the inhaler).

MDI = metered-dose inhaler.

TABLE 20–10

Key Features in the Assessment and Management of Allergic Rhinitis

CLINICAL FINDINGS	Typical onset 4–5 yr; mouth breathing, snoring, nasal speech; mucosal hyperemia to purplish pallor and edema; clear, watery to seromucoid rhinorrhea; allergic facies, horizontal crease across the lower third of nose, itching and rubbing of nose, "allergic salute"; postnasal drip, sneezing, congested cough; malocclusion if chronic
MANAGEMENT	Stepwise approach

1. *Avoidance:* Child to avoid known or suspected triggers or allergens (e.g., house dust, cats, cigarette smoke, mold). Eliminate/control environmental allergens/triggers
2. *Pharmacologic Therapy:*
   Antihistamines
   - Good for seasonal allergic rhinitis
   - Relieve itching, sneezing, and rhinorrhea; do little for nasal congestion and obstruction
   - Increase dosage of drug until relief of symptoms or side effects experienced
   - Need to rotate drugs if tolerance develops
   - If side effects with one antihistamine, switch to another in a different class or one in the same class but with different actions
   - If sedating antihistamines interfere with activities, consider nonsedating agent
   Nasal Antihistamine Spray
   - Azelastine approved for use in seasonal allergic rhinitis in children >12 yr
   Decongestants
   - May help relieve nasal congestion; other agents listed earlier are more effective
   Nasal Cromolyn
   - Used for seasonal and perennial allergic rhinitis; initiate treatment before seasonal exposure
   - 1–2 sprays in each nostril four times a day; taper with control
   Intranasal Corticosteroids (see Table 20-11)
   - Child to clear nasal passages of mucus before use
   - Use when symptoms not relieved with antihistamines or if severe symptoms
   - Effective alone or together with antihistamines
   - Can take ≥1 wk before improvement noted
   - Side effects include local burning, irritation, soreness, and/or epistaxis
3. *Immunotherapy:* If symptoms are severe and not relieved by Steps 1 and 2
   Antibiotics: Use only if secondary sinusitis present

TABLE 20–11

Intranasal Corticosteroid Preparations Used for Allergic Rhinitis: Usual Doses

DRUG	DOSE	NO. INHALATIONS OR SPRAYS & DAILY FREQUENCY	AGE
Beclomethasone (Vancenase, Beconase inhaler)	42 μg/inhalation	1 tid 1 bid–qid or 2 bid	6–12 yr ≥12 yr
Beclomethasone—aqueous inhalation (Vancenase AQ, Beconase AQ) (Vancenase AQ 84 μg)	42 μg/inhalation	1–2 bid	≥6 yr
Budesonide* (Rhinocort)	84 μg/spray 32 μg/spray	1–2 once daily 2 sprays bid or 4 sprays daily (in morning)	≥6 yr ≥6 yr
Dexamethasone (Dexacort Turbinaire, Decadron Turbinaire)	84 μg/spray	1–2 sprays bid 2 sprays bid–tid	6–12 yr ≥12 yr
Flunisolide (Nasalide, Nasarel)	25 μg/spray	1 spray tid or 2 sprays twice daily; maintenance dose is 1 spray daily 2 sprays bid	6–14 yr ≥14 yr
Fluticasone (Flonase)	50 μg/spray	1 spray daily; 2 sprays daily if severe or poor response	≥4 yr
Triamcinolone (Nasacort)	55 μg/spray	2 sprays daily 2 sprays daily; after 4–7 days may increase to 4 sprays daily or 2 sprays bid or 1 spray qid	6–11 yr ≥12yr
Triamcinolone AQ (Nasacort AQ)	55 μg/spray	2 sprays daily; maintenance dose 1 spray daily	>12 yr

* Reduce slowly every 2–4 wk to smallest effective dose.

Adapted from Taketomo CK, Hodding JH, Kraus DM: Pediatric Dosage Handbook, 5th ed. Hudson, OH, Lexi-Comp, Inc., 1998.

ATOPIC DERMATITIS

Atopic dermatitis is frequently referred to as the "itch that rashes." Assessment and management issues are summarized in Tables 20–12 and 20–13, respectively.

T A B L E 20–12

Assessment of Atopic Dermatitis

ONSET	SIGNS AND SYMPTOMS	PROGNOSIS
INITIAL PRESENTATION		
<3 mo old (⅓ of cases)	Dry skin first sign	Often not noticed
2–3 mo	Itch–scratch–itch cycle starts	
Infantile phase	Acute presentation—common in infants: intense itching; redness, papules, vesicles, edema; serous discharge and crusts; xerosis, dry hair, scalp; diaper area sparing; cheeks, forehead, scalp, extremities	⅔ of cases resolve by 2–3 yr
Childhood phase (starts 18–24 mo of age)	Involves wrists, hands, popliteal and antecubital fossa; eyebrows thin and broken off; some only have feet involved; may have allergic/atopic facies and white dermatographism	⅓ continue into teen years
Adolescent phase	Often only hand dermatitis; can involve other typical sites	New or recurrent problem
CHRONIC PRESENTATION	Common in children and teenagers; thickened, leathery, hyperpigmented skin; scratch marks	

T A B L E 20–13

Management of Atopic Dermatitis

ANTIPRURITIC AGENTS	Stop itch–scratch–itch cycle • Hydroxyzine (Atarax, Vistaril): If need during the day, give 2 mg/kg/d divided q6–8h (Taketomo et al., 1998). If itching mainly problematic at night, Atarax at 0.5–1 mg/kg at bedtime (Eichenfield & Friedlander, 1998). • Diphenhydramine hydrochloride (Benadryl) useful, especially if sedation is needed. Usual oral dose in children: 5 mg/kg/d divided doses q6–8h. • Nonsedating antihistamines in older children: cetirizine beneficial. • Do not use topical diphenhydramine (Benadryl): allergic sensitization problem.
HYDRATION	Correct skin dryness • Wet compresses if weeping, oozing lesions and signs of acute inflammation. Aluminum acetate (Burow solution 1:20 or 1:40 preparation). Solution should be tepid or body temperature. Use up to 5 d during acute stage. • Use moderately wet soft cloths; corticosteroid topical preparations can be applied either before or after compresses. • Aveeno or oatmeal baths for pruritus, followed by application of heavy cream emollient. • Bath or shower limited to 5–10 min (no soaking baths) in warm, not hot, water. Immediately after, gently pat dry and emolliate with a heavy cream.
EMOLLIENT	• Apply emollient (e.g., petrolatum [Vaseline] or Aquaphor [Beiersdorf]) before getting out of the bath water or just after while still damp. Also good time to apply topical corticosteroid preparations. • Apply emollient 2–3 times/d as needed (e.g., Eucerin cream, Crisco [plain, not butter flavored], or petroleum). If sensitive to fragrances, do not use scented creams (e.g., Nivea).
SOAPS	• Use mild soap such as Dove or Neutrogena; no drying or deodorant soaps and no oils in bath water. Cetaphil, a nondrying soap-free cleanser, can substitute for bathing. Do not wipe off after applying.

T A B L E 20–13

Management of Atopic Dermatitis *Continued*

TOPICAL CORTICOSTEROIDS (TCS)	• Mainstay of therapy. Do not use agents with propylene glycol. • If applying over large areas or if occlusion (covering with plastic wrap) is used, there is a possibility of systemic absorption, especially in infants and young children. • Apply thin layer of 1% hydrocortisone cream (acute stage) or ointment (chronic stage) to atopic dermatitis areas 3–4 times/d. • Mix TCS with Eucerin cream or Aquaphor and apply together. • If fluorinated TCS needed, consult physician; never use them on face; use only 1% hydrocortisone ointment sparingly 2–3 times/d until symptoms improve. After flare up cleared (1 to 2 wk), reduce to once daily, then every other day, to twice weekly. Do not use Class II–III TCS for longer than 5–7 d (Arndt et al., 1997).
ANTIBIOTICS	• Treat secondary skin infections (*Staphylococcus aureus* or *S. pyogenes*). Oral erythromycin (30–50 mg/kg/d), dicloxacillin (12.5–50 mg/kg/d), or cephalexin (25–50 mg/kg/d) for 10–14 d (Drolet and Esterly, 1999); if skin infections recurrent or frequent, treat for 3 wk. • Topical antibiotic preparations can be used as supplemental therapy; apply topical bacitracin, polysporin, and mupirocin (Bactroban) to excoriations and crusts.
TAR	• To help manage chronic and lichenified forms; caution about photosensitivity.
ELIMINATION	• Avoid/eliminate known or suspected offending agents (e.g., bubble bath, chlorine, fragrances, house dust). • Avoid nonbreathable fabrics, nylon, or wool; wear soft cotton clothing. • Dietary restrictions may include the elimination of cow's milk from infants predisposed to atopy. No eggs, fish, chocolate, nuts, and citrus fruits until 12 mo old.
ENVIRONMENT	• Attempt to increase environmental humidity and decrease exposure to antigens. Cool temperatures (air conditioning) help.

REFERENCES

Arndt KA, Wintroub BU, Robinson JK, LeBoit PE: Primary Care Dermatology. Philadelphia, WB Saunders, 1997.

Drolet BA, Esterly NB: Atopic dermatitis. *In* Burg FD, Ingelfinger JR, Wald ER, Polin RA (eds): Gellis and Kagan's Current Pediatric Therapy. Philadelphia, WB Saunders, 1999, pp 954–956.

Eichenfield LF, Friedlander SF: Coping with chronic dermatitis. Contemp Pediatr 15(10):53–68, 1998.

May JN: Asthma. *In* Finberg L (ed): Saunders Manual of Pediatric Practice. Philadelphia, WB Saunders, 1998, pp 905–911.

National Heart, Lung, and Blood Institute. Highlights of the Expert Panel Report 2: Guidelines for the Diagnosis and Management of Asthma (NIH Publication No. 97–4051A). Bethesda, MD: National Institutes of Health, May 1997.

Taketomo CK, Hodding JH, Kraus DM: Pediatric Dosage Handbook, 5th ed. Hudson OH: Lexi-Comp, Inc., 1998.

CHAPTER 21

Endocrine and Metabolic Diseases

INTRODUCTION

The endocrine system is a secretory feedback system that controls many bodily functions, including growth and sexual development. Primary care nurse practitioners are in a position to assess whether physical findings related to growth or sexual development are normal variants or indicators of a disease process. Metabolic disorders generally affect multiple organs and tissues. They alter metabolic processes to produce deleterious end products or produce abnormal substances. Early identification of metabolic and endocrine disorders is imperative. Referral to a pediatric endocrinologist for additional diagnostic studies and treatment generally is indicated. Routine metabolic screening of the newborn is discussed in Chapter 34 of the Pocket Reference.

COMMON ENDOCRINE AND METABOLIC DISORDERS

Newborn Screening

Important factors to consider in common endocrine and metabolic disorders detected in the newborn period are summarized in Table 21-1. Children with these disorders should be referred to specialists in genetics and pediatric endocrinology.

Short Stature

Children with poor growth or abnormal growth patterns should be carefully monitored to assess possible genetic, prenatal, endocrine,

T A B L E 21-1

Characteristics of Common Disorders Detected in the Newborn Period

DISORDER	ETIOLOGY	CLINICAL FINDINGS	ENDOCRINE/METABOLIC DISTURBANCE
Ambiguous genitalia	Varied: genetic; enzyme deficiency (CAH)	Varied degrees of either male or female genitalia	See CAH
Congenital adrenal hyperplasia (CAH)	Deficiency of 21-hydroxylase most common defect; leads to salt-losing syndrome	Virilization of genitalia; inability to maintain serum electrolytes, resulting in dehydration (low Na, Cl; high K) and vomiting	Overproduction of ACTH, excessive adrenal androgen production
Phenylketonuria (PKU)	Autosomal recessive trait	Normal at birth; if untreated, S & S of vomiting, irritability, urine with musty odor, eczematoid rash; eventually mental retardation if not treated	Deficiency of phenylalanine hydroxylase
Galactosemia	Autosomal recessive trait	Jaundice, hepatomegaly, hypotonia, cataracts; death if not treated	Deficiency of galactose-1-phosphate uridyltransferase

ACTH = adrenocorticotropic hormone; S & S = signs and symptoms; Na = sodium; Cl = chloride; K = potassium.

nutritional, metabolic, psychological, and/or systemic chronic illness. The most common cause of short stature is constitutionally delayed growth. Most children with constitutional short stature do not have growth hormone abnormalities or any other detectable alteration. Growth hormone deficiency is a rare problem. Table 21-2 differentiates these two problems.

Diabetes Mellitus

Diabetes mellitus results from defects in insulin secretion, insulin action, or both. Type 1 diabetes generally is immune mediated with β-cell destruction in the pancreas that leads to absolute insulin deficiency. Type 1 diabetes occurs most frequently in children and adolescents. Type 2 diabetes includes disorders that range from predominantly insulin resistance with relative insulin deficiency to a predominantly insulin secretory defect with insulin resistance. Type 2 diabetes is most commonly associated with obesity and sedentary lifestyle and with those with strong genetic predisposition. It can occur in children and young adults and has been called maturity-onset diabetes in youth. A summary of key findings of type 1 diabetes mellitus, an outline of the management plan, and a guide to insulin adjustment are presented in Tables 21-3, 21-4, and 21-5, respectively.

Hypothyroidism

Hypothyroidism is a deficiency in thyroid hormone that can be either congenital or acquired (juvenile hypothyroidism). Table 21-6 summarizes the diagnosis and management for both of these conditions. Newborn screening for congenital hypothyroidism is mandated in every state. Early treatment improves intellectual capacity.

Puberty: Precocious and Delayed

A diagnosis of precocious puberty is made when a child exhibits signs of genital maturation, advanced bone age, secondary characteristics of sexual development, and accelerated linear growth before the acceptable age for the emergence of puberty. Children who have isolated breast development (premature thelarche) and isolated pubic hair (premature adrenarche) often have benign conditions. Puberty also can be delayed. Because both precocious puberty and delayed puberty have many causes, refer the child to a pediatric endocrinologist for evaluation. See Table 21-7 for age guidelines.

Text continued on page 242

T A B L E 21–2

Short Stature: Characteristics of Growth Hormone Deficiency (GHD) and Constitutional Short Stature (CSS) in Children

CONDITION	ETIOLOGY	ONSET	PRESENTATION	ENDOCRINE/METABOLIC DISTURBANCE
GHD	Most cases are idiopathic; pituitary or hypothalamic disease; minor organic hypothalamic lesion; infection; radiation	Congenital or acquired	<4 cm of growth/yr with normal birth weight; S & S of increased CNS pressure; microphallus, proportional short stature; delayed bone age	Deficiency or impairment in secretion of GH-releasing hormone
CSS	Variation of normal growth; not a disease	First years of life impaired growth	Growth velocity is normal; delayed puberty and pubertal growth spurt; delayed bone age; positive family history	None—final height is appropriate for parents' heights

S & S = signs and symptoms; CNS = central nervous system.

TABLE 21-3

Type I Diabetes Mellitus: Key Clinical Findings

History	Polydipsia, polyphagia, polyuria, nocturia, blurred vision, weight loss, fatigue
Onset	Usually acute, ketones in blood and urine, high blood glucose level
Laboratory findings	Ketonuria and ketonemia
Physical findings	Signs of ketoacidosis: dehydration; slow, labored breathing or air column; flushed cheeks and face; mental confusion; lethargy; fruity odor (acetone) on breath
Diagnostic tests	1. Random plasma glucose concentration ≥200 mg/dl (11.1 mmol/L)
	2. Fasting plasma glucose ≥126 mg/dl (7.0 mmol/L)
	3. Two hours after meal, plasma glucose ≥200 mg/dl (11.1 mmol/L) during an oral glucose tolerance test (American Diabetes Association, 1998a, b)
Other tests	1. Verification of autoantibodies substantiates type 1 diabetes but is not universally recommended
	2. Glycosylated hemoglobin (HbA1c) measurements are not currently recommended for the diagnosis of diabetes; useful for follow-up monitoring

T A B L E 21–4

Management Plan for Type 1 Diabetes Mellitus

Blood glucose (BG) levels:
　Guidelines target levels of BG range from 80 to 120 mg/dl at fasting and from 80 to 180 mg/dl at other times of the day. Younger children (<6 yr) may have goals of 90 to 130 mg/dl fasting and from 90 to 200 mg/dl at other times (Porter et al., 1997).

Indicators of diabetic control:
　Diabetic control is based on glycohemoglobin (HbA1c) levels, daily log of metered glucose values, and clinical symptoms.

HbA1c:
　8–8.5% or less is acceptable for children <7 yr; for older children and teenagers, <8.0% is desirable. However, this value must be used in consideration of metered serum glucose values.

Insulin:
1. Via pump or injections (2–4 times daily) with BG monitored before meals and at bedtime.
2. See Table 26–3 in *Pediatric Primary Care* for information about various types of commercially available insulins and their peak and duration.
3. For children receiving pork NPH, generally give ⅔ dose in morning and ⅓ in evening; for those on Humulin NPH, give ½ to ½ split between morning and evening doses.
4. Total insulin dosage is 1 U/kg/d but may vary (e.g., child <5 yr). A range of 0.5–1.5 U/kg/d is acceptable and allows for individual differences. Type and schedule of insulin delivery depend on a number of factors, such as the child's routine schedule and the need for flexibility in daily routine.
5. Adjustments of the insulin dose are based on patterns of BG over several days. Parent and teenagers generally are given an algorithm of Regular or Humalog insulin doses based on before-meal BG and are taught to make adjustments in insulin based on patterns of control. Usually, a 10% adjustment in insulin can be safely made by parents. In young children, dose adjustments must be made in ½ unit increments.

Follow-up visits:
1. Visits at a minimum of 3 mo intervals
2. Glycosylated hemoglobin every 3 mo
3. Total urinary protein excretion measured once yearly if child has had diabetes for >5 yr or after puberty
4. Lipid profile if child >2 yr of age at time of diagnosis and when BG control is established (American Diabetes Association, 1998a, b)
5. Thyroid screen yearly

Emotional issues:
　Address and focus on social and emotional concerns

Exercise and medical nutritional therapy:
　Address these issues at each visit (see Chapter 26 in *Pediatric Primary Care*)

T A B L E 21–5

Considerations for Insulin Adjustments

HYPOGLYCEMIA

Is there a known reason for the hypoglycemia?
  Insufficient food; delayed meal?
  Exercise?
  Extra insulin taken?
Was hypoglycemia severe? Easily treated by mouth?
Is there a long period of time between meals and snacks?
Which insulin is most likely to be peaking at the time of hypoglycemia?

HYPERGLYCEMIA

Is there a known reason for hyperglycemia?
  Too much food; sweets?
  Meals/snacks too close together?
  Insufficient exercise?
  Less insulin given; insulin leaked out of pump if used?
Are ketones present in the urine?
Which insulin is most likely to be peaking at the time of hyperglycemia?
Does the high blood glucose follow hypoglycemia?

T A B L E 21–6

Diagnosis and Management of Congenital Hypothyroidism (CH) and Acquired Hypothyroidism (AH)

	CAUSATIVE FACTORS	CLINICAL FINDINGS	MANAGEMENT	COMPLICATIONS
CH	Failure in gland development; enzyme defect; autosomal genetic defect	Most appear normal at birth; may have prolonged jaundice; positive family history; lethargy; large posterior fontanel and tongue; hypothermia; dry, cool, scaly skin; umbilical hernia; delayed bone ossification	Synthroid (levothyroxine sodium), start at 10–15 µg/kg/d; keep T_4 level at 10–15 µg/dl range; T_4, free T_4, TSH q mo for first 6 mo; q other mo from 6 to 12 mo of age, then q3 mo; bone age at Dx and 12 mo of age; retest infant with trisomy 21 at 3 mo	Mental ratardation if not treated
AH	Autoimmune chronic lymphocytic thyroiditis (Hashimoto thyroiditis); thyroidectomy; ingestion of propylthiouracil; iodine deficiency; irradiation	Lethargy, decreased appetite, poor school performance, delayed puberty, cold intolerance, goiter, tender neck; weakness, delayed dentition, cool skin, reflexes diminished or absent	Levothyroxine sodium, range of 8–10 µg/kg/d for newborns to 100–200 µg/kg/d for adults; monitor TSH q2–3 mo after dose change and with symptoms	

Dx = diagnosis; q = every; T_4 = thyroxine; TSH = thyroid-stimulating hormone.

TABLE 21-7
Precocious and Delayed Puberty: Age Guidelines

	AGE		KEY POINTS
	Female	Male	
Precocious puberty	<8 yr	<9 yr	Girls often have no underlying pathology; boys often have central nervous system pathology
Delayed puberty	13 yr or 5 yr since first sign of puberty and menarche	14 yr or 5 yr since first signs of puberty and completion of genital growth	No signs of puberty by these ages or failure to complete puberty

◼ HYPERCHOLESTEROLEMIA AND HYPERLIPIDEMIA

Atherosclerosis begins in childhood. Selective rather than universal screening of at-risk children is recommended. The risk factors for screening children for hypercholesterolemia are

1. Family history of heart disease: If parent or grandparent at age 55 years or younger had any of the following:

- Coronary angiography for coronary atherosclerosis
- Balloon angioplasty or coronary bypass surgery
- Documented myocardial infarction, angina pectoris, peripheral vascular disease, cerebrovascular accident, or sudden cardiac death

2. Either parent has a known total cholesterol level of 240 mg/dL or higher (Schieken, 1999)

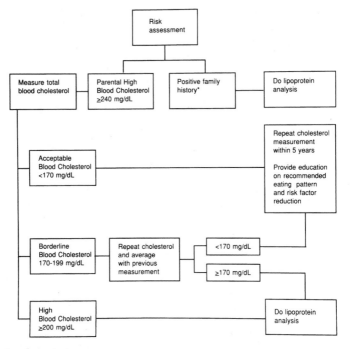

FIGURE 21-1
Risk assessment of children based on high parental blood cholesterol or a positive family history of premature atherosclerotic disease. (Reprinted from NIH Publication No. 91-2732. September 1991, p 46.)

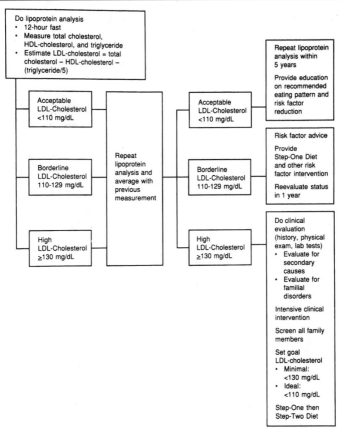

F I G U R E 21-2

Classification, education, and follow-up of patients based on low-density lipoprotein (LDL) cholesterol level. (Reprinted from NIH Publication No. 91-2732. September 1991, p 47.)

Figures 21-1 and 21-2 show the National Institutes of Health's childhood risk assessment and screening algorithm that include the classification, education, and follow-up of patients based on low-density lipoprotein (LDL) cholesterol levels.

Dietary management based on total and LDL cholesterol levels and characteristics of the Step-One and Step-Two diets are found in Tables 21-8 and 21-9.

T A B L E 21-8

Cutoff Points of Total and LDL Cholesterol for Dietary Intervention in Children and Adolescents with a Family History of Hypercholesterolemia or Premature Cardiovascular Disease

CATEGORY	TOTAL CHOLESTEROL (mg/dl)	LDL CHOLESTEROL (mg/dl)	DIETARY INTERVENTION
Acceptable	<170	<110	Recommended population eating pattern: normal diet with reduced cholesterol intake
Borderline	170–199	110–129	Step-One diet prescribed, other risk-factor intervention
High	≥200	≥130	Step-One diet prescribed, then Step-Two diet if necessary

From National Cholesterol Education Program: Report of the Expert Panel on Blood Cholesterol Levels in Children and Adolescents. National Heart, Lung, and Blood Institute. US Department of Health and Human Services. Public Health Service. NIH Publication No. 91-2732. Washington, DC: Government Printing Office, 1991.

T A B L E 21-9

Characteristics of Step-One and Step-Two Diets for Lowering Blood Cholesterol

NUTRIENT	RECOMMENDED INTAKE	
	Step-One Diet	Step-Two Diet
Total fat	Average of no more than 30% of total calories	Same
Saturated fatty acids	Less than 10% of total calories	Less than 7% of total calories
Polyunsaturated fatty acids	Up to 10% of total calories	Same
Monounsaturated fatty acids	Remaining total fat calories	Same
Cholesterol	Less than 300 mg/d	Less than 200 mg/d
Carbohydrates	About 55% of total calories	Same
Protein	About 15–20% of total calories	Same
Calories	To promote normal growth and development and to reach or maintain desirable body weight	Same

From National Cholesterol Education Program: Report of the Expert Panel on Blood Cholesterol Levels in Children and Adolescents. National Heart, Lung, and Blood Institute, US Department of Health and Human Services, Public Health Service. NIH Publication No. 91-2732. Washington, DC: Government Printing Office, 1991.

245

Promotion of a healthy lifestyle should begin in childhood, with an emphasis on exercise, weight control, prudent diet (including breastfeeding, late introduction of appropriate solids, control of salt intake, and reduced saturated fat intake), and management of stress, hypertension, and diabetes.

REFERENCES

American Diabetes Association: Nutrition recommendations and principles for people with diabetes mellitus. Diabetes Care 21 (suppl 1):32–35, 1998a.

American Diabetes Association: Standards of medical care for patients with diabetes mellitus. Diabetes Care 21 (suppl 1), 1998b.

Porter PA, Keating B, Byrne G, Jones TW: Incidence and predictive criteria of nocturnal hypoglycemia in young children with insulin dependent diabetes mellitus. J Pediatr 130:366–372, 1997.

Schieken RM: The child at risk for coronary heart disease as an adult. *In* Burg FD, Ingelfinger JR, Wald ER, Polin RA (eds): Gellis and Kagan's Current Pediatric Therapy, 16th ed. Philadelphia, WB Saunders, 1999, pp 578–582.

CHAPTER 22

Hematological Diseases

▰▰▰ INTRODUCTION

Hematological diseases involve disorders in red blood cell (RBC), white blood cell (WBC), and/or platelet and coagulation functions with resulting alteration in blood cell production, maturation, or destruction. This chapter presents information about common anemias seen in children and provides guidelines for identifying three of the more serious hematological disorders of childhood, namely, idiopathic thrombocytopenia, leukemia, and lymphoma.

Many hematological processes are inherited. Family history, nationality, and geographical origins are helpful assessment information. In addition, particular attention should be paid to the historical findings listed in Table 22-1.

T A B L E 22-1

Key Historical Information Related to the Possibility of Hematological Disease

- Episodes of jaundice (including newborn period)
- Pain in extremities or abdomen
- Pallor, petechiae, ecchymosis
- Weight loss, recent or chronic infections, drug exposures
- Changes in stool characteristics (e.g., black tarry stool)
- Travel
- Exposure to lead
- Adenopathy
- Family history of hematological disorders (e.g., glucose-6-phosphate dehydrogenase, sickle cell anemia, thalassemia)
- Bleeding tendencies

ANEMIA IN CHILDHOOD

Anemia may be suspected on the basis of clinical judgment and deviation from established hemoglobin and hematocrit norms for age (Fig. 22–1). An initial laboratory workup for anemia should include

- A complete blood count (CBC)
- Reticulocyte count
- Peripheral smear to examine morphological characteristics and staining properties of the RBC

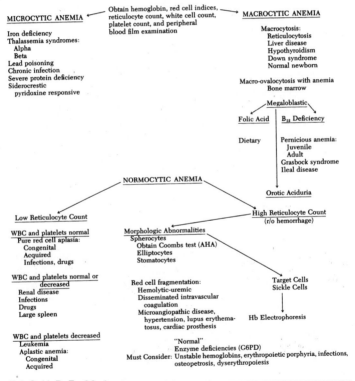

FIGURE 22–1

A diagnostic approach to anemia. AHA = acquired hemolytic anemia; G6PD = glucose-6-phosphate dehydrogenase; Hb = hemoglobin; r/o = rule out; WBC = white blood cell count. (From Nathan D, Oski FA: Hematology of Infancy and Childhood, 4th ed. Philadelphia, WB Saunders, 1993, p. 352.)

Iron deficiency is the most common cause of childhood anemia and must be differentiated from other, more serious anemias. Table 22-2 summarizes the characteristic clinical findings, screening and diagnostic tests, and treatments for the common acute anemias seen in childhood and adolescence.

Laboratory findings are important in the differentiation of the various anemias seen in infants and children. Table 22-3 identifies key laboratory tests and their expected results when an anemia is caused by iron deficiency, β-thalassemia trait, chronic inflammation, or lead intoxication.

TABLE 22-2

Acute Anemia in Childhood and Adolescence

CLASSIFICATION	HISTORY	PHYSICAL FINDINGS	SCREENING TESTS	DIAGNOSTIC TESTS	TREATMENT
I. Microcytic					
Iron-deficiency anemia	Infant and toddler Excessive cow's milk ingestion Poor solid food intake	Waxy, sallow appearance of skin	Hb: <7 g/dl MCV: <60 fl ↑ Retic: ↓ to sl ↑	Serum Fe: ↓ TIBC: ↑ % Saturation: ↓	Ferrous sulfate, 6 mg/kg/d of elemental iron Discontinue cow's milk Limit formula to <24 oz/d and encourage solid foods that are iron rich
Homozygous thalassemia (Cooley anemia)	Infant and toddler Growth failure Ethnic background consistent	Hepato-splenomegaly Frontal bossing	Hb: var ↓ MCV: 50–60 fl		
II. Macrocytic			See III. Normocytic		
Diamond-Blackfan anemia					
Megaloblastic anemia	Variable, depending on etiology	Variable, depending on etiology	Hb: var ↓ MCV: ↑ Retic: ↓ Platelets and WBC: ↓ Hypersegmented polys	Bone marrow: megaloblastic Vitamin B$_{12}$ Folate Others	Variable, depending on etiology

III. Normocytic

	Clinical Features	Laboratory	Bone Marrow / Other	Treatment
A. Productive defect				
Diamond-Blackfan anemia	Age: 65% <6 mo; 90% <1 yr; Insidious onset; 25% with physical abnormalities	Hb: 2-3 g/dl; MCV: ↑ in 30% (100% after treatment); Retic: <1%	Bone marrow: erythroid hypoplasia and lymphocytosis; Hb F: ↑; RBCi antigen: ↑	Prednisone: 2 mg/kg/d in 3-4 doses until Hb >10 g/dl
Transient erythroblastopenia of childhood	1-3 yr of age; Viral illness in preceding 3 mo; None	Hb: 3-9 g/dl; MCV: normal; Retic: <1%	Bone marrow: erythroid hypoplasia	Supportive
Aplastic crisis of hemolytic anemia	Underlying hemolytic anemia; Viral syndrome in preceding 1-3 wk; Sudden exacerbation of pallor; Splenomegaly	Hb: <7 g/dl; Retic: <1%; Smear: abnormalities of chronic anemia	Bone marrow: erythroid hypoplasia	Supportive
Marrow infiltration	Variable, depending on etiology; Bleeding; Infection; Petechiae, purpura; Infection; Hepatosplenomegaly	Hb: var ↓; Retic: ↓ to nl; Platelets: ↓; WBC: ↓ or ↑; Smear: variable	Bone marrow: infiltration by non-hematopoietic cells	Variable, depending on etiology (e.g., leukemia, neuroblastoma)
Aplastic anemia	Bleeding; Infection; Petechiae, purpura; Infection; Multiple anomalies possible with Fanconi anemia	Hb: var ↓; MCV: ↑ in Fanconi anemia; Retic: ↓; Platelets and WBC: ↓	Bone marrow: hypoplasia of all hematopoietic elements	Variable

T A B L E 22-2
Acute Anemia in Childhood and Adolescence Continued

CLASSIFICATION	HISTORY	PHYSICAL FINDINGS	SCREENING TESTS	DIAGNOSTIC TESTS	TREATMENT
B. Hemolytic Autoimmune hemolytic anemia	Jaundice Gastrointestinal symptoms Dark/red urine	Icterus Hepato-splenomegaly	Hb: var ↓ Retic: ↑ (occ ↓) Smear: microspherocytes	Direct Coombs test: positive	Corticosteroids: prednisone or intravenous equivalent: 2–6 mg/kg/d Transfusion indicated
Hemolytic-uremic syndrome	Infant and toddler Viral prodrome Gastrointestinal bleeding in 20% Sudden pallor, purpura ± Central nervous system symptoms	Purpura Hypotension ± Central nervous system abnormalities	Hb: 7–8 g/dl Retic: ↑ Platelets: ↓ Smear: microangiopathy	None Renal failure—supportive	Supportive: early dialysis ? Plasma infusion/exchange ? Antiplatelet drugs
C. Blood loss Splenic sequestration crisis of sickle cell (SS) disease (internal blood loss)	SS disease: 5 mo to 2 yr of age Hb SC or S-thalassemia: all ages Sudden weakness, dyspnea, abdominal distention Shock	Hypotension Massive splenomegaly	Hb: <4 g/dl Retic: ↑ Smear: sickle cells	None	Plasma expanders: whole or reconstituted blood

Fe = iron; Hb = hemoglobin; MCV = mean corpuscular volume; nl = normal; occ = occasionally; polys = polymorphonuclear leukocytes; RBCi = red blood cell i antigen; Retic = reticulocytes; sl = slightly; TIBC = total iron-binding capacity; var = variably; WBC = white blood cell count.
Adapted from Green M, Haggerty R: Ambulatory Pediatrics IV. Philadelphia, WB Saunders, 1990, pp 378–379.

TABLE 22-3

Laboratory Findings in Anemia of Infants and Children

DIAGNOSIS	LABORATORY TEST	EXPECTED RESULTS
Iron deficiency	Serum ferritin	Low <25 μg/dl
	Serum iron and total iron-binding capacity	Low/high
	% Iron saturation	Low <15%
	Bone marrow iron stores	Absent
	Stool for occult blood	Absent
	Urine for blood, hemoglobin, or hemosiderin	Present (if renal loss)
	MCV/RBC ratio	>13
		Basophilic stippling
β-Thalassemia trait	Blood film	
	Hemoglobin electrophoresis	Increased A$_2$ or F hemoglobin
	Biosynthetic β/α-globin chain ratio	<1
	MCV/RBC ratio	<13
	Family studies	Hb/Hct decreased
		Blood film
		Anisocytosis
		Poikilocytosis
		Basophilic stippling
		MCV <70 fl/cell

Table continued on following page

T A B L E 22–3

Laboratory Findings in Anemia of Infants and Children Continued

DIAGNOSIS	LABORATORY TEST	EXPECTED RESULTS
Chronic inflammation	Nonspecific tests	
	Erythrocyte sedimentation rate	Increased
	Acute-phase reactants	Increased
	C-reactive protein	
	Fibrinogen	
	Haptoglobin	
	Serum ferritin	Increased
	Serum iron and total iron-binding capacity	Low/low
	% Iron saturation	Low
	Bone marrow iron stores	Increased
	Bone marrow sideroblasts	Decreased
	Blood film	Basophilic stippling
	Erythrocyte protoporphyrin	Increased
Lead intoxication	Blood lead	Increased

MCV = mean corpuscular volume; RBC = red blood cell; Hb/Hct = hemoglobin/hematocrit.
From Segel GB: Anemia. Pediatr Rev 10:77–88, 1988.

CHAPTER **23**

Neurological Diseases

INTRODUCTION

Neurological conditions are not generally independently diagnosed and treated by nurse practitioners. Most conditions are potentially quite serious. Additionally, problems in other body systems may affect the neurological system. Nurse practitioners do, however, have an important role in the identification of children with neurological conditions and in the management and monitoring of diagnosed children.

ASSESSMENT

The assessment of the nervous system includes history, general physical examination, and added neurological assessment of the cerebrum, cerebellum, cranial nerves, and peripheral nervous system. Assessment of child development provides essential data about nervous system functioning.

Although the 12 cranial nerves are only one part of this body system, their functions and assessment techniques and possible disorders are summarized in Table 23-1.

Assessment of the primitive reflexes (Tables 23-2 and 23-3) of infants provides information about the development of the nervous system in the critical first years of life.

NEUROLOGICAL CONDITIONS

Cerebral Palsy

Cerebral palsy is a relatively common neurological condition that presents with different movement abnormalities. The classification of

Cranial Nerves

NO.	NAME	FUNCTIONS	EXAMINATION	DISORDERS
I	Olfactory	S—smell	Child closes eyes. Occlude one nostril. Present odors for identification.	Smell impaired.
II	Optic	S—vision	Test visual acuity, visual fields, examine fundus of eye.	Vision impaired.
III	Oculomotor	M—eye muscles	III, IV, and VI are tested together. Test extraocular movements by having child follow finger or toy in all quadrants of vision. Pupils should also constrict together when light is shined in one only. Eyelids should be symmetrical.	Ptosis, dilated pupil, cannot turn eye in.
IV	Trochlear	M—superior oblique eye muscle	See III.	Cannot turn eye out and down.
V	Trigeminal	S—face and head M—chewing muscles	S—Light touch, pressure, prick to forehead, cheeks, jaws. M—Child should clench teeth tightly. Corneal branch can be tested by blowing air on cornea with insufflator bulb. Both eyes should close.	Jaw paralysis. Trigeminal neuralgia.
VI	Abducens	M—lateral rectus eye muscle	See III.	Cannot turn eye outward. Strabismus.

VII	Facial	S—taste, lacrimal, salivary glands M—facial expression	S—Eyes tear? Taste salt, sugar. M—Ask child to smile, grimace, puff cheeks, raise eyebrows.	Facial paralysis. Bell's palsy.
VIII	Acoustic	S—hearing, balance	S—Auditory testing.	Deafness, vertigo.
IX	Glossopharyngeal	S—posterior 1/3 of tongue, tonsils, pharynx M—swallowing	IX and X tested together. Elicit gag reflex or have child say "ah" to raise palate symmetrically. Hoarseness or pooled secretions also related.	Swallowing and dysarthria.
X	Vagus	S and M—enervate most abdominal and chest organs. Cardiac inhibitor and bronchial constrictor	See IX.	Difficulty swallowing (M). Loss of taste, vomit, gag, carotid body reflex, carotid sinus reflex (S).
XI	Accessory	M—trapezius and sternocleidomastoid muscles	Have child "shrug" shoulders against pressure. Have child turn head against pressure. Have child stick tongue out.	
XII	Hypoglossal	M—tongue movements	Movement should be smooth, not lolling to side, no tremors. Have child push against tongue blade on side of tongue.	

S = sensory tract; M = motor tract.

257

T A B L E 23–2

Primitive Reflex Timing

REFLEX	AGE APPEARS	AGE DISAPPEARS
Newborn Reflexes		
Rooting	Birth	3–4 mo
Sucking	Birth	3–4 mo
Asymmetrical tonic neck	Birth	4–6 mo
Palmar grasp	Birth	3–6 mo
Trunk incurvation (Galant's)	Birth	2 mo
Stepping	Birth	6–8 wk
Moro's	Birth	4 mo
Crossed extension	0–4 mo	Never
Plantar grasp	Birth	10 mo
Later Reflexes		
Landau	3 mo	15 mo–2 yr
Neck righting	6 mo	2 yr
Parachute	6–8 mo	Never

cerebral palsy types is summarized in Table 23-4. Care of children with cerebral palsy is most often multidisciplinary.

Seizures

Seizures represent problems of cerebral functioning. The type of seizure guides the search for etiology, the prognosis, and the management strategies, including medications. Table 23-5 is an annotated table of seizure types, and Table 23-6 lists commonly used anticonvulsants, the mainstay of seizure management.

Febrile Seizures

Febrile seizures are considered relatively benign and are limited to early childhood. Differentiating the child with seizures due to meningitis or other serious problems from the child with a febrile seizure is important. Table 23-7 will help the clinician with this diagnosis and its management.

Headaches in Children

Headaches in children may be benign or a symptom of stress, infection, tumor, or intracranial pressure. Thus, accurate assessment is essential. Table 23-8 will assist the clinician with the differential

Text continued on page 271

T A B L E 23–3
Primitive Reflex Description

REFLEX	DESCRIPTION	RESPONSE	NOTES
Newborn Reflexes			
Rooting	Head midline, stroke perioral area	Infant opens mouth and turns head to stimulated side	Absence indicates severe CNS disease or depressed infant; sleeping infant may not respond
Sucking	Place nipple or finger 3–4 cm into mouth	Suck should be strong, push finger up and back; note rate	Absence indicates CNS depression; satiated or sleeping baby may not respond well
Asymmetrical tonic neck	With baby supine, rotate head to one side. Hold 15 s	Arm and leg extend on facial side, arm and leg on other side flex	Obligatory response when child can't get out of position is abnormal; persistence beyond 4–6 mo indicates CNS lesion (e.g., CP)
Palmar grasp	Place finger into infant's palm and press against palm	Infant flexes all fingers around examiner's finger	Grasps should be strong and symmetrical
Trunk incurvation (Galant)	Suspend baby prone; stroke 2–3 cm from spine with fingernail	Baby flexes toward stimulus	Asymmetry is significant; tests for spinal cord lesions. Should not persist after 6 mo
Stepping	Infant is held as though weight bearing with feet on surface	Infant steps along, raising one foot at a time	Tests brain stem, spinal column; absence indicates paralysis or depressed baby

Table continued on following page

T A B L E 23-3

Primitive Reflex Description Continued

REFLEX	DESCRIPTION	RESPONSE	NOTES
Moro	Present loud noise or allow infant's head to drop slightly	Arms spread and fingers extend and then flex, then arms come toward each other; cry is possible	Asymmetry indicates paralysis or fractured clavicle; absence indicates brain stem problem, usually severe; persistence also abnormal
Crossed extension	Passively extend one leg and press knee to table; prick sole of that foot with pin	Other leg should slightly extend and adduct	
Plantar grasp	Place finger firmly against base of toes	Toes should curl down	Tests S1-S2 spinal nerves. Suspect after 4 mo
Later Reflexes			
Landau	Suspend infant prone by supporting abdomen	Infant should lift both head and legs	Abnormal if arm tone increased with internal rotation or held at side or does not lift as noted
Neck righting	With infant supine, turn head to one side	Infant's trunk rotates in direction of head	Absent or decreased can indicate spasticity; can also rotate trunk and then look for head to follow; tests midbrain
Parachute	Suspend infant prone and lower quickly toward table	Infant should extend arms, hands, fingers	Response should be symmetrical as well as "protective"

CNS = central nervous system; CP = cerebral palsy.

TABLE 23-4

Classification of Cerebral Palsy Types

TYPE	DESCRIPTION	COMMENTS
Spastic	Increased tone. Toe walks. Fisted hands and other signs	70–80% frequency. Diplegia most common in preterm babies. Usually hypertonic but may be hypotonic early or in some positions. Often shows after 4–6 mo
Diplegic	Affects both legs	
Quadriplegic	Affects all 4 extremities. Scissors	
Hemiplegic	Affects one side of the body. One hand fisted, toe walks on affected side	
Dyskinetic	Problems with voluntary movements	10–15% frequency
Athetoid	Continuous, writhing movements	
Dystonic	Problems with tone	
Choreic	Disorganized tone	
Ballismic	Violent, jerky movements	
Tremulous	Involuntary, rhythmic movements of opposing muscles	
Rigid	Stiffness	5% frequency. Associated with severe decerebrate lesions
Ataxic	Balance problems. Wide-based gait, clumsiness	1% frequency. Often not identified until child walks
Mixed		10–15% frequency

T A B L E 23-5

International Classification of Seizures

SEIZURE TYPE	AGE	PATTERN	COMMENTS
I. Partial seizures			
A. Simple partial			
1. With motor symptoms	Any age	Begin locally Consciousness not impaired Any part of body: includes jacksonian seizures	Affect one hemisphere Lasts 10–20 s Birth trauma, inflammation, cerebrovascular accident; tumor if new or with progressive neurological symptoms
2. With sensory or somatosensory symptoms	Any age	"Pins and needles," numb; auras include lights, tastes, sounds	
3. With autonomic symptoms	Any age	Recurrent abdominal pain, headache, sweat, laugh, cry, tachycardia, dilated pupils	May have migraine quality; family history of migraine or seizures
4. Compound forms	Any age		
B. Complex partial	Any age; may be hard to recognize in young child	Consciousness impaired: complex symptoms and interesting automatisms	Lasts 1–2 min
1. Impaired consciousness only		Staring spell	
2. With cognitive symptoms		May have confusion	
3. With affective symptoms		Aura of fear	
4. With "psychosensory" symptoms		May have odd smell/taste; visual or auditory hallucination	
5. With "psychomotor" symptoms		Automatisms; facial, tongue, or swallow movements	
6. Compound forms			

TABLE 23-5

International Classification of Seizures

SEIZURE TYPE	AGE	PATTERN	COMMENTS
C. Partial seizures secondarily generalized		Seizure begins in one part of body but then generalizes	Aura can let person seek safe position
II. Generalized seizures			
A. Absence	4–8 yr most common	Petit mal; 5–30-s lapses of consciousness; can have associated movements; no falling; no aura	Hyperventilation for 3–4 min can trigger; blinking lights can trigger
B. Myoclonic	Infancy	Head drops or sudden flexing; may cry out	Hypsarrhythmia on EEG with no normal background activity; difficult to treat
C. Clonic		Rhythmic jerking	
D. Tonic		Intense muscle contraction	
E. Tonic-clonic	Any age: most common type	Grand mal; begins with loss of consciousness; stiffens, then jerks violently; postictal phase of sleep and confusion; 15% incontinent	Aura in some; may have abdominal pain or headache; life-threatening if continues, producing hypercarbia, respiratory acidosis, lactic acidemia; some occur in sleep
F. Atonic		Similar to myoclonic	Child often falls

EEG = electroencephalogram; s = seconds.

263

TABLE 23-6

Anticonvulsant Medication Therapy for Children

DRUG	HALF-LIFE (hr)	ORAL DOSE* (mg/kg/24 hr)	FREQUENCY (doses/24 hr)	BLOOD LEVELS (μg/ml)	SEIZURE TYPE	SIDE EFFECTS	LABORATORY MONITORING*
Carba-mazepine (Tegretol)	8–20	10 to start; 20–30	2–3	4–12	Partial, tonic-clonic	Vertigo, diplopia, drowsiness, hepatotoxicity, anemia, leukopenia	CBC: baseline, at 6–12 wk, then annually Blood levels
Phenytoin (Dilantin)	10–40	4–8	1–2	10–20	Partial, tonic-clonic	Drowsiness, gum hyperplasia, rash, Stevens-Johnson syndrome, anemia, behavioral and cognitive problems, hirsutism	None recommended Blood levels
Phenobarbital	50–150	4–8	1–2	10–40	Partial, tonic-clonic	Sedation, irritability, hyperkinesis, ataxia, slurred speech, nystagmus, Stevens-Johnson syndrome, attention, memory, learning	None recommended

Drug							
Ethosuximide (Zarontin)	20–60	10–20 to start; 20–50	2–3	50–100	Absence, myoclonic	Gastric upset, drowsiness, hematological problems	None recommended
Valproic acid (Depakene)	6–12	10 to start; 15–50	3–4	50–150	Partial, tonic-clonic, absence, myoclonic	Nausea/vomiting, weight gain, transient alopecia, tremor, hepatic failure, hematological problems	Baseline (and after 1 mo) AST, ALT, ammonia, prothrombin, partial thromboplastin
Primidone (Mysoline)	6–18	1–2 to start; 5–10 maximum	3–4	5–12	Partial, tonic-clonic, myoclonic	Drowsiness, ataxia, vertigo, anorexia, nausea/vomiting, rash, aggression	None recommended
Vigabatrin	5–7	30–40 to start; 80–100 maximum	1–2	1.4–14	Partial, myoclonic, infantile spasms	Agitation, depression, drowsiness, abdominal pain, weight gain, dizziness, headache, ataxia	
Felbamate (Felbatol)	14–22	15–45	3–4	Not determined	Partial, Lennox-Gastaut syndrome	Drowsiness, lethargy, nausea, vomiting, aplastic anemia, hepatitis, anorexia, ataxia	ALT, AST, bilirubin, CBC with differential, platelet, reticulocyte count weekly

Table continued on following page

265

TABLE 23-6

Anticonvulsant Medication Therapy for Children Continued

DRUG	HALF-LIFE (hr)	ORAL DOSE* (mg/kg/24 hr)	FREQUENCY (doses/24 hr)	BLOOD LEVELS (µg/ml)	SEIZURE TYPE	SIDE EFFECTS	LABORATORY MONITORING*
Gabapentin (Neurontin) (add-on therapy)	5-7	300 to start; 900-1200 maximum	3	Not monitored	Complex partial, secondarily generalized	Somnolence, dizziness, ataxia, headache, tremor, vomiting, nystagmus, fatigue	
Lamotrigine (add-on therapy)	7-45; up to 6 d with valproic acid	5-15, 1-5 with valproic acid	2	1-4	Lennox-Gastaut syndrome, partial tonic-clonic	Rash (Stevens-Johnson syndrome), drowsiness, headache, blurred vision, vomiting	

ALT = alanine aminotransferase; AST = aspartate aminotransferase; CBC = complete blood count.

*Data from Burg F, Ingelfinger J, Wald E, et al: Gellis & Kagan's Current Pediatric Therapy, 16th ed. Philadelphia, WB Saunders, 1999. Other data from Burg F, Ingelfinger J, Wald E: Gellis & Kagan's Current Pediatric Therapy. Philadelphia, WB Saunders, 1993; Haslam R: Nonfebrile seizures. Pediatr Rev 18:39–49, 1997. Russell J & Parles B: Anticonvulsant medications. Pediatr An 28:238–245, 1999. Calli J & Farrington E: Vigabatrin. Pediatr Nurs 24:357–361, 1998.

Consult a more specific reference for information on initial dosing, adult doses, and maximum doses.

T A B L E 23-7

Febrile Seizures

CHARACTERISTICS	MANAGEMENT
Fever, little postictal confusion, lasts less than 15 min, does not recur within 24 hr, generalized clonic or tonic-clonic type	Protect child during seizure
	Reduce fever with acetaminophen
Occurs in children ages 3 mo to 7 yr. Not related to crying/tantrum episode	Lumbar puncture for child less than 1 yr with first seizure
	Provide family education, explaining seizures and providing reassurance that no long-term effects persist, and first aid information if another seizure occurs
	Follow up with family in about 1 wk

T A B L E 23–8

Differential Diagnosis of Headaches

CHARACTERISTICS	VASCULAR (MIGRAINE)	TENSION	TRACTION AND INFLAMMATORY (INCREASED INTRACRANIAL PRESSURE)
Time course	Acute, paroxysmal, recurrent	Chronic, recurrent, nonprogressive	Chronic or intermittent but with increasing frequency and severity
Prodrome	Yes; aura in older children	No	No
Description	Intense, pulsating, unilateral in older children; frontotemporal Infants: irritability, pallor, sleepiness, and/or vomiting	Diffuse, band-like, tight, dull, bifrontal or occipital; mild to moderate intensity	Diffuse, can be localized to one area (e.g., occipital)
Predisposing factors	Positive family history (75%), head trauma	Problems at home, school, or with peers common	No
Associated findings	Transient neurological signs, sleep relief, nausea/vomiting in older children; older children can have visual changes, abdominal pain	Depression, inadequacy, anxiety; school avoidance common. Sleep may help. Nausea/vomiting rare	Positive neurological signs such as ataxia, weakness, lethargy, decreased intellectual functioning, visual disturbances, sensory abnormalities, behavior/mood alterations. Papilledema, worse in morning (with vomiting); straining increases pain, diplopia

TABLE 23-9

Medications for Migraine and Tension Headaches in Children

ANALGESIC DRUG	DOSAGE
Acetaminophen	10–15 mg/kg not to exceed 5 doses/day and 5 consecutive days of treatment
NSAIDs:	
Ibuprofen (DOC)	5–10 mg/kg per dose (200–800 mg/dose q6–8 hr; maximum, 40 mg/kg per d)
Naproxen	10 mg/kg per d (250–500 mg bid)
Naproxen sodium (Anaprox, Aleve)	220–550 mg 1st dose; maximum dose, 825 mg/d

ABORTIVE PHARMACOLOGY FOR MIGRAINE HEADACHE

Ergotamine tartrate	2 mg dose SL. Maximum, 6 mg/d or 10 mg/wk to avoid chronic ergotism, dependency, withdrawal symptoms
	Contraindications: heart disease, hypertension, pregnancy (uterine stimulant, teratogen)
Dihydroergotamine (DHE)	0.5–1.0 mg IM; can be repeated in 1 hr
	No associated dependence/withdrawal symptoms
	Side effects: nausea/vomiting
	Contraindications: heart disease, hypertension, pregnancy (uterine stimulant, teratogen)
	Give metoclopramide or prochlorperazine as pretreatment for nausea
Metoclopramide (Reglan)	5–10 mg (up to 1 mg/kg)
	Side effects: sedation, dizziness, confusion
Prochlorperazine (Compazine)	2.5–5.0 mg/kg q4hr (up to 0.1 mg/kg in younger children)
Sumatriptan (Imitrex)	6 mg SC, 100 mg PO, or 10–20 mg nasal spray. May repeat injection in 1 hr
	Contraindications: do not give with ergotamine derivatives
	Side effects: irritation at site, flushing, tachycardia, disorientation, chest tightness for several minutes after parenteral administration

Table continued on following page

269

T A B L E 23–9

Medications for Migraine and Tension Headaches in Children *Continued*

ANALGESIC DRUG	DOSAGE
PROPHYLACTIC MEDICATIONS FOR MIGRAINE HEADACHE	
Propranolol (Inderal)	1–2 mg/kg/d in 2–3 divided doses; maximum, 320 mg/d
	Contraindications: asthma, arrhythmia, depression, diabetes
Amitriptyline (Elavil)	Adolescents: 0.1 mg/kg at bedtime (may be increased q2wk to 0.5–2 mg/kg)
	Contraindications: not recommended for children younger than 12 yr
Cyproheptadine (Periactin)	Children: 0.2–0.5 mg/kg per d in 2–3 divided doses; 2–6 yr: 12 mg/d; 7–14 yr: 16 mg/d; adults: 32 mg/d
	Contraindications: none
Nortriptyline (Pamelor)	10 mg/d hs
	Contraindications: may cause sudden death with prolonged QT interval syndrome; less sedation than amitriptyline; not recommended for children younger than 12 yr

DOC = drug of choice; hs = at bedtime; IM = intramuscularly; NSAIDs = nonsteroidal anti-inflammatory drugs; SC = subcutaneously; SL = sublingually.
From Graf W, Riback P: Pharmacologic treatment of recurrent pediatric headache. Pediatr Ann 24:477–484, 1995.

diagnosis of vascular, tension, and traction/inflammatory types of headaches.

Migraine and tension headaches are common in children and adolescents. Table 23-9 summarizes the variety of medications used to treat these conditions.

CHAPTER 24

Eye Problems

ASSESSMENT OF THE EYE

Optimal functioning of the eyes plays an important role in the ongoing growth and development of a child. Normal visual developmental milestones are listed in Table 24-1.

Visual acuity testing should be performed on all children every time they present for a routine check-up, when there is a concern related to visual acuity, and when eye trauma occurs. Visual acuity normal values are listed in Table 24-2.

Other methods of visual screening include the red reflex, inspection, fix and follow, alternate occlusion, corneal light reflex, stereoacuity, and the cover test. Figure 24-1 illustrates the corneal light reflex and cover test.

TABLE 24-1

Normal Visual Developmental Milestones

Birth to 2 wk: Infant sees and responds to change in illumination; refuses to reopen eyes after exposure to bright light; increasing alertness to objects; fixes on contrasts (e.g., black and white).

2–4 wk: Infant fixes on an object.

By 1 mo: Infant fixes and follows an object.

By 3–4 mo: Infant recognizes parent's smile; looks from near to far and focuses close again; beginning development of depth perception; follows 180-degree arc; reaches toward toy.

By 4 mo: Color vision near that of an adult; tears are present.

By 6–10 mo: Infant fixes and follows toy in all directions.

By 12 mo: Vision is close to fully developed.

T A B L E 24–2
Visual Acuity Norms

AGE	VISUAL ACUITY	VISUAL RANGE
Birth	20/100	45°
6 wk	20/100	90°
4 mo	20/80	180°
1 yr	20/40	180°
3–4 yr	20/30	180°
6 yr	20/25 or 20/20	180°

Table 24-3 identifies screening methods for various age groups and criteria that can be used to indicate need for referral. Other indications that should alert the nurse practitioner to the need for a comprehensive eye evaluation are listed in Table 24-4.

CORRECTION OF REFRACTIVE ERRORS

Children often receive corrective lenses (eyeglasses or contacts) to correct refractive errors. Recommendations for use of these lenses are listed in Table 24-5.

PREVENTION OF EYE INJURY

Injuries to the eye are common, many resulting in some loss of vision. It is estimated that 90% of injuries could be prevented (Hoffman, 1997). Educating parents and children about the prevention of eye injury is an important role of the nurse practitioner. Key concepts to include are listed in Table 24-6.

EYE INFECTIONS AND INJURY

Eye infections and eye injuries are common issues that the nurse practitioner must be prepared to deal with. Diagnosis and management of various types of conjunctivitis are discussed in Table 24-7, and the diagnosis and management of other common eye infections are discussed in Table 24-8.

CORNEAL LIGHT REFLEX

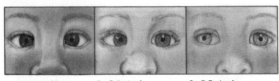

A **Pseudostrabismus**   B   R Esotropia   C   R Exotropia

Symmetric Corneal Light Reflex

A. *Pseudostrabismus* has the appearance of strabismus due to epicanthic fold but is normal for a young child.

Asymmetric Corneal Light Reflex

Strabismus is true disparity of the eye axes. This constant malalignment is also termed tropia and is likely to cause amblyopia.

B. Esotropia—inward turn of the eye.

C. Exotropia—outward turn of the eye.

COVER TEST

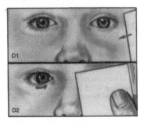

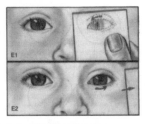

D   **Right, uncovered eye is weaker**

D. Uncovered eye—if it jumps to fixate on designate point, it was out of alignment before (i.e., when you cover the stronger eye, the weaker eye now tries to fixate).

Phoria—mild weakness, apparent only with the cover test and less likely to cause amblyopia than a tropia but still possible.

E   **Left, covered eye is weaker**

E. Covered eye—if this is the weaker eye, once macular image is suppressed it will drift to relaxed position.

As eye is uncovered—if it jumps to re-establish fixation, weakness exists.

Esophoria—nasal (inward) drift.

Exophoria—temporal (outward) drift.

FIGURE 24–1

Extraocular muscle dysfunction as measured by the corneal light reflex and cover test. (From Jarvis C: Physical Examination and Health Assessment, 2nd ed. Philadelphia, WB Saunders, 1996, p. 340.)

Pediatric Eye Evaluation Screening Recommendations for Primary Care Providers, Nurses, Physician's Assistants, and Trained Lay Personnel

RECOMMENDED AGE FOR SCREENING	SCREENING METHOD	CRITERIA FOR REFERRAL TO AN OPHTHALMOLOGIST
Newborn to 3 mo	Red reflex*	Abnormal or asymmetrical
	Inspection	Structural abnormality
6 mo to 1 yr	Fix and follow with each eye	Failure to fix and follow in cooperative infant
	Alternate occlusion	Failure to object equally to covering each eye
	Corneal light reflex	Asymmetrical
	Red reflex*	Abnormal or asymmetrical
	Inspection	Structural abnormality
3 yr (approximately)	Visual acuity†	20/50 or worse or 2 lines of difference between eyes
	Corneal light reflex/cover-uncover	Asymmetrical ocular refixation movements
	Red reflex*	Abnormal or asymmetrical
	Inspection	Structural abnormality

Table continued on following page

T A B L E 24–3

Pediatric Eye Evaluation Screening Recommendations for Primary Care Providers, Nurses, Physician's Assistants, and Trained Lay Personnel *Continued*

RECOMMENDED AGE FOR SCREENING	SCREENING METHOD	CRITERIA FOR REFERRAL TO AN OPHTHALMOLOGIST
5 yr (approximately)	Visual acuity† Corneal light reflex/cover-uncover Stereoacuity‡ Red reflex* Inspection	20/40 or worse or 2 lines of difference between eyes Asymmetrical/ocular refixation movements Failure to appreciate stereopsis Abnormal or asymmetrical Structural abnormality
Older than 5 yr	Visual acuity† Corneal light reflex/cover-uncover Stereoacuity‡ Red reflex* Inspection	20/30 or worse or 2 lines of difference between eyes Asymmetrical/ocular refixation movements Failure to appreciate stereopsis Abnormal or asymmetrical Structural abnormality

Note: These recommendations are based on expert opinion.

*Physician or nurse responsibility.

†Figures, letters, "tumbling E," or optotypes.

‡Optional: Random Dot E Game (RDE), Titmus Stereograms (Titmus Optical, Inc. Petersburg, VA), Randot Stereograms (Stereo Optical Company, Inc, Chicago).

Reprinted with permission from the American Academy of Ophthalmology: Pediatric Eye Evaluations Preferred Practice Pattern®, © 1997, American Academy of Ophthalmology, Inc.

T A B L E 24-4
Indications for a Comprehensive Eye Evaluation by an Ophthalmologist

INDICATION	SPECIFIC EXAMPLES
Abnormalities on screening evaluations	Decreased visual attentiveness or acuity (monocular or binocular)*
	Strabismus
	Leukokoria or opacities of ocular media (emergency referral)
	Behavior indicating difficulty (straining, squinting)**
Signs or symptoms of eye problems by history or intuitive concerns of family members†	Defective ocular fixation development or visual interactions (bonding or contact)
	Misaligned eyes (strabismus)
	Light sensitivity
	Ocular discharge
	Persistent redness
	Tearing
	Nystagmus (shaking of eyes)
	Abnormal light reflex (including both the corneal light reflections and the "red" fundus reflection)
	Reading difficulty or complaints of eye fatigue, blurry vision**
General health problems, systemic disease, or use of medications that are known to be associated with eye disease and visual abnormalities	Diabetes present for 5 yr
	Juvenile rheumatoid arthritis
	Neurodegenerative disease
	Neurodevelopmental delay
	Prematurity (born at 28 wk or less gestational age or weighing 1500 g or less; first examination due at chronological age of 4–6 wk or at 31–33 wk postconceptional age)‡
	Systemic steroid therapy
	Systemic syndromes with ocular manifestations

Table continued on following page

T A B L E 24–4

Indications for a Comprehensive Eye Evaluation by an Ophthalmologist *Continued*

INDICATION	SPECIFIC EXAMPLES
A family history of conditions that cause or are associated with eye or vision problems	Glasses in preschool children
	Strabismus
	Amblyopia
	Retinoblastoma
	Presenile cataract
	Infantile or childhood glaucoma
	Retinal dystrophy/degeneration
	Systemic syndromes with ocular manifestations
Health and developmental problems that make screening by the primary care provider difficult or inaccurate	Developmental delay

Note: These recommendations are based on expert opinion.

*Approximately 5% of school-age children have refractive errors.

†"Headache" is not included because it is rarely caused by eye problems in children. This complaint should first be evaluated by the primary care provider.

‡American Academy of Pediatrics, American Association for Pediatric Ophthalmology and Strabismus, American Academy of Ophthalmology: Screening Examination of Premature Infants for Retinopathy of Prematurity. Information Statement. San Francisco, American Academy of Ophthalmology, 1996.

**Inserted by authors.

Reprinted with permission from the American Academy of Ophthalmology: Pediatric Eye Evaluations Preferred Practice Pattern®. © 1997, American Academy of Ophthalmology, Inc.

T A B L E 24–5

Recommendations for Use of Corrective Lenses

EYEGLASSES

Plastic frames, lightweight yet sturdy, with spring hinges, and rounded temporal pieces that hug the back of the ear are best.

In infants, the temples can be shortened and an elastic strap attached that goes around the back of the head to allow movement without dislodging the glasses.

Rolled or flared nose pads help prevent glasses from sliding down the nose.

Tinted lenses can be used for photosensitivity.

Remove eyeglasses with both hands.

Do not lay eyeglasses directly on any surface.

Clean glasses daily with liquid soap and a soft cloth. Do not use paper towels, toilet tissue, or facial tissues.

CONTACT LENSES

Child or adolescent is able to demonstrate ability to cleanse, insert, and remove lenses.

Protective gear should be worn when participating in contact sports.

Lenses should not be worn when eye is inflamed or when topical ophthalmic medications are being used.

Adapted from MacDonald MA: Refractive errors and corrective lenses in children and adolescents. J Pediatr Health Care 10(3):121–123, 1996.

T A B L E 24–6

Eye Injury Prevention

Fundamental concepts
- Do not run with or throw sharp objects
- Store harmful chemicals and sharp objects out of the reach of small children
- Limit and supervise use of BB guns, air rifles, darts, and fireworks
- Use protective eyewear when hammering or using power tools
- Use eye wash fountains when indicated
- Use orthodontic headwear that breaks away if force is applied
- Do not shine laser pointers in eyes

Sunglasses
- Large framed, wraparound lenses with side shields
- Nonbreakable plastic
- Adequate UV protection indicated by one of the following: blocks 99% of UV rays, UV absorption to 400 nm, special purpose, meets ANSI UV requirement

Protective goggles
- Mandatory for all functionally one-eyed individuals or for any athlete who has had eye surgery or trauma or whose ophthalmologist recommends eye protection
- Highly recommended for basketball and baseball or softball
- Also recommended for pool activities, racquet sports, football, soccer, hockey, lacrosse, and squash
- Use in shop class, laboratories, or when working with high-velocity projectiles (e.g., hammer on metal, power tools, or lawn mowers)
- Properly fitted with 2–3 mm plastic blend polycarbonate lens set deeply in grooved frames with padding or rubber bridges around the nose. A headband or wraparound earpieces should be used to secure the goggles

ANSI = American National Standards Institute; UV = ultraviolet.

TABLE 24-7

Types of Conjunctivitis

TYPE	POPULATION AND ETIOLOGY	CLINICAL FINDINGS	DIAGNOSIS	MANAGEMENT
Ophthalmia neonatorum	Neonates *Chlamydia, Neisseria gonorrhoeae* (GC), herpes simplex virus (HSV) Silver nitrate reaction occurs in 10% of neonates	Erythema, chemosis, purulent exudate	Cultures Gram stain R/O GC, *Chlamydia*	Saline irrigation to eyes until clear, followed by erythromycin ointment GC: ceftriaxone or cefotaxime *Chlamydia:* erythromycin PO HSV: IV antivirals
Bacterial conjunctivitis	Preschoolers and sexually active teens *Haemophilus influenzae* (nontypable), *Streptococcus pneumoniae*, GC, enterococci	Erythema, chemosis, itching, burning, mucopurulent exudate, matted eyelashes	Cultures Gram stain Chocolate agar R/O pharyngitis, GC, AOM, URI, seborrhea	Sulfacetamide sodium 10% ophthalmic solution Chloramphenicol 1% ophthalmic ointment Erythromycin 0.5% ophthalmic ointment Augmentin oral suspension if concurrent AOM Warm soaks to eyes tid until clear No sharing towels, pillows No school until treatment begins *Table continued on following page*

TABLE 24-7

Types of Conjunctivitis *Continued*

TYPE	POPULATION AND ETIOLOGY	CLINICAL FINDINGS	DIAGNOSIS	MANAGEMENT
Chronic bacterial conjunctivitis	School-aged children and teens *Staphylococcus aureus*	As for bacterial conjunctivitis; foreign body sensation	Cultures R/O dacryostenosis, blepharitis	Gentamicin 0.3% ophthalmic solution/ointment Erythromycin 0.5% ophthalmic ointment Lacrimal duct massage tid-qid, 10 strokes Refer to M.D. if no improvement in 3 d
Inclusion conjunctivitis	Neonates and sexually active teens	Erythema, chemosis, clear or mucoid exudate, palpebral follicles	Cultures R/O sexual activity	Erythromycin PO for 2-3 wk Tetracycline PO (adolescents only)
Viral conjunctivitis	More common in children older than 6 yr Adenovirus 3, 4, 7, HSV, herpes zoster, enterovirus	Erythema, chemosis, tearing HSV and herpes zoster: unilateral photophobia, fever Zoster: nose lesion	Cultures R/O corneal infiltration	Refer to ophthalmologist if herpes lesions or photophobia present Cool compresses tid-qid
Allergic and vernal conjunctivitis	Atopy sufferers, seasonal (warm)	Erythema, chemosis, clear or mucoid exudate, palpebral follicles, headache, rhinitis	Eosinophilia in exudate	Vasocon 0.1%, 0.012%, 0.03% ophthalmic solution Refer to allergist

AOM = acute otitis media; IV = intravenous; PO = oral; qid = four times a day; R/O = rule out; tid = three times a day; URI = upper respiratory tract infection.

Common Eye Infections

CONDITION	CLINICAL FINDINGS	MANAGEMENT	PREVENTION
Blepharitis	Swelling, erythema of eyelid margins and palpebral conjunctiva, pruritus, flaking	Cleanse eyes, warm compresses, antibiotic drops or ointment	New eye makeup, clean contacts and glasses, hygiene
Hordeolum	Tender, red, swollen furuncle at eyelid margin	Warm compresses, remove eyelash, antibiotic drops or ointment	Hygiene
Chalazion	Initially, mild erythema and slight swelling; later, slow-growing, round painless mass	As for hordeolum plus treat cellulitis if present	Hygiene
Nasolacrimal duct obstruction (dacryostenosis)	Tearing or mucus, continuous or intermittent, blepharitis; express thin mucopurulent discharge from punctum	Daily massage, antibiotic ointment with inflammation or infection, normal saline for nasal congestion	Massage duct, minimize nasal congestion
Nasolacrimal duct infection (dacryocystitis)	Tenderness and swelling over lacrimal duct, edema and erythema of tear sac, excoriation of skin; express purulent discharge from punctum	Warm compresses, massage, oral antibiotic	As above
Periorbital cellulitis	Acute onset, pain, swelling and erythema; temperature >39°C, systemic symptoms	Outpatient systemic antibiotic therapy with close follow-up or hospitalization if moderate to severe infection, nonresponsive, or younger than 1 yr	HIB vaccine, hygiene, thorough cleansing of any skin disruption around eye, prompt treatment of sinusitis

HIB = *Haemophilus influenzae* type b.

Common Eye Injuries

INJURY	CLINICAL FINDINGS	TREATMENT
Corneal injury (abrasion)	Sensation or evidence of foreign body, pain, photophobia, tearing and blepharospasm, decreased vision, positive fluorescein staining	Rest and patch for 24 hr, topical antibiotics and cycloplegics, oral analgesics, follow-up in 24 hr
Foreign body	Vertical striation on cornea, pain, tearing, sensation of foreign body, irregular or peaked pupil, perforating wound	*Do not* remove intraocular foreign body; irrigate eye to remove; topical antibiotic and patch for 5–7 d; to ophthalmologist immediately
Burns Chemical Thermal UV radiation	Pale, necrotic appearance to skin and eyelids, opaque cornea, visual impairment, photophobia, tearing, pain with UV injury only	*Chemical:* emergency: continuous irrigation for 20–30 min; to ophthalmologist immediately with ongoing irrigation *Thermal:* as for abrasion *UV:* topical antibiotic, patch, analgesics; heal in 1–2 d
Hyphema	Pain, tearing, photophobia; blood in anterior chamber, hazy iris, or inability to detect red reflex; change in visual acuity	Refer to ophthalmologist immediately; restrict intake, place eye shield; increased risk if child has sickle cell trait or disease

UV = ultraviolet.

Common eye injuries that the nurse practitioner sees include abrasions, foreign bodies, burns, and hyphema. These are discussed in Table 24-9.

REFERENCES

American Academy of Ophthalmology: Pediatric Eye Evaluations Preferred Practice Patterns. San Francisco: American Academy of Ophthalmology, Inc., 1997.

Hoffman RO: Evaluating and treating eye injuries. Contemp Pediatr 14(4):74-98, 1997.

Jarvis C: Physical Examination and Health Assessment, Philadelphia, WB Saunders, 1996.

MacDonald MA: Refractive errors and corrective lenses in children and adolescents. J Pediatr Health Care 10(3):121-123, 1996.

CHAPTER 25

Ear Disorders

ASSESSMENT OF THE EAR

Developmental milestones can be used to assess a child's hearing. These are listed in Table 25-1.

TABLE 25-1

Developmental Milestones Used to Assess Hearing

Birth to 3 mo
  Startles (Moro reflex) to loud noise
  Awakens to sounds
  Blinks or widens eyes to noises
3–6 mo
  Quiets to parent's voice
  Stops activity to listen to new sound
  Looks for source of sound
  Reciprocates vocally and initiates sounds
6–12 mo
  Coos and gurgles with inflection
  Responds to simple phrases
  Turns to localize sound in any plane
  Responds to own name
12–18 mo
  Points to unexpected sound or familiar objects when asked
  Follows simple direction without cues
  Imitates some sounds, first words by 12–15 mo
18–24 mo
  Points to body parts when asked
  Has expressive vocabulary of 20–50 words
  50% of speech intelligible to strangers

T A B L E 25–2
Evaluation of Audiometric Results

AVERAGE THRESHHOLD AT 500–2000 Hz (dB)	DESCRIPTION	SIGNIFICANCE
− 10 to + 15	Normal	
16–25	Slight loss	Difficulty hearing faint speech, slight verbal deficit
26–40	Mild loss	Auditory learning dysfunction, language or speech problems
41–55	Moderate loss	Trouble hearing conversational speech, may miss 50% of class discussion
56–70	Moderately severe loss	
71–90	Severe loss	Educational retardation, learning disability, limited vocabulary
90 +	Profound loss	

Audiometry is the most commonly used technique to measure hearing thresholds via bone or air conduction, or both, in decibles at varying frequencies. Evaluation of audiometric results is outlined in Table 25-2. Pneumatic otoscopy and tympanometry assess the mobility of the tympanic membrane. These techniques are especially helpful for persistent otitis media with effusion or when there is a questionable finding during physical examination of the eardrum.

OTITIS EXTERNA, ACUTE OTITIS MEDIA, AND OTITIS MEDIA WITH EFFUSION

Otitis externa (OE), acute otitis media (AOM), and otitis media with effusion (OME) are common issues that the nurse practitioner faces. OE is an inflammatory reaction of the external auditory canal. Table 25-3 discusses this issue.

AOM often following eustachian tube dysfunction accounts for over half the office visits for ill children in the United States. Diagnosis and management of AOM are outlined in Figure 25-1.

Your patient has recently had a viral upper respiratory tract infection and now has an earache, fever, and some degree of hearing loss. You suspect acute otitis media.

↓

Confirm the diagnosis with pneumatic otoscopy. Consider tympanometry as an adjunct to confirm the presence of fluid in the middle ear. If the diagnosis is uncertain or the child is seriously ill or toxic, consider tympanocentesis and culture of the exudate.

↓

Is any statement true? — **NO**
- The child has had six episodes by age 6.
- The child has had five episodes in 1 year.
- The child has had three episodes in 6 months.

↓ **YES**

Diagnose recurrent acute otitis media. Treat the current episode as indicated. Consider prophylaxis with amoxicillin or sulfisoxazole and examine regularly for an asymptomatic effusion. If the child is allergic to these drugs, prophylaxis fails to prevent recurrence, or hearing loss or other complications develop, consider tympanostomy tube insertion. Depending on age and individual circumstances, other options include adenoidectomy, pneumococcal vaccine, and influenza vaccine.

NO → Is the child allergic to penicillin? — **YES**

↓ **NO**

Prescribe a 10-day course of amoxicillin or ampicillin.

Is any statement true?
- You suspect or confirm a β-lactamase-producing pathogen.
- The incidence of resistant strains in the community is high.
- The patient previously failed to respond to amoxicillin or ampicillin.

↓ **YES**

Consider a 10-day course of amoxicillin/clavulanate potassium if there is β-lactam resistance. Other choices include cefaclor, cefuroxime, axetil, cefixime, cefprozil, loracarbef, and cefpodoxime proxetil.

Consider tympanocentesis and culture of the exudate. Consider switching to another antibiotic. Examine the child every 2 to 4 weeks until the infection resolves. Monitor for suppurative complications and concurrent infection such as meningitis.

↑ **NO**

Has the infection resolved by the end of the antibiotic course? — **YES**

↓ **YES**

Schedule a follow-up visit for two to three weeks afterward to confirm that the infection has resolved and most of the liquid has dissipated

YES → Consider a 10-day course of erythromycin ethylsuccinate/sulfisoxazole acetyl. An alternative is trimethoprim/sulfamethoxazole (TMP/SMX).*

→ Recommend warm compresses for the ear and an analgesic-antipyretic such as acetaminophen. Consider prescribing eardrops containing antipyrine and benzocaine for pain relief. Instruct the parent to return if symptoms do not significantly improve within 48–72 h.

Do symptoms significantly improve within 48–72 hours?

↓ **NO**

Consider switching to another antibiotic. If amoxicillin or ampicillin was used, consider amoxicillin/clavulanate potassium, cefaclor, or another suitable cephalosporin. If a cephalosporin was used, consider switching to a different one. Cephalosporins should be used cautiously in children with penicillin sensitivity because of cross-hypersensitivity among β-lactam antibiotics. Consider also tympanocentesis and culture of the exudate.

*TMP/SMX is associated with rare but severe adverse reactions, including Stevens-Johnson syndrome, toxic epidermal necrolysis, fulminant hepatic necrosis, agranulocytosis, and aplastic anemia and other blood dyscrasias.

F I G U R E 25–1
See legend on opposite page

T A B L E 25–3

Management of Otitis Externa

Clinical findings	Simple infection with edema, discharge, and erythema
	Furuncles or small abscesses in hair follicles
	Impetigo or infection of superficial layers
Treatment	Remove any foreign body
	Irrigate with saline or Burow solution
	Instill antibiotic with steroid drop—use wick if significant swelling
	Administer analgesics as needed
	If furuncle is present, lance
	If impetigo is present, clean with antiseptic and apply antibiotic ointment
	If mycotic infection is present, clean with 5% boric acid in ethanol solution, followed by antifungal cream
Prevention	Avoid water in ears
	Use 50% acetic or boric acid and 50% alcohol solutions after swimming
	Avoid scratching, persistent cleaning, or prolonged use of ceruminolytics

Medications approved by the Food and Drug Administration to treat AOM are listed in Table 25-4. Amoxicillin is the first-line drug choice for AOM. Children with AOM who have high fever most likely have *Streptococcus pneumoniae* in their middle ear fluid and might benefit from high-dose amoxicillin therapy (80-90 mg/kg/d, Dowell et al., 1999; 60-80 mg/kg/d, Fitzgerald, 1998). Children at low risk for drug-resistant *Streptococcus pneumoniae* (DRSP) (no antimicrobial exposure in the previous 3 months, no day care attendance, over 2 years of age) are still appropriate for the 40-45 mg/kg/day dosage (Dowell et al., 1999). If the child is allergic to amoxicillin, erythromycin/sulfisoxazole is recommended as second line. The DRSP therapeutic working group (Dowell et al., 1999) recommends amoxicillin-clavulanate (70-90 mg/kg/d given twice a day, with the clavulanate component at 10 mg/kg/d), cefuroxime axetil, or intramuscular ceftri-

Text continued on page 294

F I G U R E 25–1

Diagnosing and managing otitis media. (From Eden AN, Fireman P, Stool SE: Managing acute otitis: A fresh look at a familiar problem. Contemp Pediatr 12[3]:80, 1996.)

T A B L E 25-4

Medications Approved by the Food and Drug Administration to Treat Acute Otitis Media as of 1999

DRUG	DOSE	COMMENTS
Amoxicillin	40–90 mg/kg per d given t.i.d.	First choice unless contraindicated
TMP-SMX	0.5 ml/kg per d given b.i.d.	Potent side effect profile
Erythromycin-sulfisoxazole (Pediazole)	50 mg/kg per d and 150 mg/kg per d given t.i.d. or q.i.d.	Broad spectrum of activity but a higher cost than for amoxicillin or TMP-SMX
Clarithromycin (Biaxin)	15 mg/kg per d given b.i.d.	Children older than 6 mo
Azithromycin (Zithromax)	10 mg/kg per d on day 1, then 5 mg/kg per d on days 2–5 given q.d.	Children older than 6 mo, 5-d treatment course
Cefaclor (Ceclor)	40 mg/kg per d given b.i.d. or t.i.d.	Broad spectrum but poor *Haemophilus influenzae* coverage and costly; risk of erythema multiforme; 2nd generation; not recommended; rarely used
Amoxicillin-clavulanate (Augmentin)	40–90 mg/kg per d given b.i.d.; clavulanate ≤10 mg/kg per d	Good β-lactamase coverage; costly and more likely to cause diarrhea
Cefixime (Suprax)	8 mg/kg per d given q.d. or b.i.d.	Good β-lactamase coverage but poor *Streptococcus pneumoniae* coverage and very costly; 3rd generation
Cefuroxime (Ceftin)	30 mg/kg per d given b.i.d. 125 mg b.i.d. if younger than 2 yr 250 mg b.i.d. if 2–12 yr old 250–500 mg b.i.d. if older than 12 yr	Broad spectrum of coverage, costly; 2nd generation
Cefprozil (Cefzil)	30 mg/kg per d given b.i.d.	Broad spectrum of coverage, cost similar to that of other cephalosporins; 2nd generation
Cefpodoxime (Vantin)	10 mg/kg per d given b.i.d.	Broad spectrum of coverage, costly; 3rd generation
Loracarbef (Lorabid)	30 mg/kg per d given b.i.d.	Broad spectrum of coverage, costly; 2nd generation
Ceftibuten (Cedax)	9 mg/kg given q.d. in one dose	Children older than 6 mo; active against β-lactamase; 3rd generation
Ceftriaxone (Rocephin)	50–75 mg/kg per d IM in 1 dose (may be given q.d. up to 5 d)	Costly; 3rd generation

IM = intramuscularly; TMP-SMX = trimethoprim-sulfamethoxazole.

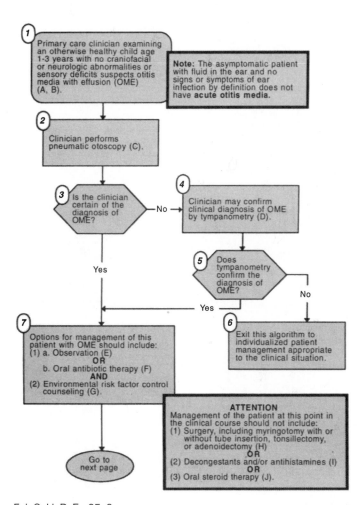

F I G U R E 25–2
Illustration continued on following page

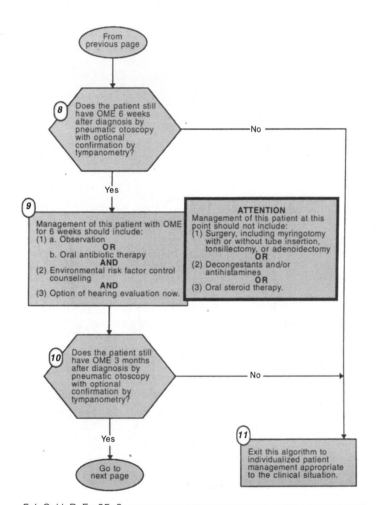

8 Does the patient still have OME 6 weeks after diagnosis by pneumatic otoscopy with optional confirmation by tympanometry?

No

Yes

9 Management of this patient with OME for 6 weeks should include:
(1) a. Observation
OR
b. Oral antibiotic therapy
AND
(2) Environmental risk factor control counseling
AND
(3) Option of hearing evaluation now.

ATTENTION
Management of this patient at this point should not include:
(1) Surgery, including myringotomy with or without tube insertion, tonsillectomy, or adenoidectomy
OR
(2) Decongestants and/or antihistamines
OR
(3) Oral steroid therapy.

10 Does the patient still have OME 3 months after diagnosis by pneumatic otoscopy with optional confirmation by tympanometry?

No

Yes

Go to next page

11 Exit this algorithm to individualized patient management appropriate to the clinical situation.

F I G U R E 25–2
See legend on opposite page

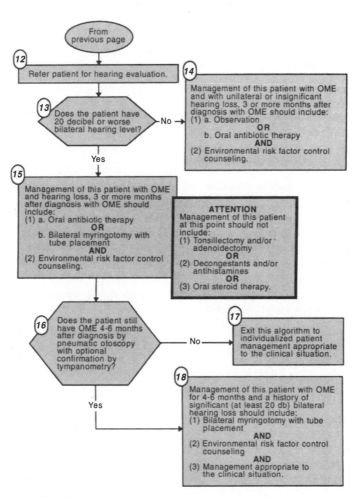

F I G U R E 25–2
Management of otitis media with effusion. (From Agency for Health Care Policy and Research: Quick Reference Guide for Clinicians: Managing Otitis Media With Effusion in Young Children. AHCPR Publication No. 94-0623. Rockville, MD: Agency for Health Care Policy and Research, 1994.)

T A B L E 25-5

Indications for Tympanostomy and the Insertion of Pressure-Equalizing Tubes

Otitis media with effusion lasting more than 3 mo or with language delay, hearing loss, severe retraction pocket, vertigo, tinnitus, or frequent superimposed acute otitis media

Recurrent otitis media (if the child has 2 or more infections despite prophylaxis, or instead of prophylaxis if avoidance of long-term antibiotics is desired, or with language delay, hearing loss, or multiple drug allergies)

Severe eustachian tube dysfunction (persistent ear popping, pain, vertigo, tinnitus, or fluctuating hearing loss)

Complications of otitis media present or suspected (mastoiditis, facial nerve paralysis, brain abscess, labyrinthitis)

Adapted from Pizzuto MP, Volk MS, Kingston LM: Common topics in pediatric otolaryngology, Pediatr Clin North Am 45:973–991, 1998.

axone (50 mg/kg daily as single dose or three daily doses) as useful alternative agents for clinical treatment failure. Bullous myringitis should be treated with an erythromycin/sulfisoxazole combination for *Haemophilus influenzae* and mycoplasma coverage.

OME is characterized by an accumulation of fluid in the middle ear and a decrease in the mobility of the tympanic membrane. Management of OME is outlined in Figure 25-2.

Factors that should alert the nurse practitioner to the need for tympanostomy and the insertion of pressure-equalizing tubes are listed in Table 25-5.

REFERENCES

Agency for Health Care Policy and Research: Quick Reference Guide for Clinicians: Managing Otitis Media with Effusion in Young Children. AHCPR Publication No. 94-0623. Rockville, MD, Agency for Health Care Policy and Research, 1994.

Dowell SF, Butler JC, Giebink GS, et al: Acute otitis media: Management and surveillance in an era of pneumococcal resistance—a report from the Drug-Resistant Streptococcus Pneumonia Therapeutic Working Group [published erratum appears in Pediatr Infect Dis J 18(4):341, 1999. Pediatr Infect Dis J 18:1–9, 1999.

Eden AN, Fireman P, Stool SE: Managing acute otitis: A fresh look at a familiar problem. Contemp Pediatr 12(3):80, 1996.

Fitzgerald M: Reducing antibiotic angst. Ensuring that your therapy choice is effective. Adv Nurse Pract 6(3):43–46, 1998.

Pizzuto MP, Volk MS, Kingston LM: Common topics in pediatric otolaryngology. Pediatr Clin North Am, 45(4):973–991, 1998.

CHAPTER 26

Cardiovascular Problems

INTRODUCTION

Most cardiovascular problems in the pediatric population are due to congenital heart disease (CHD), although high blood pressure and chest pain become increasingly common in adolescence. This chapter addresses all three conditions.

CARDIAC ASSESSMENT AND HEART MURMURS

Cardiac auscultation is a skill the nurse practitioner must develop. Determination of heart rate (normal values are listed in Table 26–1) and rhythm followed by identification of heart sounds and detection of murmurs should occur in all five areas of the heart.

A murmur is an extra heart sound that may be detected during

TABLE 26–1

Normal Heart Rates (bpm) in Infants and Children

AGE	RESTING (AWAKE)	RESTING (ASLEEP)	EXERCISE/ FEVER
Newborn	100–180	80–160	Up to 220
1 wk–3 mo	100–220	80–200	Up to 220
3 mo–2 yr	80–150	70–120	Up to 200
2 y–10 yr	70–100	60–90	Up to 200
10 yr-adult	55–90	50–90	Up to 200

examination of the heart and may be heard in 50 to 90% of children at some point. Less than 5% denote pathology (Feit, 1997; Smith, 1997). Table 26-2 outlines criteria that are helpful in assessing a heart murmur.

Functional or innocent heart murmurs are quite common in children, are usually asymptomatic, and are usually classic in quality (Table 26-3). Four common innocent heart murmurs are described in Table 26-4.

All murmurs should be thoroughly evaluated to determine an accurate diagnosis. As with functional heart murmurs, pathologic heart

T A B L E 26-2

Assessment of a Heart Murmur

1. Intensity or grade. Murmurs are reported as I/VI, II/VI, etc. Intensity of the murmur does not necessarily indicate severity of the problem.
   Intensity may be altered with position change from supine to sitting:
   Grade I: Barely audible. Heard faintly after a period of attentive listening
   Grade II: Soft but easily audible
   Grade III: Moderately loud, no thrill
   Grade IV: Loud, thrill present
   Grade V: Loud, audible with stethoscope barely on the chest
   Grade VI: Loud, audible without stethoscope
2. Timing within the cardiac cycle:
   Systolic
   Diastolic
   Continuous
3. Location defines area on chest where the murmur is loudest:
   Aortic
   Pulmonic
   Mitral tricuspid
4. Transmission or radiation to other locations:
   To back
   To apex
   To carotids
5. Quality:
   Musical
   Vibrating
   Harsh
   Blowing
6. Duration: point of onset and how long during systole and diastole murmurs last
7. Pitch:
   Low
   Middle
   High

T A B L E 26–3

Characteristics of Innocent Murmurs

Usually grade I–II/VI in intensity and localized
Changes with position (sitting to lying)
May vary in loudness or presence from visit to visit
May increase in loudness (intensity) with fever, anemia, exercise, or anxiety
Musical or vibratory in quality
Systolic in timing except for venous hum, which is continuous
Duration is short
Best heard in LLSB or pulmonic area (except for venous hum)
Rarely transmitted
May disappear with Valsalva maneuver, position, or gentle jugular pressure
Vital signs are normal
ECG is normal
General health status is good

ECG = electrocardiogram; LLSB = left lower sternal border.

T A B L E 26–4

Common Innocent Heart Murmurs

Still murmur is the most common type of innocent murmur heard. It is a
systolic ejection murmur that is vibratory or musical in quality and heard
best at the apex or the lower left sternal border. The murmur is of low
frequency and grade I–II/VI and may change with respiration or position.

Pulmonary flow murmur is commonly heard in a newborn but may also be
heard in children. This murmur is a soft, blowing systolic murmur that is
grade I–II/VI in intensity. It is heard best in the pulmonic area or the upper
left sternal border and is related to high velocity of flow in the pulmonary
artery. An important characteristic of this murmur is that it disappears with
the Valsalva maneuver.

Venous hum is a murmur consisting of a soft, low-frequency, continuous
sound heard best at the upper left or right sternal borders or clavicles and
may be mistaken for a patent ductus arteriosus. This murmur is caused by
turbulent flow in the veins draining the superior vena cava. It is loudest in
the sitting position and should disappear when lying down. It may also
disappear with very light, gentle pressure on the right or left external
jugular vein. Turning the head to "flatten" the vessels can also decrease
the sound.

Peripheral pulmonic stenosis is a short systolic murmur heard best in the
axillae and back that usually disappears during infancy as the pulmonary
arteries enlarge.

T A B L E 26–5
Characteristics of Pathological Murmurs That Merit Referral

Significant history
Loud, harsh quality or continuous murmur
Diastolic or late systolic murmur
Holosystolic or pansystolic murmur
Associated abnormalities in cardiac findings (e.g., loud single S_2 gallop, decreased femoral pulses, ejection click, cyanosis)
Associated failure to thrive, congestive heart failure, other systemic illness
Murmur not changing or diminishing in different positions and possibly becoming more intense (e.g., mitral valve murmur intensifying in the squatting position)

Data from Feit LR: The heart of the matter: Evaluating murmurs in children. Contemp Pediatr 14:97–122, 1997; Smith KM: The innocent heart murmur in children. J Pediatr Health Care 11:207–214, 1997; McCrindle BW, Shaffer KM, Kan JS, et al: Cardinal clinical signs in the differentiation of heart murmurs in children. Arch Pediatr Adolesc Med 150:169–174, 1996.

murmurs have some classic characteristics. These are outlined in Table 26–5.

CONGESTIVE HEART FAILURE

Congestive heart failure (CHF) refers to a set of clinical signs and symptoms that indicate myocardial dysfunction most commonly due to congenital heart disease. Seventy-five to 80% of CHF in children occurs before their first birthday, often in the first 2 months of life (Lamb, 1994). The nurse practitioner must be watchful for the following signs and symptoms:

- Tachypnea, rales/wheezing, cough
- Tachycardia and cardiomegaly
- Hepatomegaly and periorbital edema
- Poor feeding, poor weight gain, and diaphoresis

CONGENITAL HEART DEFECTS

Review of the family, maternal, fetal, neonatal, and infant medical history, as well as growth and development, is helpful in the cardiac evaluation of a newborn or child with a suspected cardiac abnormality (see Table 26–6 for risk factors).

T A B L E 26-6

Risk Factors for Congenital Heart Disease

Perinatal risk factors
   Maternal infections and exposures (CMV, rubella, other viral syndromes)
   Maternal use of tobacco, alcohol, street drugs, or prescription drugs
   Maternal health diseases (CHD, lupus, diabetes)
   Maternal age at child's birth (increase in chromosomal abnormalities after 40 yr of age)
   Maternal pregnancy history (excessive weight gain, history of gestational diabetes)
Neonatal risk factors
   Fetal or newborn distress (aspiration, hypoxia, cyanosis)
   Prematurity (increased incidence of CHD in premature infants)
   Presence of associated anomalies (genetic or chromosomal abnormalities or syndromes)
   Neonatal infections (GABHS)
   Birth weight (term infants, <2500 g; SGA, <2 SD from the mean for gestational age)
Newborn risk factors
   Murmur at birth or early infancy
   Hypertension (at birth or beyond)
   Feeding difficulty (SOB, easily fatigued, diaphoresis, poor intake)
   Poor weight gain (failure to regain birth weight by 2 wk, continued poor growth)
   Cyanosis (increases with crying, feeding, exertion)
   Tachypnea (persistent, with crying, feeding)
Toddler, school-aged, or teenage risk factors
   Deviation from normal growth and development (normal milestone development, following own growth curve)
   Deviation from activity level appropriate for chronological age (keeps up with peers; able to run, ride bike)
   Frequent respiratory tract infections (pneumonia, URIs that last longer than normal)
   Prior murmurs, blue spells
   Documented GABHS infection
   Hypertension (documented on a minimum of 3 separate visits)
   Chest pain with exertion
   SOB with exertion (beyond normal peers)
   Syncope or dizziness (especially associated with noted heart rate change)
   Tachycardia or bradycardia (fluttering in chest, racing heart)
   Diet (excessive caffeine usage, obesity)
   Alcohol, drug, or tobacco use
   Other health factors (disease state, general health status)
Family history risk factors
   CHD (especially siblings, parents, first-degree relatives)
   Sudden death or premature myocardial infarction (before age 50)
   Hypertension
   Rheumatic fever
   Genetic syndromes
   Hypercholesterolemia

CHD = congenital heart disease; CMV = cytomegalovirus; GABHS = group A β-hemolytic streptococcus; SGA = small for gestational age; SOB = shortness of breath; URIs = upper respiratory infections.

Congenital heart defects may be classified into three major categories. *Acyanotic* defects such as atrial septal defect, ventricular septal defect, and patent ductus arteriosus are characterized by increased pulmonary blood flow. Table 26-7 provides a quick differential diagnosis for these defects.

Cyanotic defects, characterized by decreased pulmonary blood flow or mixed blood flow, include transposition of the great vessels, tetralogy of Fallot, and tricuspid atresia. Table 26-8 differentiates these defects.

Congenital heart defects characterized as *obstructive* lesions include aortic stenosis, pulmonic stenosis, and coarctation of the aorta. A differential of these defects can be found in Table 26-9.

▥ BACTERIAL ENDOCARDITIS PREVENTION

Prevention of bacterial endocarditis is recommended by the American Heart Association for all nonrepaired defects with the exception of a small isolated atrial septal defect (Dajani et al., 1997). Patent ductus arteriosus and ventricular septal defect require prophylaxis until 6 months after repair. Table 26-10 gives antibiotic prophylactic dosing recommendations.

▥ HYPERTENSION

Hypertension, defined as systolic and/or diastolic blood pressure at the 95th percentile or higher for age, sex, and height on at least three consecutive occasions, requires early identification and prompt evaluation. Figure 26-1 shows an algorithm for identifying these children. Tables 26-11 and 26-12 give normal blood pressure values for the 90th and 95th percentiles for boys and girls.

▥ CHEST PAIN

Chest pain is a common complaint in the pediatric population. Although not often due to a cardiac problem, it causes great anxiety for children, adolescents, and their parents. Table 26-13 outlines the diagnosis and management of chest pain.

Text continued on page 312

Differential Diagnosis of Acyanotic Congenital Heart Defects

FEATURE	ATRIAL SEPTAL DEFECT	VENTRICULAR SEPTAL DEFECT	PATENT DUCTUS ARTERIOSUS
Age at initial presentation	Variable: may be asymptomatic into adulthood	Variable depending on size. Large by 4–8 wk; small by 6 mo	Neonate to 3 mo
Clinical findings	Murmur on preschool examination	CHF or murmur	CHF or murmur
Auscultation	Midsystolic murmur at ULSB with wide-split 2nd heart sound	Holosystolic murmur at LLSB	Continuous murmur under left clavicle, refers to back
Radiological findings	May have mild cardiomegaly	Normal or cardiomegaly	Cardiomegaly
Pulmonary vasculature	Normal to slightly increased	Normal or increased	Increased markings
ECG	May have RsR1 in V₁, right atrial enlargement	Combined ventricular hypertrophy	Combined ventricular hypertrophy
Treatments	Surgical closure	Observation, digoxin, and/or diuretics; if large, surgical closure	Surgical closure if large Indomethacin may be given to premature infants

CHF = congenital heart failure; ECG = electrocardiogram; LLSB = left lower sternal border; ULSB = upper left sternal border.

Differential Diagnosis of Cyanotic Congenital Heart Defects

FEATURE	TRANSPOSITION OF THE GREAT VESSELS	TETRALOGY OF FALLOT	TRICUSPID ATRESIA
Age at initial presentation	Immediately at birth	Usually by 6 mo	Usually newborn
Clinical findings	Cyanosis	Cyanosis	Cyanosis
Auscultation	Usually no murmur	Early systolic ejection murmur at 2nd left intercostal space, holosystolic murmur at LLSB	ASD murmur may be associated with PDA
Radiological findings	Egg-shaped heart	Boot-shaped heart	Cardiomegaly
Pulmonary vasculature	May have increased markings or be normal	Decreased pulmonary vascularity	Decreased pulmonary markings
ECG	RV hypertrophy	RV hypertrophy	Right atrial enlargement, absent RV voltage
Treatments	Newborn PGE, septostomy, arterial switch (Jatene)	Tetralogy repair, BT shunt	Shunt and surgical repair

ASD = atrial septal defect; BT = Blalock-Taussig; ECG = electrocardiogram; LLSB = left lower sternal border; PDA = patent ductus arteriosus; PGE = prostaglandin E; RV = right ventricular.

Differential Diagnosis of Obstructive Congenital Heart Defects

FEATURE	AORTIC STENOSIS	PULMONIC STENOSIS	COARCTATION OF THE AORTA
Age at initial presentation	Depends on severity; critical in newborn	Depends on severity; newborn to school aged	First weeks of life or 3–5 yr
Clinical findings	Murmur, CHF; older child, chest pain	Cyanosis or murmur	CHF in newborn; hypertension in preschooler
Auscultation	Systolic ejection murmur at URSB, constant systolic click at apex with bicuspid valve	Late systolic ejection murmur at ULSB, intermittent systolic ejection click	Systolic ejection murmur in left intraclavicular region with transmission to back
Radiological findings	Normal	Normal	Rib notching
Pulmonary vasculature	Normal	Decreased in severity	Normal
ECG	LV hypertrophy	RV hypertrophy	RV hypertrophy
Treatments	Catheter valvulotomy or surgical repair	Catheter valvuloplasty or surgery	Surgical repair or balloon dilation

CHF = congenital heart failure; ECG = electrocardiogram; LV = left ventricular; RV = right ventricular; ULSB = upper left sternal border; URSB = upper right sternal border.

TABLE 26-10

Prophylactic Regimens for Dental, Oral, Respiratory Tract, or Esophageal Procedures (No Follow-Up Dose Recommended)

SITUATION	AGENT	REGIMEN*
Standard general prophylaxis	Amoxicillin	Adults: 2.0 g; children: 50 mg/kg PO 1hr before procedure
Unable to take oral medications	Ampicillin	Adults: 2.0 g IM or IV; children: 50 mg/kg IM or IV within 30 min before procedure
Penicillin-allergic	Clindamycin or Cephalexin† or cefadroxil† or Azithromycin or clarithromycin	Adults: 600 mg; children: 20 mg/kg PO 1 hr before procedure Adults: 2.0 g; children: 50 mg/kg PO 1 hr before procedure Adults: 500 mg; children: 15 mg/kg PO 1 hr before procedure
Penicillin-allergic and unable to take oral medications	Clindamycin or Cefazolin†	Adults: 600 mg; children: 20 mg/kg IV within 30 min before procedure Adults: 1.0 g; children: 25 mg/kg IM or IV within 30 min before procedure

IM = intramuscular; IV = intravenous; PO = oral.

*Total children's dose should not exceed adult dose.

†Cephalosporins should not be used by individuals with immediate type hypersensitivity reaction (urticaria, angioedema, or anaphylaxis) to penicillins.

From American Heart Association Committee on Rheumatic Fever, Endocarditis, Kawasaki Disease: Prevention of bacterial endocarditis. JAMA 277:1794–1801, 1997. Copyright 1997, American Medical Association.

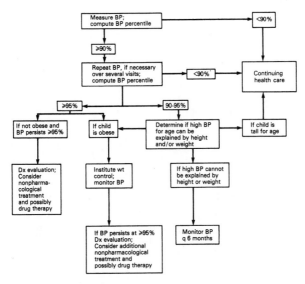

F I G U R E 26–1

Algorithm for identifying children with high blood pressure (BP). Note: Whenever BP measure is stipulated, the average of at least two measurements should be used. (Reproduced by permission of Pediatrics, Vol. 79, page 7, copyright 1987.)

T A B L E 26–11

Blood Pressure Levels for the 90th and 95th Percentiles of Blood Pressure for Girls Aged 1 to 17 yr by Percentiles of Height

AGE	BP*	SYSTOLIC BP (mm Hg) AT HEIGHT PERCENTILE† OF							DIASTOLIC BP (mm Hg) AT HEIGHT PERCENTILE† OF						
		5%	10%	25%	50%	75%	90%	95%	5%	10%	25%	50%	75%	90%	95%
1	90th	97	98	99	100	102	103	104	53	53	53	54	55	56	56
	95th	101	102	103	104	105	107	107	57	57	57	58	59	60	60
2	90th	99	99	100	102	103	104	105	57	57	58	58	59	60	61
	95th	102	103	104	105	107	108	109	61	61	62	62	63	64	65
3	90th	100	100	102	103	104	105	106	61	61	61	62	63	63	64
	95th	104	104	105	107	108	109	110	65	65	65	66	67	67	68
4	90th	101	102	103	104	106	107	108	63	63	64	65	65	66	67
	95th	105	106	107	108	109	111	111	67	67	68	69	69	70	71
5	90th	103	103	104	106	107	108	109	65	66	66	67	68	68	69
	95th	107	107	108	110	111	112	113	69	70	70	71	72	72	73
6	90th	104	105	106	107	109	110	111	67	67	68	69	69	70	71
	95th	108	109	110	111	112	114	114	71	71	72	73	73	74	75
7	90th	106	107	108	109	110	112	112	69	69	69	70	71	72	72
	95th	110	110	112	113	114	115	116	73	73	73	74	75	76	76

Age	BP Percentile*	Systolic BP by Height Percentile†							Diastolic BP by Height Percentile†						
8	90th	108	109	110	111	112	113	114	70	70	71	71	72	73	74
	95th	112	112	113	115	116	117	118	74	74	75	75	76	77	78
9	90th	110	110	112	113	114	115	116	71	72	72	73	74	74	75
	95th	114	114	115	117	118	119	120	75	76	76	77	78	78	79
10	90th	112	112	114	115	116	117	118	73	73	73	74	75	76	76
	95th	116	116	117	119	120	121	122	77	77	77	78	79	80	80
11	90th	114	114	116	117	118	119	120	74	74	75	75	76	77	77
	95th	118	118	119	121	122	123	124	78	78	79	79	80	81	81
12	90th	116	116	118	119	120	121	122	75	75	76	76	77	78	78
	95th	120	120	121	123	124	125	126	79	79	80	80	81	82	82
13	90th	118	118	119	121	122	123	124	76	76	77	78	78	79	80
	95th	121	122	123	125	126	127	128	80	80	81	82	82	83	84
14	90th	119	120	121	122	124	125	126	77	77	78	79	79	80	81
	95th	123	124	125	126	128	129	130	81	81	82	83	83	84	85
15	90th	121	121	122	124	125	126	127	78	78	79	80	80	81	82
	95th	124	125	126	128	129	130	131	82	82	83	84	84	85	86
16	90th	122	122	123	125	126	127	128	79	79	79	80	81	82	82
	95th	125	126	127	128	130	131	132	83	83	83	84	85	86	86
17	90th	122	123	124	125	126	128	128	79	79	79	80	81	82	82
	95th	126	126	127	129	130	131	132	83	83	83	84	85	86	86

*Blood pressure percentile determined by a single measurement.
†Height percentile determined by standard growth curves.

T A B L E 26-12

Blood Pressure Levels for the 90th and 95th Percentiles of Blood Pressure for Boys Aged 1 to 17 yr by Percentiles of Height

		SYSTOLIC BP (mm Hg) AT HEIGHT PERCENTILE† OF							DIASTOLIC BP (mm Hg) AT HEIGHT PERCENTILE† OF						
AGE	BP*	5%	10%	25%	50%	75%	90%	95%	5%	10%	25%	50%	75%	90%	95%
1	90th	94	95	97	98	100	102	102	50	51	52	53	54	54	55
	95th	98	99	101	102	104	106	106	55	55	56	57	58	59	59
2	90th	98	99	100	102	104	105	106	55	55	56	57	58	59	59
	95th	101	102	104	106	108	109	110	59	59	60	61	62	63	63
3	90th	100	101	103	105	107	108	109	59	59	60	61	62	63	63
	95th	104	105	107	109	111	112	113	63	63	64	65	66	67	67
4	90th	102	103	105	107	109	110	111	62	62	63	64	65	66	66
	95th	106	107	109	111	113	114	115	66	67	67	68	69	70	71
5	90th	104	105	106	108	110	112	112	65	65	66	67	68	69	69
	95th	108	109	110	112	114	115	116	69	70	70	71	72	73	74
6	90th	105	106	108	110	111	113	114	67	68	69	70	70	71	72
	95th	109	110	112	114	115	117	117	72	72	73	74	75	76	76
7	90th	106	107	109	111	113	114	115	69	70	71	72	72	73	74
	95th	110	111	113	115	116	118	119	74	74	75	76	77	78	78

Age	BP* percentile	Systolic BP by height percentile†							Diastolic BP by height percentile†						
8	90th	107	108	110	112	114	115	116	71	71	72	73	74	75	75
	95th	111	112	114	116	118	119	120	75	75	76	77	78	79	80
9	90th	109	110	112	113	115	117	117	72	73	73	74	75	76	77
	95th	113	114	116	117	119	121	121	76	77	77	78	80	80	81
10	90th	110	112	113	115	117	118	119	73	73	74	74	76	77	78
	95th	114	115	117	119	121	122	123	77	78	78	79	80	81	82
11	90th	112	113	115	117	119	120	121	74	74	75	76	77	78	78
	95th	116	117	119	121	123	124	125	78	79	79	80	81	82	82
12	90th	115	116	117	119	121	123	123	75	75	76	77	78	78	79
	95th	119	120	121	123	125	126	127	79	79	80	81	82	83	83
13	90th	117	118	120	122	124	125	126	75	76	76	77	78	79	80
	95th	121	122	124	126	128	129	130	79	80	81	82	83	83	84
14	90th	120	121	123	125	126	128	128	76	76	77	78	79	80	80
	95th	124	125	127	128	130	132	132	80	81	81	82	83	84	85
15	90th	123	124	125	127	129	131	131	77	77	78	79	80	81	81
	95th	127	128	129	131	133	134	135	81	81	82	83	84	85	86
16	90th	125	126	128	130	132	133	134	79	79	80	81	82	82	83
	95th	129	130	132	134	136	137	138	83	83	83	84	85	86	87
17	90th	128	129	131	133	134	136	136	81	81	81	82	83	84	85
	95th	132	133	135	136	138	140	140	85	85	85	86	87	88	89

*Blood pressure percentile determined by a single measurement.
†Height percentile determined by standard growth curves.

TABLE 26-13

Chest Pain

ETIOLOGY	CLINICAL FINDINGS	DIAGNOSTIC WORKUP	TREATMENT	COMMENTS
Musculoskeletal (costochondritis, strains)	• Common in growing preadolescents and adolescents • Often related to sports or casual athletic activity • History of trauma or muscle strain • Tenderness over ≥1 costochondral joint	• Chest (lungs, heart) and abdominal examinations	• Nonsteroidal anti-inflammatory medications • Rest	
Respiratory (asthma, pneumonia, embolism, pneumothorax, exercise-induced asthma [EIA], foreign bodies)	• Sternal pain ± • Rales, wheezing, tachypnea, decreased breath sounds • History of OC use • May have history of foreign body ingestion or choking	• Chest radiograph • Pulmonary function test if suspect EIA	• May require referral • Refer to Chapters 20 and 27 on management of asthma and respiratory diseases	• Differential diagnoses: sickle cell crisis, aortic abdominal aneurysm, pleural effusion

Gastrointestinal (reflux, foreign body)	• Burning, substernal pain, worse with reclining and spicy foods • Pain may awaken	• Complete chest and abdominal examination • Diet history	• Antacids • Elevate head of bed	• See above
Chronic (psychogenic anxiety, hyperventilation)	• Vague in nature • Occurs over many months and in variety of circumstances, particularly stressful events • Patient appears well • Often associated with anxiety and hyperventilation	• Complete chest and abdominal examination • Psychosocial history	• Reassure • Counseling related to issues • Request follow-up • Mental health referral if persistent	• Adolescent less likely to have cardiorespiratory etiology
Cardiac disease	• Syncope • Exertional dyspnea • Irregular heart rhythm • ± murmurs, rubs, clicks	• 24 hr Holter monitor and/or stress test • ECG	• Refer	• Usually those with true cardiac pain describe a very specific history with details consistent from event to event • Young children more likely to have a cardiorespiratory etiology

ECG = electrocardiogram; OC = oral contraceptive.

311

REFERENCES

Dajani AS, Taubert KA, Wilson W, et al: Prevention of bacterial endocarditis: Recommendations by the American Heart Association. JAMA 277:1794–1801, 1997.

Feit LR: The heart of the matter: Evaluating murmurs in children. Contemp Pediatr 14(10):97–122, 1997.

Lamb F: Heart failure. *In* Oski FA, DeAngelis CD, Feigin RE, McMillan JA, Warshaw JB (eds): Principles and Practice of Pediatrics, 2nd ed. Philadelphia, JB Lippincott, 1994, pp 1561–1564.

McCrindle BW, Shaffer KM, Kan JS, et al: Cardinal clinical signs in the differentiation of heart murmurs in children. Arch Pediatr Adolesc Med 150:169–174, 1996.

Smith KM: The innocent heart murmur in children. J Pediatr Health Care 11:207–214, 1997.

CHAPTER 27

Respiratory Disorders

INTRODUCTION

Respiratory diseases are leading causes of illness in children and a major reason for health care visits. This chapter discusses key points for the nurse practitioner to focus on in the diagnosis and management of common viral and bacterial infections of the upper and lower respiratory tracts. Because inflammation, foreign body, or mucus secretion easily obstructs the airways of young infants and children, parents must be carefully counseled about signs and symptoms of respiratory distress, when to bring their child in for evaluation, and the home management of these children.

COUGH

The characteristics of a child's cough are often the significant key to the diagnosis of the type or cause of a respiratory illness. Obtaining a thorough history of the cough assists the nurse practitioner in analyzing the potential differential diagnoses (Table 27–1).

COMMON UPPER RESPIRATORY INFECTIONS, PURULENT RHINORRHEA, AND SINUSITIS

Children have an average of six to eight upper respiratory tract infections (URIs) a year. Nasopharyngitis, the typical URI, is often caused by viral agents and treated with supportive care. Complications of

313

TABLE 27-1

Key Characteristics of Cough, Common Causes, and Questions to Ask in a Pediatric History

Purpose	A cough is a protective reflex to ensure airway patency
Characteristics	
Age factor	Infants have a weak, nonproductive cough
Quality	Staccato-like, brassy, barking (LTB), whooping (pertussis), weak, honky (psychogenic)
Duration	Acute (most causes are infectious), recurrent (associated with allergies and asthma), or chronic (e.g., cystic fibrosis); continuous or intermittent. A chronic cough is defined as coughing that lasts more than 3-4 wk
Productive	Mucus producing or nonproductive
Timing	During the day, night (associated with asthma), or both
Associated symptoms	Fever—may indicate bacterial infection
	Rhinorrhea, sneezing, wheezing, atopic dermatitis—associated with asthma and allergic rhinitis
	Malaise, sneezing, watery nasal discharge, mild sore throat, no or low fever, not ill appearing—typical of URI
	Tachypnea—pneumonia or bronchiolitis in infants (infants may not have a cough)
Causes	
Congenital anomalies	Tracheoesophageal fistula, laryngeal cleft, vocal cord paralysis, pulmonary malformations and tumors, tracheobronchomalacia, congenital heart disease, congestive heart failure
Infectious agents	Viral (respiratory syncytial virus, adenovirus, parainfluenza, HIV), bacterial (tuberculosis, group A β-hemolytic streptococci, pertussis), fungal, and others (*Chlamydia* and *Mycoplasma*)
Allergic conditions	Allergic rhinitis, asthma
Other	Foreign body aspiration, gastroesophageal reflux, psychogenic cough, environmental triggers (air pollution, tobacco smoke, wood smoke, glue sniffing, volatile chemicals), cystic fibrosis, drug induced

HIV = human immunodeficiency virus; LTB = laryngotracheobronchitis; URI = upper respiratory infection.

Adapted from Noble JE: Cough. In Berkowitz C (ed): Pediatrics: A Primary Care Approach. Philadelphia, WB Saunders, 1996, pp 226–239; Guilbert TW, Taussig LM: Chronic cough. Contemp Pediatr 15:155–172, 1998.

URI include otitis media, conjunctivitis, and lower respiratory tract infections. URIs are often associated with purulent rhinorrhea. Persistent (>10 days) purulent rhinorrhea indicates a likely or possible secondary sinusitis. Bilateral nasal drainage is associated with sinusitis; unilateral purulent nasal discharge is commonly due to a foreign body. The sinuses become clinically significant sites of infection as follows:

- Maxillary and ethmoid sinuses as early as infancy
- Sphenoid sinuses around the third and fourth years of life
- Frontal sinuses around the sixth to tenth years of life

Table 27–2 presents information on the differentiation of the common URI from purulent rhinorrhea and sinusitis and their management.

▓▓▓ TONSILLOPHARYNGITIS

Viral agents (e.g., adenovirus, enteroviruses [coxsackievirus, echovirus], herpesvirus, and Epstein-Barr) also are responsible for most cases of tonsillopharyngitis in children. Classic features of viral tonsillopharyngitis infection include

- Hoarseness
- Cough
- Coryza
- Conjunctivitis

The diagnosis and management of group A β-hemolytic streptococcus (GABHS) are summarized in Table 27–3.

▓▓▓ BRONCHIOLITIS, LARYNGOTRACHEOBRONCHITIS, AND FOREIGN BODY OBSTRUCTION

Table 27–4 identifies the assessment and management of bronchiolitis, laryngotracheobronchitis, and foreign body obstruction of the airways, three respiratory tract problems associated with wheezing and/or stridor.

▓▓▓ PNEUMONIA

Pneumonia causes inflammation of the parenchyma of the lung. Viral pneumonia is the most frequently seen type in children. Bacterial

Text continued on page 322

TABLE 27-2

Differentiation of Common Upper Respiratory Infections in Children

SITE OF INFECTION	SYMPTOMS	DURATION OF SYMPTOMS (d)	ETIOLOGICAL AGENT	MANAGEMENT	DURATION OF TREATMENT	COMMENTS
The common cold (viral URI)	Malaise, sneezing, watery nasal discharge, mild sore throat, may have a fever, not ill appearing	0–10	Rhinoviruses (cause 40% of URIs), RSV, parainfluenza, enteroviruses, adenoviruses	No antibiotics; symptomatic Rx, e.g., saline nose drops, increased fluids; for infants, bulb-syringe the nose before meals and bedtime; for older children, cough suppression at night if unable to sleep; humidifier		If lasts longer than 10–14 d, consider other diagnosis (e.g., sinusitis)
Acute purulent rhinorrhea	Thick, yellow nasal discharge (often associated with URI)	>3	Part of the natural history of URI; superinfection by *Streptococcus pneumoniae*, *Haemophilus influenzae*, β-hemolytic streptococci	Symptomatic care; a wait-and-see approach for antibiotics; if >10- to 14-d duration, treat with amoxicillin or dicloxacillin if staphylococci suspected	Best approach, *wait and see;* if a persistent cycle of symptoms is seen in an occasional child, consider a 3-d course of amoxicillin (Abbasi & Cunningham, 1996)	Avoid indiscriminate and frequent use of antibiotics (development of antibiotic resistance)

	Clinical features	Duration (d)	Organisms	Rx	Duration of Rx	Comments
Acute purulent sinusitis	Persistent nasal symptoms for more than 10 d with URI, nasal drainage, cough, recalcitrant asthma	10–30	S. pneumoniae, Moraxella catarrhalis, nontypable H. influenzae	Amoxicillin, trimethoprim-sulfamethoxazole, or amoxicillin-clavulanate	10–14 d	By 7 d should be asymptomatic; change antibiotics 48–72 hr after start of treatment if no response
Subacute sinusitis	Same as above but persistent for at least 30 d	30–120	Same as above; may be β-lactamase producing	Amoxicillin-clavulanate		Initial acute infection did not clear; need to switch antibiotics
Chronic/recurrent sinusitis	Malaise, easy fatigability, unilateral or bilateral nasal discharge, postnasal discharge, nasal obstruction if middle turbinate significantly obstructed	>120	Same as above plus α-hemolytic streptococci and Staphylococcus aureus	Amoxicillin-clavulanate, azithromycin, cefixime, clindamycin	3–6 wk	May need endoscopic sinus surgery if chronic sinusitis does not respond to prolonged medical management, including antibiotic prophylaxis; investigate differential diagnoses

RSV = respiratory syncytial virus; Rx = medication; URI = upper respiratory infection.

T A B L E 27–3

Group A β-Hemolytic Streptococcus (GABHS)-Tonsillopharyngitis: Assessment and Management

History

Most common ≥5–11 yr; uncommon <2 yr; abrupt onset; no nasal S & S; fever, malaise, sore throat, dysphagia; nausea, GI discomfort, vomiting, headache

Physical findings

Petechiae, beefy-red uvula, red tonsillopharyngeal tissue, tonsillar exudate, tender anterior cervical lymph nodes, scarlatiniform rash

Diagnostic tests

Rapid strep test: positivity confirms GABHS; if negative, must culture to dx; culture is test of choice to confirm dx (picks up carrier states); ASO for past infection

Management

Antimicrobial therapy: One of the following (American Academy of Pediatrics, 1997):
- Benzathine penicillin G IM (600,000 units if <60 lb; 1.2 million units for larger children and adults)
- Potassium penicillin V PO (250 mg 2–3 times/d for 10 d for children; 500 mg 2–3 times/d for 10 d for adolescents)
- Erythromycin estolate (20–40 mg/kg/d in 2–4 divided doses for 10 d) or erythromycin ethyl succinate (40 mg/kg/d in 2–4 divided doses) if allergic to penicillin
- A 10 d course of oral cephalosporin (first generation) is acceptable, particularly if allergic to penicillin
- If penicillin resistance is present, use β-lactamase-resistant antibiotic (e.g., amoxicillin-clavulanate or dicloxacillin)

Supportive care: Antipyretics, fluids, rest

Reculture: Generally not needed unless necessary to ensure eradication of GABHS

Treatment failure: If due to noncompliance with medications, give injection of benzathine penicillin. If patient compliant, treat with any of the following drugs: erythromycin, a penicillinase-resistant penicillin, amoxicillin-clavulanate, a cephalosporin, dicloxacillin, or other macrolides (American Academy of Pediatrics 1997). If clinical relapse occurs, give second course of antibiotic. If recurrent infection is a problem, culture family. Toothbrushes or orthodontic devices may harbor GABHS.

Return to school: When afebrile and has taken antibiotics ≥24 h

ASO = antistreptolysin O; Dx = diagnosis; S & S = signs and symptoms; GI = gastrointestinal; IM = intramuscular; PO = oral.

Diagnosis and Management of LTB, Foreign Body, and Bronchiolitis

	LTB	FOREIGN BODY	BRONCHIOLITIS
Peak age	3-60 mo	Toddlers	Infancy to 2 yr of age
Onset	Gradual/acute onset and worse at night, can have recurrent (spasmodic) LTB	Acute symptoms or gradual onset (depends on where foreign body is lodged)	URI for several days with gradual development of respiratory distress
Common findings	URI, seal-bark cough, may improve in few hr	Coughing/choking episode, dyspnea, wheezing, cyanosis, S & S of secondary infection	URI S & S to paroxysmal cough and wheezing, nasal flaring, retractions, cyanosis, prolonged expiration, decreased appetite
Respiratory efforts	Rate generally <50	Minor to significant distress	Rate ranging from 60 to 80; minor to moderate to severe distress
Fever	Common—low grade	Normal to low grade	Moderate to 102°F
CBC	Generally normal	Normal unless secondary infection	Generally normal
Organism(s)	Usually viral—parainfluenza, adenovirus, RSV		RSV (50% of cases), parainfluenza (type 3), mycoplasma, adenovirus
Specific laboratory tests	None	None	Pulse oximetry: O_2 saturations decreased

Table continued on following page

319

Diagnosis and Management of LTB, Foreign Body, and Bronchiolitis *Continued*

	LTB	FOREIGN BODY	BRONCHIOLITIS
Radiographic findings	Lateral or AP of neck: subglottic narrowing	May see localized hyperinflation, mediastinal shift, atelectasis	Hyperinflation, increased AP diameter, some scattered consolidation due to atelectasis or inflammation of alveoli
Treatment	Humidification, corticosteroids in selected cases	Remove foreign body, treat secondary infection/bronchospasm	Maintain hydration (fluids) needs, antipyretics for fever, small frequent feedings, hospitalization if severe respiratory distress or if infant less than 2 mo of age and requires O_2
Intubation	Rare	Endoscopy to remove foreign body	May be necessary in young infants with severe distress (prematures)
Prevention	None	Education on child proofing home and monitoring child	Synagis vaccine for high risk infants

LTB = laryngotracheobronchitis; URI = upper respiratory infection; CBC = complete blood count; AP = anteroposterior; S & S = signs and symptoms; RSV = respiratory syncytial virus.

Differentiating Various Forms of Pneumonia in Infants, Young Children, and Adolescents

CHARACTERISTIC	BACTERIAL	VIRAL	MYCOPLASMAL	CHLAMYDIAL
Common age	All ages	All ages	>5 yr	3-19 wk
Onset	Acute; gradual	Acute; gradual	Slow	Gradual
Clinical findings	Depend on age; start with URI, cough, dyspnea, tachypnea, rales, decreased breath sounds, grunting, retractions, toxic look	Depend on age; cough, coryza, hoarseness, crackles, wheezing	Persistent cough, malaise, headache	Tachypnea, staccato cough, crackles, wheezing rare, 50% have signs or history of conjunctivitis
Fever	Acute onset of fever (≥39°C)	Present	>39°C	Afebrile
CBC	WBCs often elevated >15,000/ μl	Normal/slight elevation	Normal	Eosinophilia in 75% of cases
Organism(s)	90% caused by *Streptococcus pneumoniae*	RSV, parainfluenza, influenza (types A and B)	*Mycoplasma pneumoniae*	*Chlamydia trachomatis*
Radiographic findings	Lobar consolidation	Transient lobar infiltrates	Varies, interstitial infiltrates	Hyperinflation, infiltrates
Treatment	Depends on bacteria; penicillin, methicillin, cefuroxime, gentamicin, vancomycin	Supportive care	Erythromycin/ clarithromycin	Erythromycin

CBC = complete blood count; RSV = respiratory syncytial virus; URI = upper respiratory infection; WBCs = white blood cells.

TABLE 27-6

Parental Education for At Home Care of the Child with a Respiratory Tract Infection: Issues to Discuss

- Fluid: Give guidelines on amount and frequency of fluids child should take
- Humidification: For laryngotracheobronchitis, take the child out into the cold night air, open a freezer door, or turn on the shower at home. In dry climates, humidifiers help in respiratory illnesses; instruct about cleaning of nebulizers and humidifiers
- Bulb syringe: Instruct to use the bulb syringe gently and intermittently and to obstruct one nostril while suctioning the other
- Normal saline nose drops or spray: Use before feedings and when mucus is thick or crusted. Follow by suctioning nares with bulb syringe
- Other educational issues to cover
  - Indications for immediate reevaluation of the child
  - Signs and symptoms of respiratory distress
  - Other indicators of worsening of illness (e.g., toxic appearance, malaise, feeding difficulty)
  - Information on when to expect improvement in the child's symptoms and, if symptoms do not improve as expected, what to do next
  - Clear instructions about medications—how much to give, when to give, side effects to watch for, how long to give, and to complete the course of antibiotics
  - Infection control information if needed
  - Instructions on next return visit

pneumonias are usually secondary infections following a viral respiratory infection. Most children managed in the primary care setting do not need chest radiographs unless there is an unusual presentation, a complication, no response to treatment, or a recurrent pneumonia. Table 27-5 differentiates the various types of childhood pneumonias by infecting agent.

GENERAL MANAGEMENT MEASURES

Table 27-6 summarizes general management measures for the treatment of respiratory infections.

REFERENCES

Abbasi S, Cunningham AS: Are we over treating sinusitis? Contemp Pediatr 13(10):49–62, 1996.

American Academy of Pediatrics Committee on Infectious Diseases: 1997 Red

Book: Report of the Committee on Infectious Diseases, 24th ed. Elk Grove Village, IL: American Academy of Pediatrics, 1997.

Guilbert TW, Taussig LM: Chronic cough. Contemp Pediatr 15(3):155–172, 1998.

Noble JE: Cough. *In* Berkowitz C (ed): Pediatrics: A Primary Care Approach. Philadelphia, WB Saunders, 1996, pp 226–239.

CHAPTER 28

Gastrointestinal Disorders

Dehydration, gastroesophageal reflux, colic, acute, chronic, and recurrent abdominal pain, infectious diarrhea, and intestinal parasites are the common gastrointestinal conditions addressed in this chapter.

DEHYDRATION

Dehydration often follows episodes of vomiting or diarrhea. Table 28-1 can help the nurse practitioner determine the extent of dehydration based on clinical signs.

Treatment of dehydration is based on the extent of dehydration. Guidelines for oral and intravenous rehydration are outlined in Table 28-2.

Oral rehydration is an important part of the treatment of dehydration. The electrolyte compositions of commercial solutions are outlined in Table 28-3, and recipes for "homemade" solutions are given in Table 28-4.

GASTROESOPHAGEAL REFLUX

Gastroesophageal reflux may be physiological, functional, or pathological. Management strategies include manipulation of feedings, positioning, and the use of medications. These strategies are included in Table 28-5.

COLIC

Colic is characterized by persistent crying in infants younger than 3 months of age for more than 4 hours a day for no known reason.

T A B L E 28-1

Estimation of Dehydration

CHARACTERISTIC	EXTENT OF DEHYDRATION			
	Mild	Moderate	Severe	Shock
Weight loss—infants (%)	3–5	5–10	10–15	>15
Weight loss—children (%)	3–4	6–8	10	
Pulse	Normal	Slightly increased	Very increased	Rapid and weak
Blood pressure	Normal	Normal to orthostatic, >10-mm Hg change	Orthostatic to shock	
Behavior	Normal	Irritable, more thirsty	Hyperirritable to lethargic	Difficult to awaken/ unresponsive. Too weak to stand; very dizzy
Thirst	Slight	Moderate	Intense	
Mucous membranes*	Normal	Dry	Parched	

Table continued on following page

T A B L E 28–1

Estimation of Dehydration Continued

CHARACTERISTIC	EXTENT OF DEHYDRATION			
	Mild	Moderate	Severe	Shock
Tears	Present	Decreased	Absent; sunken eyes	
Anterior fontanel	Normal	Normal to sunken	Sunken	
External jugular vein	Visible when supine	Not visible except with supraclavicular pressure	Not visible even with supraclavicular pressure	
Skin* (S & S less useful in children >2 yr of age)	Capillary refill <2 s	Slowed capillary refill, 2–4 s (decreased turgor)	Very delayed capillary refill (>4 s) and tenting; skin cool, acrocyanotic, or mottled*	Capillary refill time >4 s. Cold/ acrocyanotic
Urine production	Slight decrease	>8 hr since last void in infants or >12 hr in children	Very decreased or absent	Anuria
Urine specific gravity	>1.020	>1.020; oliguria	Oliguria or anuria	

S & S = signs & symptoms.
*These signs are less prominent in patients who have hypernatremia.
From Jospe N, Forbes G: Fluids and electrolytes: Clinical aspects. Pediatr Rev 17:395–403, 1996.

TABLE 28-2

Treatment of Dehydration

REHYDRATION (with increased sodium concentration)

Mild	ORS	40–50 ml/kg over 4 hr (10 ml/kg per hr)
Moderate	ORS	60–100 ml/kg over 4–6 hr (20 ml/kg per hr)
Severe	IV fluids	Ringer's lactate or normal saline, 20-ml/kg bolus over 1 hr; may repeat bolus if needed (until pulse, perfusion, mental status are normal)
		Follow with 5% dextrose with NaCl and KCl added (once the child has voided) for maintenance fluids and abnormal loss replacement (see later); if severe dehydration, give ½ amount over 8 hr, the other ½ over the next 16 hr; include bolus amounts in the 24-hr total
		Begin ORS as soon as possible

MAINTENANCE

Total water volume	0–10 kg	100 ml/kg per 24 hr
	10–20 kg	1000 ml + 50 ml/kg for each kg over 10 kg/24 hr
	>20 kg	1500 ml + 20 ml/kg for each kg over 20 kg/24 hr

May give up to 150 ml/kg in first 24 hr

REPLACEMENT OF FLUID LOSSES (if continued, heavy losses)

10 ml/kg or 4–8 oz of ORS for each diarrhea stool (1 to 1½ times the amount of stool)

REFEEDING

Reintroduce age-appropriate diet within 24 hr. Avoid fatty foods and foods high in simple sugars.
Encourage complex carbohydrates, lean meats, yogurt, bananas, and applesauce.
Formula-fed infants should have full-strength formula. If that is not tolerated, use lactose-free or soy formula.
Breastfeeding infants should continue to breastfeed with shorter duration and more frequent feedings.
Use regular milk for older children.

IV = intravenous; ORS = oral rehydration solution.
Data from Lasche J, Duggan C: Managing acute diarrhea. Contemp Pediatr 16(2):74–83, 1999; Jospe N, Forbes G: Fluids and electrolytes: Clinical aspects. Pediatr Rev 17(11):395–403, 1996; Northrup RS, Flanigan TP: Gastroenteritis. Pediatr Rev 15(12):461–472, 1994.

327

T A B L E 28-3

Rehydration Solutions

SOLUTION	SODIUM*	CHLORINE*	POTASSIUM*	BASE Type	BASE Concentration*	CARBOHYDRATE Type	CARBOHYDRATE Concentration (g/L)	OSMOLALITY
STOOL†								
Pediatric diarrheal stool	50–100	75–90	25–35	HCO_3	25–40	—	—	250–300
ORAL REHYDRATION SOLUTIONS								
Recommended:								
WHO ORS	90	80	20	Citrate	30	Glucose	20	300
WHO recommendations for ORS solutions	60–90	50–80	20–30	Citrate	25–35	Glucose	20	<300
Pedialyte (Ross)	45	35	20	Citrate	30	Glucose	25	264
Rehydralyte (Ross)	75	65	20	Citrate	30	Glucose	25	327
Cereal-based ORS	60–90	—‡	—‡	—‡	—‡	Starch§	50	200–225
Infalyte (Mead-Johnson)	50	45	25	Citrate	34	Rice syrup solids	30	170–230
Home sugar-salt solution	30–60	30–60	—	—	—	Sucrose	40	170–230

Other solutions:								
Soft drinks, cola, etc.	2	(—)¶	0.1	HCO_3	13	F/G	50–150	550
Apple juice	3	(—)¶	32	—	0	F/G/S	63	700
Chicken broth	250	(—)¶	5	—	0	—	0	450
Gatorade	20	(—)¶	3	HCO_3	3	G/others	45	330

INTRAVENOUS SOLUTIONS

Recommended:								
Ringer's lactate	135	90	4	Lactate	49	—	—	278
Normal saline	135	135	0	—	0	—	—	270
5% Dextrose in saline	135	135	0	—	0	Glucose	50	545
Not recommended:								
5% Dextrose in water	0	0	0	—	0	Glucose	50	275

F = fructose; G = glucose; ORS = oral rehydration solution; S = sucrose; WHO = World Health Organization.

*In millimoles or milliequivalents per liter.

†Values included for comparison.

‡Variable.

§From various cereals: rice, wheat, sorghum, etc.

¶Value not reported.

From Northrup RS, Flanigan TP: Gastroenteritis. Pediatr Rev 15(12):461–472, 1994.

T A B L E 28-4
Oral Rehydration Solutions (Homemade)

Option 1*:	½ cup dry precooked baby rice cereal
	2 cups water
	¼ teaspoon salt (level measure)
Option 2†:	200 ml water
	2 teaspoons sugar
	⅛ teaspoon salt

CAUTION: HAVING PARENTS PREPARE THEIR OWN REHYDRATION SOLUTION IS DISCOURAGED BECAUSE OF CONCERN ABOUT ACCURATE MEASUREMENT

*From Meyers A: Modern management of acute diarrhea and dehydration in children. Am Fam Phys 51:1103–1113, 1995.
†From Northrup RS, Flanigan TP: Gastroenteritis. Pediatr Rev 15(12):468, 1994.

Colic is a diagnosis of exclusion. It is important that the nurse practitioner rule out gastrointestinal problems, temperament, neurological immaturity, or other etiologies as causes of the infant's crying. Colic is frustrating for the parent. Table 28-6 gives practical strategies to help families with a colicky infant.

ACUTE ABDOMINAL PAIN

Acute abdominal pain can be due to multiple etiologies and is frightening for parent and child alike. Figure 28-1 illustrates a decision tree with differential diagnoses the nurse practitioner will find helpful when working with children with acute abdominal pain.

CHRONIC ABDOMINAL PAIN

Chronic abdominal pain can likewise be due to multiple etiologies. Figure 28-2 illustrates a decision tree with differential diagnoses that should be helpful when working with children with chronic abdominal pain.

RECURRENT ABDOMINAL PAIN

Recurrent abdominal pain is defined as a minimum of three episodes of abdominal pain occurring over a 3-month period. It is differentiated

T A B L E 28-5
Treatment of Gastroesophageal Reflux

1. For infants, use small, frequent feedings, burp frequently during feedings, continue breastfeeding, thicken formula with 1 tablespoon of rice cereal per ounce of formula, and avoid formula changes. It is also helpful to have the head of the bed elevated 10–15 degrees after feedings (up to 30 degrees with moderate to severe reflux). Avoid the "scrunched over" or slouched position that puts pressure on the abdomen.
2. For older children, avoid chocolate, caffeine, high-fat foods, spicy foods, alcohol, and bedtime snacks.
3. Medications can be helpful when the above measures have failed to give relief (see below).
4. Follow growth parameters closely to ensure adequate weight gain.
5. Refer for Nissen fundoplication or similar surgical procedures if the GER is severe, not well medically managed, or is causing significant secondary morbidity.

MEDICATION	DOSAGE	COMMENTS
Ranitidine (Zantac)	1.5–2.3 mg/kg/dose bid	Inhibits histamine at H_2-receptor sites and decreases gastric acid secretion
Cimetidine (Tagamet)	20–40 mg/kg/d q6h	Inhibits histamine at H_2-receptor sites and decreases gastric acid secretion
Metoclopramide (Reglan)	0.1 mg/kg/dose up to qid	Hastens gastric emptying High range of side effects Give 30 min before meals
Bethanechol	0.1–0.2 mg/kg/dose up to qid	Questionable effectiveness in GER

NOTE: A combination of an H_2-inhibitor and an agent that promotes gastric emptying is often an effective regimen.

GER = gastroesophageal reflux.

331

T A B L E 28–6

Management Strategies for Infantile Colic

Acknowledge the importance of the concern.

Provide support for the parents.

Affirm the baby's good health.

Remind the parents that colic is temporary.

Reinforce parents' efforts to comfort their infant.

Encourage parents to take time off from child care by finding assistance from family or friends.

Inform parents that the stress they feel is sensed by the infant, which may cause more crying.

Allow parents to express feelings of anger, guilt, and frustration.

Inform parents of equipment sold to soothe babies (vibrating infant seats and cribs).

Share anecdotal reports of using noise from hair dryers or vacuum cleaners or a ride in the car to calm the infant.

Implement strategies to calm the infant (decrease in environmental stimulation, swaddling the infant, carrying the infant, firm and gentle pressure to the abdomen, rocking, swinging).

Ensure proper feeding (e.g., correct latch-on, frequent burping, avoid early addition of solids, change diet if lactose intolerance or milk allergy is a problem).

Have the parents keep a diary of the baby's crying for analysis by the health care provider; a diary may assist in identifying patterns that can lead to interventions.

Data from Dihigo S: New strategies for the treatment of colic: Modifying the parent/infant interaction. J Pediatr Health Care 12(5):256–262, 1998; Fleisher D: Coping with colic. Contemp Pediatr 15(6):144–156, 1998; Cervisi J, Chapman M, Niklas B, et al: Office management of the infant with colic. J Pediatr Health Care 5:184–190, 1991.

from chronic abdominal pain because each episode of recurrent abdominal pain is distinct, separated by periods of wellness. Table 28-7 lists signs, or "red flags," that should alert the nurse practitioner to some other pathological episode occurring in the child who presents with recurrent abdominal pain.

▨ DIARRHEA

Acute diarrhea occurs when there is excessive loss of fluids and electrolytes in the stool. Table 28-8 outlines signs, symptoms, and treatments for the seven most common causes of diarrhea in children. Table 28-9 details laboratory findings associated with each of these conditions.

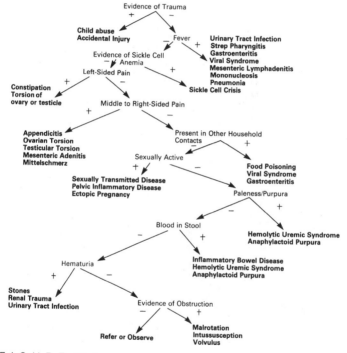

ACUTE ABDOMEN
Differential Diagnosis

Accidental Injury
Accidental Ingestion
Anaphylactoid Purpura
Appendicitis
Child Abuse
Constipation

Ectopic Pregnancy
Food Intolerance
Gastroenteritis
Hemolytic Uremic Syndrome
Mechanical Obstruction
Mononucleosis

Pneumonia
Renal Stones
Sickle Cell Anemia
Tortion of Ovary or Testicle
Trauma
Urinary Tract Infection
Viral Syndrome

Evidence of Trauma

+   −

Child abuse
Accidental Injury

− Fever +

Urinary Tract Infection
Strep Pharyngitis
Gastroenteritis
Viral Syndrome
Mesenteric Lymphadenitis
Mononucleosis
Pneumonia

Evidence of Sickle Cell
− Anemia

Left-Sided Pain   +

Sickle Cell Crisis

+   −

Constipation
Torsion of
ovary or testicle

Middle to Right-Sided Pain

+   −

Appendicitis
Ovarian Torsion
Testicular Torsion
Mesenteric Adenitis
Mittelschmerz

Present in Other Household
Contacts   +

Sexually Active   −

Food Poisoning
Viral Syndrome
Gastroenteritis

+

Sexually Transmitted Disease
Pelvic Inflammatory Disease
Ectopic Pregnancy

Paleness/Purpura

−   +

Blood in Stool

−   +

Hemolytic Uremic Syndrome
Anaphylactoid Purpura

Hematuria

+   −

Inflammatory Bowel Disease
Hemolytic Uremic Syndrome
Anaphylactoid Purpura

Stones
Renal Trauma
Urinary Tract Infection

Evidence of Obstruction

−   +

Refer or Observe

Malrotation
Intussusception
Volvulus

FIGURE 28–1

Decision tree for differential diagnosis of acute abdominal pain. (From Schwartz WM (ed): Pediatric Primary Care: A Problem-Oriented Approach. St. Louis, Mosby, 1997, p 188.)

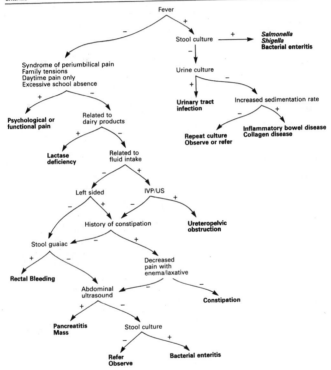

Decision tree for differential diagnosis of chronic abdominal pain (From Schwartz WM (ed): Pediatric Primary Care: A Problem-Oriented Approach. St. Louis, Mosby, 1997, p 193.)

T A B L E 28-7

"Red Flags" to Consider in Recurrent Abdominal Pain

Positive family history of GI problems (not recurrent abdominal pain)
No stressful life events
No school absences
No evidence of need to be high achiever
Anorexia
Diarrhea
Pain related to mealtimes
Vomiting/bloody emesis
Extraintestinal symptoms (rash, joint pain, dysuria)
Sleepiness following pain
Night awakening
Change in bowel habits, dysuria, polyuria, menstrual problems
Sexual activity
Weight loss
Growth deceleration
Child keeping eyes open during examination
Localized pain away from umbilicus
Anemia
Elevated ESR
Abnormal UA/UC
Blood in stool

ESR = erythrocyte sedimentation rate; GI = gastrointestinal; UA = urinalysis; UC = urine culture.

Data from Pearl RH, Irish MS, Caty MG, et al: The approach to common abdominal diagnoses in infants and children, part 2. Pediatr Clin North Am 45(6):1287–1326, 1998; Boyle JT: Recurrent abdominal pain: An update. Pediatr Rev 18(9): 310–320, 1997; Pierce C: What not to do for a child with recurrent abdominal pain. Pediatr News March 25, 1995.

▨ INTESTINAL PARASITES

Although there are multiple organisms that cause parasitic infections in children, giardia, pinworms, roundworms, and tapeworms are the four most commonly seen parasites in children. Table 28-10 outlines signs, symptoms, and treatment for these parasitic infections. Table 28-11 details laboratory findings associated with each of these conditions.

▨ DIFFERENTIAL DIAGNOSIS OF ABDOMINAL PAIN

The most common gastrointestinal causes of abdominal pain are outlined in Table 28-12, along with differential criteria that are helpful to use in determining a diagnosis.

Text continued on page 345

T A B L E 28–8

Infectious Diarrhea: Signs, Symptoms, and Treatment

CAUSE	DIARRHEA	BLOODY STOOL	ABDOMINAL PAIN	VOMITING	FEVER	OTHER	TREATMENT
Campylobacter jejuni	+++ Foul smelling		+	+	+		Erythromycin, 40 mg/kg per d in 3 divided doses for 5–7 d Decreases fecal excretion in 24–48 hr Illness lasts 7–12 d
Clostridium difficile	++	+	+				Discontinue antibiotic Metronidazole, 30 mg/kg per d in 4 divided doses for 7–10 d, or Vancomycin, 40 mg/kg per d in 4 divided doses for 7–10 d Cholestyramine helps bind the toxin and decrease diarrhea
Yersinia entercolitica	+ Green/malodorous	+	+ RLQ pain		+		Usually resolves spontaneously in 3–4 d. If septic, TMP-SMZ, 8 mg TMP/kg per d in 2 divided doses for 7–10 d, or Chloramphenicol, 50–75 mg/kg per d in 4 divided doses for 7–10 d, or Tetracycline, 25–50 mg/kg per d in 4 divided doses for 7–10 d (older teens only)

| Salmonella | ++ | + | + | + Rebound tenderness | + | Sepsis Bacteremia | No treatment if uncomplicated; usually resolves spontaneously |

No treatment if uncomplicated; usually resolves spontaneously

Antibiotics can prolong the carrier state

Antibiotics indicated for children younger than 1 yr who are at risk for bacteremia and for patients who are immunosuppressed, have cardiac or valvular disease, lymphoproliferative diseases, sickle cell disease, or hemolytic anemias

If indicated, use amoxicillin, 40 mg/kg per d in 3 divided doses for 7–10 d, or

TMP-SMZ, 8 mg TMP/kg per d for 7–10 d in 2 divided doses, or

Chloramphenicol, 50–75 mg/kg per d in 4 divided doses for 7–10 d

Steroids and prostaglandins may be necessary for severe illness

Table continued on following page

337

T A B L E 28–8

Infectious Diarrhea: Signs, Symptoms, and Treatment *Continued*

CAUSE	DIARRHEA	BLOODY STOOL	ABDOMINAL PAIN	VOMITING	FEVER	OTHER	TREATMENT
Shigella	+++ (initially) + (after 1–3 d)	+	+		+	Irritability Listlessness Patulous rectum	Need susceptibility information Resistance is common TMP-SMZ, 8 mg TMP/kg per d in 2 divided doses for 5 d, *or* Cefixime, 8 mg/kg per d for 5 d
Escherichia coli	++	+	+ Cramps and abdominal pain	–/+	+	Hemolytic-uremic syndrome	TMP-SMZ, 8 mg TMP/kg per d in 2 divided doses for 7–10 d if diarrhea is moderate to severe Do CBC, platelets, and kidney function tests
Virus	+++ Watery	+ Cramps	+	+/–		Symptomatic treatment and maintenance of fluids	

CBC = complete blood count; RLQ = right lower quadrant; TMP-SMZ = trimethoprim-sulfamethoxazole; + = mild; ++ = moderate; +++ = severe; +/– = may or may not be present.

TABLE 28-9
Laboratory Findings Associated with Infectious Diarrhea

CAUSE	BLOODY STOOL	WBCs IN STOOL	STOOL CULTURE	CBC	OTHER
Campylobacter jejuni	+ Gross	+	+	↑ WBC	Darting and motility on microscopy
Clostridium difficile	+ Gross	+	For toxin	Slightly ↑ WBCs ESR nl	
Yersinia enterocolitica	Gross or occult	+	+		
Salmonella	+ Gross	+	+	↓, nl, or slightly ↑ WBCs with left shift	
Shigella	+ Gross	+	+	nl or slightly ↑ WBCs with left shift	
Escherichia coli	+ Gross	−	+		Hemolytic-uremic syndrome as a complication
Virus	−	−	±*		

CBC = complete blood count; ESR = erythrocyte sedimentation rate; nl = normal; WBCs = white blood cells; + = present; − = not a clinical finding.
*If virus suspected, consider studying stool for reducing substances, Clinitest, heme test, and pH. Can test stool using enzyme-linked immunosorbent assay (ELISA) and latex agglutination assay for rotavirus.

Intestinal Parasite Infestation: Signs, Symptoms, and Treatment

PARASITE	GI SYMPTOMS	DIARRHEA	WEIGHT LOSS	OTHER	TREATMENT
Giardia lamblia	+ Abdominal cramps, flatulence, bloating	+ + Rarely bloody, watery, greasy, foul smelling	+		Treat all positive stool cultures with Furazolidone, 5–8 mg/kg per d in 4 divided doses for 7–10 d, or Metronidazole, 40 mg/kg per d in 3 divided doses for 7–10 d Can repeat either if treatment fails
Enterobius vermicularis (pinworm)	−	−	−	Perirectal/vaginal itching	Mebendazole, 100-mg tablet for 1 dose, then repeat in 2 wk, or Pyrantel pamoate, 11 mg/kg (max, 1 g) for 1 dose, then repeat in 2 wk Simultaneously treat family members Vaginitis is self-limiting
Ascaris lumbricoides (roundworm)	Worms in stool or vomit Bowel or biliary obstruction	−	+ Malnutrition		Pyrantel pamoate, 11 mg/kg for 1 dose (max, 1 g), or Mebendazole, 100-mg tablet per d for 3 d If intestinal obstruction present, piperazine citrate, 75 mg/kg per d (max, 3.5 g) for 2 d; makes worms flaccid and easier to pass
Taenia (tapeworm)	Worms in stool, abdominal pain, excessive appetite	−	−		Praziquantel, 20 mg/kg per d in 4 divided doses for 1 d

+ = present; − = not a clinical finding; + + = moderate; GI = gastrointestinal.

T A B L E 28-11

Laboratory Findings Associated with Intestinal Parasite Infestation

PARASITE	STOOL FINDINGS	STOOL FOR OVA AND PARASITES	STOOL CULTURE	CBC	DUODENAL ASPIRATE	OTHER
Giardia lamblia		−	+ Three cultures over 1 wk		May be necessary to continue	EIA for *Giardia*
Enterobius vermicularis (pinworm)						Transparent tape test during night
Ascaris lumbricoides (roundworm)	Worms in stool	+	−	Marked eosinophilia		
Taenia (tapeworm)		+ Ova in stool				

CBC = complete blood count; EIA = enzyme immunoassay; + = present; − = not a clinical finding; ± = may or may not be present.

T A B L E 28-12

Differential Diagnosis of Gastrointestinal Causes of Abdominal Pain in Children

DISEASE AND AGE OF ONSET	MAJOR SYMPTOMS AND SIGNS	EXCRETA	TESTS
Appendicitis Frequency increases with age, peaking between 15 and 30 yr	Fever, anorexia, vomiting; process evolves over 12 hr Diffuse then localized to right-sided tenderness, guarding maximal pain over McBurney's point	Constipation or diarrhea, rare blood and pus	CBC = neutrophils UA = pyuria Abdominal x-ray = *may* show fecalith Ultrasound = *may* be abnormal
Foreign body Highest incidence between 14 mo and 6 yr	Children may be asymptomatic *or* Coughing, choking, gagging, pain in throat or chest, anorexia, pain with swallowing May have salivation, refusal to swallow, respiratory symptoms; normal abdominal examination	May see passage of FB	Chest x-ray if respiratory symptoms Abdominal x-ray if FB not seen to pass in stool or signs of abdominal pain/obstruction
Gastroenteritis, viral or bacterial Any age	Vomiting, diarrhea General abdominal tenderness	Watery, bilious (green) vomitis, may or may not have blood in stool	Stool = *may* show bacteria, WBCs, blood, mucus

Gastroesophageal reflux (chalasia) Common 0–24 mo with 60–80% spontaneous resolution; can occur in specific disease disorders and in older children and adolescents	Regurgitation, vomiting, irritability Infants: gastric distention, effortless regurgitation during or after feedings, FTT, strider, apnea, recurrent pneumonia, bronchospasm Older children: vomiting, abdominal pain, burning sensation in substernal area; chronic nocturnal cough, wheezing, pneumonia; dysphagia; nausea, FTT	Barium swallow with fluoroscopy 24-hr esophageal pH probe study Esophageal manometry Endoscopy for esophageal biopsy
Intussusception 70% <2 yr, with peak incidence at 5 mo and 3 yr; as age of onset increases, there is often further pathology	Episodic, cyclic abdominal pain with vomiting Tender, sausage-shaped mass RUQ, distention, legs drawn up at time of pain followed by periods of lethargy, absence of bowel sounds in RLQ; these "classic" symptoms occur in <50% of cases	Blood-tinged mucus ("currant jelly" stool); this occurs as a late sign Abdominal ultrasound 100% reliable (abdominal x-ray misses diagnosis in 33–55% of cases) Barium enema
Irritable bowel 5–15 yr	Recurrent diarrhea or crampy abdominal pain Intense thirst, fluctuating abdominal distention, bowel sounds; history of others in family with recurrent abdominal pain related to social stimulation, travel, holidays, trauma; healthy appearance; borborygmus and flatus in school-aged and older children; vague tenderness RLQ, LLQ, and epigastrium; pain usually not related to eating or defecation; occasional pallor and nausea	Rare hematemesis Watery, malodorous stools First stool of the day may be formed followed by very watery through the day CBC, ESR, urinalysis, stools for O&P and occult blood Abdominal ultrasound Upper GI with small bowel follow-through

Table continued on following page

Differential Diagnosis of Gastrointestinal Causes of Abdominal Pain in Children *Continued*

DISEASE AND AGE OF ONSET	MAJOR SYMPTOMS AND SIGNS	EXCRETA	TESTS
Lactose intolerance 5–15 yr, rare in infancy; prominent in some ethnic groups	Bloating, gaseousness, crampy abdominal pain Pain and diarrhea within hours of lactose ingestion; may have history of recent severe viral gastroenteritis In infants: vomiting, distention, abdominal pain after lactose-containing formula or bovine milk ingestion by breastfeeding mother	Acidic diarrhea	Breath hydrogen test after lactose challenge Reducing substances in stool Lack of normal increase in blood glucose after ingestion of lactose

Table developed by Catherine Blosser with information from Burg F et al (1996); Teitelbaum SJ et al (1999); Behrman RE, Kliegman RM (1998); Finberg L (1998); Irish MS et al (1998); Kaye R et al (1988).

CBC = complete blood count; ESR = erythrocyte sedimentation rate; FB = foreign body; FTT = failure to thrive; GI = gastrointestinal; LLQ = left lower quadrant; O&P = ova and parasites; RLQ = right lower quadrant; RUQ = right upper quadrant; UA = urinalysis; WBCs = white blood cells.

REFERENCES

American Academy of Pediatrics Provisional Committee on Quality Improvement: Subcommittee on Acute Gastroenteritis: Practice parameter: The management of acute gastroenteritis in young children. Pediatrics 97:424–436, 1996.

Behrman RE, Kliegman RM: Nelson Essentials of Pediatrics, 3rd ed. Philadelphia, WB Saunders, 1998.

Boyle JT: Recurrent abdominal pain: An update. Pediatr Rev 18(9):310–320, 1997.

Burg F, Ingelfinger J, Wald E, et al: Gellison & Kagan's Current Pediatric Therapy, 15. Philadelphia, WB Saunders, 1996.

Cervisi J, Chapman M, Niklas B, et al: Office management of the infant with colic. J Pediatr Health Care 5:184–190, 1991.

Dihigo S: New strategies for the treatment of colic: Modifying the parent/infant interaction. J Pediatr Health Care 12(5):256–262, 1998.

Finberg L: Saunders Manual of Pediatric Practice. Philadelphia, WB Saunders, 1998.

Fleisher D: Coping with colic. Contemp Pediatr 15(6):144–156, 1998.

Irish MS, Pearl MH, Caty MG, et al: The approach to common abdominal diagnosis in infants and children. Pediatr Clin North Am 45:729–772, 1998.

Jospe N, Forbes G: Fluids and electrolytes: Clinical aspects. Pediatr Rev 17(11):395–403, 1996.

Kaye R, Odki F, Barness L: Core Textbook of Pediatrics. New York: Lippincott, 1988.

Lasche J, Duggan C: Managing acute diarrhea. Contemp Pediatr 16(2):74–83, 1999.

Meyers A: Modern management of acute diarrhea and dehydration in children. Am Fam Phys 51:1103–1113, 1995.

Northrup RS, Flanigan TP: Gastroenteritis. Pediatr Rev 15(12):461–472, 1994.

Pearl RH, Irish MS, Caty MG, et al: The approach to common abdominal diagnoses in infants and children, part 2. Pediatr Clin North Am 45(6):1287–1326, 1998.

Pierce C: What not to do for a child with recurrent abdominal pain. Pediatr News March 25, 1995.

Schwartz WM [ed]: Pediatric Primary Care: A Problem-Oriented Approach. St. Louis, Mosby, 1997.

Teitelbaum SJ, Leichtner AM, Tunnessen WW: "Read my lips": Abdominal pain in a 14 year old. Contemp Pediatr 16(3):31–41, 1999.

CHAPTER 29

Dental and Oral Diseases

Nurse practitioners are involved daily in assessing a child's oral health and providing parents with oral health counseling. Knowing the usual eruption sequence (Table 29-1) is often helpful in both of these areas.

CARIES

Dental caries is a major, almost entirely preventable infectious disease in children. The body's demineralization-remineralization process can be used to help ensure healthy dentition. Counseling parents about children's eating habits and the use of fluoride are two important strategies to prevent caries. Use of a milk bottle in bed or as a pacifier, and the uncontrolled use of a sippy cup containing milk or fruit juice place the child at risk for early childhood caries. Older children who are "nibblers and sippers" rather than "wolfers and gobblers" also have a higher risk for caries. Use of both a fluoride toothpaste in small amounts from the time teeth erupt and a fluoride supplement as indicated (Table 29-2) should be emphasized.

MALOCCLUSION

Malocclusion, defined as crowded, irregular, or protruding teeth, is another common problem. Malocclusion increases the likelihood of injury and interfers with dental-oral function and aesthetics. The following are primary preventive measures to use when managing a child with malocclusion:

- Refer for space maintenance devices whenever a tooth is lost prematurely

T A B L E 29–1

Eruption Sequence

DENTITION	AGE AT ERUPTION
PRIMARY	
Maxillary	
Central incisor	7½ mo
Lateral incisor	9 mo
Cuspid	18 mo
First molar	14 mo
Second molar	24 mo
Mandibular	
Central incisor	6 mo
Lateral incisor	7 mo
Cuspid	16 mo
First molar	12 mo
Second molar	20 mo
PERMANENT	
Maxillary	
Central incisor	7–8 yr
Lateral incisor	8–9 yr
Cuspid	11–12 yr
First bicuspid	10–11 yr
Second bicuspid	10–12 yr
First molar	6–7 yr
Second molar	12–13 yr
Mandibular	
Central incisor	6–7 yr
Lateral incisor	7–8 yr
Cuspid	9–10 yr
First bicuspid	10–12 yr
Second bicuspid	11–12 yr
First molar	6–7 yr
Second molar	11–13 yr

Adapted from Logan WHG, Kronfeld R: The chronology of human dentition. J Am Dent Assoc 20, 1933 (slightly modified by McCall & Schour). Copyright 1933. Reprinted by permission of ADA.

T A B L E 29–2

Fluoride Supplementation Regimen*

AGE	CONCENTRATION OF FLUORIDE IN WATER		
	<0.3 ppm (mg)	0.3–0.6 ppm (mg)	>0.6 ppm (mg)
Birth to 6 mo	0	0	0
6 mo to 3 yr	0.25	0	0
3–6 yr	0.50	0.25	0
6 yr up to at least 16 yr	1.0	0.50	0

Fluoride comes in the following formulations:
- Drops 0.5 mg/ml or 0.125 mg drop
- Tablets (dissolve or chew) 0.25, 0.5, and 1 mg; nonchewable tablets 1 mg
- In combination with multivitamins.

*Recommended daily dosage of fluoride in mg/day; 1 mg of fluoride is equivalent to 2.2 mg of sodium fluoride; ppm = parts per million.

Differentiating Oral Herpes Simplex Infection, Gingivitis, and Aphthous Ulcers

	ETIOLOGY AND AGE	CLINICAL FINDINGS	TREATMENT
Herpes simplex (HSV)	HSV type 1 primary infection is gingivostomatitis, which usually occurs before 5 yr of age; recurrent infection is herpes labialis and occurs at any age	Gingivostomatitis—erythematous soft mucosa of the mouth with vesicles that ulcerate and form white plaques on mucous membranes Herpes labialis—burning, itching cluster of small clear vesicles with an erythematous base that become crusty, usually near the mouth	Lesions heal spontaneously. Encourage fluids. Oral analgesics, oral anesthetics in older children. Occasional use of acyclovir (Zovirax) in severely ill children. Exclusion from day care if drooling
Gingivitis	Retention of bacterial plaque in the soft tissue at the neck of the tooth; most prevalent in young children because of poor hygiene	Early—mild erythema and inflammation at the margins of gum tissue Moderate—red, glazed bleeding gums Severe—spontaneously bleeding gums, fetid breath, enlarged gums	Antibacterial mouth rinses with chlorhexidine, 0.12%, if the child can expectorate. Improved oral hygiene. Refer to a dentist if severe
Aphthous ulcers	Idiopathic in origin, precipitated by trauma, stress, sun, allergies, and certain chronic disorders; most common in adolescents	Tingle or burn before lesion occurs, pain with the lesion. Single or multiple small circular lesions with an erythematous halo and pale center on the alveolar and buccal mucosa, tongue, soft palate, and floor of the mouth	Resolves spontaneously. Oral analgesics, topical anesthetics, antibacterial rinse as above. Topical steroids if severe. Refer to a dentist if duration >14 d

T A B L E   29-4

Traumatic Dental Injuries that Require Immediate Attention by a Dental Professional

INJURY	CLINICAL PRESENTATION	TREATMENT ACTION
Fractured jaw	Facial asymmetry, swelling, pain, limitation of movement	Radiographic diagnosis, immobilization
Dental alveolar bone fracture	Mobility of segments of teeth rather than individual teeth	Radiographic diagnosis, intra-arch stabilization
Dental crown fractures involving exposure of the pulpal tissues	Pulp tissue visible in tooth fracture site	Pulp capping and coverage of fracture to prevent bacterial infection of pulp, dental abscess, and endodontics
Root fractures	Mobility of one or more teeth >2 mm in any direction	Radiographic diagnosis, intra-arch stabilization
Intruded tooth	Tooth is completely or partially intruded or jammed into its socket	Radiographic diagnosis, primary tooth allowed to re-erupt followed by pulpotomy; permanent tooth requires orthodontic repositioning and endodontics
Partial avulsions (extrusions)	Tooth dislodged from its socket and will not remain stable or has >2 mm mobility	Radiographic diagnosis to rule out root fracture Primary teeth: extract if severely mobile or intra-arch stabilization and pulpotomy Permanent tooth: intra-arch stabilization and endodontics
Complete avulsion	Entire tooth displaced from the dental socket intact	Radiographic confirmation Primary tooth: stop bleeding, do not reimplant Permanent tooth: gently clean root surface, re-implant immediately to maintain intra-arch stabilization; transport tooth in saline, milk, or cold water to dental office if necessary
Toothache accompanied by swelling	Cellulitis or localized facial erythema Broken or carious tooth	Confer with pediatric dentist about antibiotic choice Start antibiotic therapy

Traumatic Dental Injuries That Require Attention by a Dental Professional Within 1 to 3 Days

INJURY	CLINICAL FEATURES	TREATMENT ACTION
Bumped deciduous incisors	Dark discolored anterior deciduous or permanent tooth	Radiographic diagnosis, pulpectomy, endodontics
Toothache not accompanied by swelling	Painful carious or fractured tooth often accompanied by mobility or a draining fistula	Start antibiotics/analgesics, insist on professional dental follow-up
Simple crown fractures	Fractures of enamel and/or dentin that do not expose the pulp	Restore the tooth to function and aesthetics as convenient
Broken braces, wires, dental appliances	Dental appliances loose or irritating to the child	Dental appointment as soon as possible; remove the appliance
Minor bumps	Teeth slightly loosened in their sockets with <2 mm mobility and stable in the dental arch	Insist on professional dental follow-up

- Counsel about the use of mouthguards for bruxism
- Discourage the use of thumb/finger or pacifier sucking after 24 to 30 months of age, especially if the habit is frequent and intense

ORAL LESIONS

Herpes simplex gingivostomatitis, gingivitis, and aphthous ulcers are common conditions seen by the nurse practitioner. Gingivitis is a sign of poor oral hygiene that increases caries activity. The gingivostomatitis caused by herpes simplex and aphthous ulcers is sometimes confused with gingivitis. Table 29-3 differentiates the diagnosis and management of these three entities.

TRAUMA

Traumatic injuries to a child's mouth and teeth are common. Immediate management of trauma seeks to prevent the aesthetic disfigurement of tooth loss, future pain or infection, and expensive dental treatment. Tables 29-4 and 29-5 outline the clinical presentation and treatment needed for injuries that require immediate attention as well as injuries that require attention within 1 to 3 days.

REFERENCE

Logan WHG, Kronfeld R: The chronology of human dentition. J Am Dent Assoc 20, 1933.

CHAPTER 30

Genitourinary Disorders

Hematuria, proteinuria, renal failure, and urinary tract infection (UTI) are genitourinary problems the nurse practitioner must be prepared to handle. These diseases range from common (UTI) to rare (renal failure) and can be subtle in presentation.

▮▮▮ ASSESSMENT AND INTERPRETATION OF THE URINE

Urine dipsticks are commonly used as a first-line assessment of genitourinary function, with abnormalities providing clues to the need for further evaluation. Chemical characteristics of urine are outlined in Table 30-1.

Microscopic examination of a fresh urine sample provides equally important information:

- Red blood cells (RBCs)—more than 2 to 5 per high power field (hpf) ($\times 40$) in unspun urine or more than 2 to 10/hpf in spun urine is thought to be abnormal (Roy, 1998; Finberg, 1998; Cruz & Spitzer, 1998; Feld et al., 1997; Opas, 1999)
- White blood cells (WBCs)—fewer than 2 WBCs/hpf is normal; more than 10 WBCs often accompany a symptomatic infection; if between 2 and 10 WBCs/hpf, urine culture or other workup is indicated
- Bacteria and leukocytes in an *unspun* sample are associated with colony counts on culture of 100,000
- Casts—RBC, hyaline, waxy, epithelial, leukocyte, or fatty casts are seen in various disease states

TABLE 30-1

Chemical Characteristics of Urine

CONSTITUENT	POSITIVES INDICATE	FALSE POSITIVES CAUSED BY	FALSE NEGATIVES CAUSED BY
Glucose	Metabolic problem (e.g., diabetes), recent high glucose intake, galactosemia	Antibiotics, delay in reading, myoglobin, oxidizing contaminants	Ascorbic acid intake, ketones, high specific gravity
Ketones	Dehydration, starvation, strenuous exercise, stress, fever, metabolic problems (e.g., diabetes)		If urine left standing, acetone evaporates
Protein	Renal disease, orthostatic proteinuria	Exercise, fever, dehydration, alkaline or concentrated urine (SG >1.020), semisynthetic penicillin, oxidizing cleansing agents	Dilute or acidic urine

Blood (hemoglobin)	If microscopic examination is negative for RBCs: Free hemoglobin secondary to chemicals, illness, or drugs; myoglobin secondary to burns, muscle trauma, physical child abuse, myositis, strenuous exercise; If microscopic examination is positive for RBCs: Renal problems	Menses, oxidizing cleansing agents, dilute urine	Ascorbic acid
Nitrite	Bacteria causing urinary tract infection	Rare	Common; urine should be in bladder at least 4 hr
Leukocyte esterase	Pyuria (WBCs in urine); inflammation from irritation or infection of vulva, vagina, or urethra; inflammation of bladder or kidneys with or without infection	Oxidizing agents	Immunocompromised status

RBCs = red blood cells; SG = specific gravity; WBCs = white blood cells.

- Crystals, if amorphous, are not unusual; calcium oxalate, cystine, tyrosine, leucine, cholesterol, or sulfa crystals are abnormal

HEMATURIA

Hematuria refers to blood in the urine that may be persistent, recurrent, or transient. It is a sign of disease or injury to the urinary system. Table 30-2 outlines a differential diagnosis for hematuria.

A progressive approach to evaluating hematuria should be undertaken with the goal of not overlooking serious, preventable conditions while avoiding unnecessary studies. Figures 30-1 and 30-2 illustrate the management of macroscopic and microscopic hematuria.

PROTEINURIA

Proteinuria is considered positive if a level of 1+ (30 mg/dl) is found. Proteinuria may be transient, recurrent, or fixed. A differential diagnosis of proteinuria is included in Table 30-3. Figure 30-3 illustrates the evaluation of proteinuria.

CHRONIC RENAL FAILURE

Although chronic renal failure is not a common diagnosis in pediatrics, its devastating effects make it essential for the nurse practitioner to be familiar with the signs and symptoms that warrant further evaluation. Table 30-4 lists seven "red flag" symptoms to be aware of.

URINARY TRACT INFECTION

Not only are UTIs frequently seen in primary care, they are the most commonly seen serious bacterial infection in young febrile children without obvious source of infection. Because young children have limited symptoms, a high degree of suspicion must be maintained. The clinical findings of UTIs in various aged children are listed in Table 30-5.

Diagnosis of a UTI depends on the method of urine collection, the sex of the child, and the colony count. Table 30-6 outlines criteria

Text continued on page 367

T A B L E   30–2

Differential Diagnosis of Hematuria

Five patterns of hematuria have been identified and may be helpful when considering the differential diagnosis of hematuria (Boineau & Lewy, 1989):

- Type 1—microscopic and persistent
- Type 2—microscopic and intermittent
- Type 3—persistent macroscopic
- Type 4—intermittent or recurrent macroscopic
- Type 5—intermittent or recurrent macroscopic with persistent microscopic

Types 1 and 2 account for most pediatric cases of hematuria. Type 3 is common with urological and nephrological disorders such as UTI, glomerulonephritis, hemoglobinopathies, renal stones, and trauma. Types 4 and 5 occur with immunoglobulin A (IgA) nephropathy, hypercalciuria, and benign recurrent hematuria.

Other differential diagnoses to consider include the following:

- *Pseudohematuria* occurs when there is a false-positive dipstick reading but the microscopic examination finds no RBCs. The two most common causes are myoglobinuria and hemoglobinuria (see Table 30–1).
- *Extrarenal hematuria* is common with systemic bleeding disorders and is evidenced by macroscopic and microscopic hematuria.
- The presence of RBC casts or proteinuria or both manifest *glomerular hematuria* such as occurs in acute or chronic glomerulonephritis.
- *Idiopathic hypercalciuria* is an inherited tubulointerstitial disorder with excessive urinary calcium excretion in the presence of macroscopic and microscopic hematuria. It is the most frequently seen isolated hematuria in children, occurring more commonly in the southeastern United States and southern Canada. It occurs in 5% of healthy white children, comprising 30% of all hematuria (Roy, 1998; Fitzwater & Wyatt, 1994). Diagnosis is made by laboratory examination of urine. The calcium/creatinine ratio done on a random urine is elevated (>0.18–0.21 mg/dl). An elevated 24-h calcium excretion (>4 mg/kg/24 hr) confirms the diagnosis. Although rare, renal stones (nephrolithiasis) or calcification (nephrocalcinosis) can occur. If suspected, a renal ultrasound can be included as part of the workup. Idiopathic hypercalciuria and Berger's disease (see section on nephritis) are responsible for 50% or more of cases of isolated hematuria in children.
- *Exercise-induced hematuria* occurs when hematuria is present after vigorous exercise but not at other times.
- Hematuria due to *viral* or *bacterial illnesses* is not uncommon, with adenovirus known to cause hemorrhagic cystitis (Cruz & Spitzer, 1998).
- *Renal trauma* can result in hematuria, but its absence does not rule out damage to the renal system.

RBCs = red blood cells; UTI = urinary tract infection.

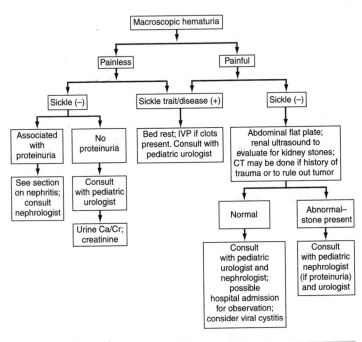

Management of macroscopic hematuria. IVP = intravenous pyelogram; CT = computed tomography; hx = history; r/o = rule out; Ca/Cr = calcium creatinine ratio. (Adapted from Dershewitz RA (ed): Ambulatory Pediatric Care, 3rd ed. Philadelphia, JB Lippincott, 1999.)

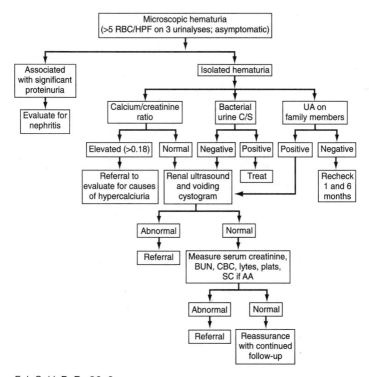

F I G U R E 30–2

Management of asymptomatic microscopic hematuria. C/S = culture/sensitivity; RBC/HPF = red blood cells per high-power field; BUN = blood urea nitrogen; CBC = complete blood count; plats = platelets; SC = sickle cell; AA = African American. (Adapted from Dershewitz RA (ed): Ambulatory Pediatric Care, 3rd ed. Philadelphia, JB Lippincott, 1999.)

T A B L E   30–3

Differential Diagnosis of Proteinuria

Four groups of proteinuria exist: isolated, transient or functional, glomerular, and tubulointerstitial.

- Orthostatic proteinuria and persistent asymptomatic proteinuria comprise the first group, termed *isolated proteinuria,* and are the most common.
    - *Orthostatic proteinuria* accounts for up to 60% (75% in adolescents) of proteinuria (Finberg, 1998; Opas, 1999). In this condition, the child excretes abnormal amounts of protein when upright but normal amounts when lying down. This is demonstrated by collecting a urine specimen immediately on arising and comparing it with a specimen collected after several hours of activity. The child must have voided before sleep to obtain accurate results. A typical result yields negative to trace in the overnight specimen but 1+ or greater in the daytime specimen. If this is equivocal, back-to-back urine specimens (from arising to bedtime and bedtime to arising) to quantify protein are evaluated.
    - *Persistent asymptomatic proteinuria* is a common, transient phenomenon in which an otherwise healthy child has an abnormally high level of protein in the urine but a normal clinical and laboratory workup.
- The second group of proteinuria is *transient* or *functional proteinuria* due to various stressors.
    - *Exercised-induced proteinuria* is documented by collecting a urine sample, having the patient exercise vigorously for several minutes, and then collecting another sample. The postexercise sample is usually strongly positive.
    - *Fever-induced proteinuria* can accompany any febrile state and usually subsides with resolution of the fever. Other stress-related causes include cold exposure, infection, congestive heart failure, and seizures. This proteinuria usually resolves in 1–2 wk and does not require workup.
- The third and fourth groups, *glomerular proteinuria,* typified by glomerulonephritis, and *tubulointerstitial proteinuria* are least common and are identified by high levels of proteinuria. Some authorities believe persistent proteinuria in childhood even at low levels should be placed in this category with a high index of suspicion for an underlying, progressive renal disorder.
- *Pseudoproteinuria* can be caused by semisynthetic penicillins or benzalkonium chloride.

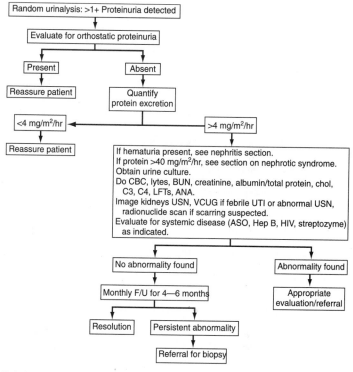

F I G U R E 30–3

Evaluation of proteinuria. alb/TP = albumin/total protein; ASO = antistreptolysin O; BUN = blood urea nitrogen; C3 = complement 3; C4 = complement 4; CBC = complete blood count; chol = cholesterol; Cr = creatinine; FANA = fluorescent antinuclear antibody; F/U = follow-up; HepB = hepatitis B; lytes = electrolytes. (Adapted from Dershewitz RA (ed): Ambulatory Pediatric Care, 3rd ed. Philadelphia, JB Lippincott, 1999.)

T A B L E 30–4
Seven Red Flags for Chronic Renal Failure

1. Failure to thrive (poor growth, fatigue, anorexia, nausea, gastroesophageal reflux, vomiting)
2. Chronic anemia (normochromic, normocytic), nonresponsive to medication
3. Complicated enuresis (daytime frequency, urgency, incontinence, chronic constipation, encopresis, infrequent voiding, straining to void, recurrent urinary tract infection)
4. Prolonged, unexplained vomiting or nausea (especially in the morning), anorexia, weight loss without diarrhea
5. Hypertension
6. Unusual bone disease (rickets, valgus deformity, fracture with minor trauma)
7. Poor school performance (headache, fatigue, inattention, withdrawal from family activity)

Adapted from Vogt BA: Identifying kidney disease: Simple steps can make a difference. Contemp Pediatr 14(3):115–127, 1997.

TABLE 30-5

Clinical Findings of Urinary Tract Infection in Children of Various Ages

NEONATES	INFANTS	TODDLERS AND PRESCHOOLERS	SCHOOL AGE AND ADOLESCENTS
Jaundice	Malaise	Altered voiding pattern	"Classic dysuria" with frequency, urgency, and discomfort
Hypothermia	Irritability	Malodor	Malodor
Failure to thrive	Difficulty feeding	Abdominal/flank pain*	Enuresis
Sepsis	Poor weight gain	Enuresis	Abdominal/flank pain*
Vomiting or diarrhea	Fever*	Vomiting or diarrhea*	Fever/chills*
Cyanosis	Vomiting or diarrhea	Malaise	Vomiting or diarrhea*
Abdominal distention	Malodor	Fever*	Malaise
Lethargy	Dribbling	Diaper rash	
	Abdominal pain/colic		

*Findings especially likely with pyelonephritis.

T A B L E 30-6

Criteria for Diagnosis of Urinary Tract Infections

METHOD OF COLLECTION	COLONY COUNT (PURE CULTURE)	PROBABILITY OF INFECTION (%)
Suprapubic aspiration	Any organism	>99
Catheterization	>10^5	95
	10^4–10^5	Infection likely, especially if obstruction or if frequent voider
	10^3–10^4, single organism	Suspicious, repeat
	<10^3	Infection unlikely
Clean voided		
Boy	>10^4, single organism	Infection likely
Girl	Three specimens >10^5	95
	Two specimens >10^5	90–95
	One specimen >10^5	80–90
	5×10^4–10^5	Suspicious, repeat
	10^4–5×10^4	Symptomatic; suspicious, repeat
	10^4–5×10^4	Asymptomatic; infection unlikely
	<10^4	Infection unlikely

Modified from Feld LG, Greenfield SP, Ogra PL: Urinary tract infections in infants and children. Pediatr Rev 11:72, 1989; updated from Rushton HG: UTI in children: Epidemiology, evaluation & management. Pediatr Clin North Am 44:1139–1169, 1997; Hoberman A, Wald ER: UTI in young children: New light on old questions. Contemp Pediatr 14(11):140–156, 1997; Heldrich FJ: UTI diagnosis: Getting it right the first time. Contemp Pediatr 12(2):110–133, 1995; Opas LM: UTI: Burning issues (unpublished manuscript), Los Angeles, CA, 1999.

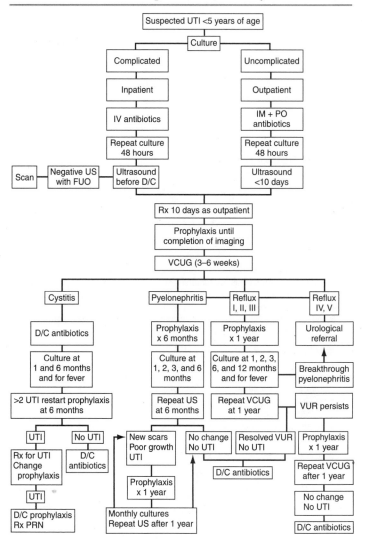

F I G U R E 30–4

Treatment of urinary tract infection (UTI). US = ultrasound; FUO = fever of unknown origin; D/C = discharge; IM = intramuscular; PO = oral; Rx = prescribe; VCUG = voiding cystourethrogram; VUR = vesiculoureteral reflux. (Reproduced with permission from Opas LM: UTI—Burning Issues, Unpublished Manuscript, Los Angeles, CA, 1999.)

T A B L E 30-7

Radiological Workup and Prophylaxis for Urinary Tract Infections

WHY DO A WORKUP?

1. To identify any structural or functional abnormality of the urinary tract
2. To identify any renal scarring or damage

WHO REQUIRES A WORKUP?

Recommendations vary among experts. Those who recommend the most aggressive workup (all children after any infection) do so to identify scarring early and prevent further damage.

1. Infants or any child <5 yr old (Opas, 1999).
2. Any child <8 yr with *acute* symptoms, especially fever or toxicity (at least 50% have reflux or obstructive lesions)
3. Any child with pyelonephritis
4. Males with a first infection; females after a second infection if no other criteria are met
5. Any child with suspicious factors (e.g., high blood pressure, abnormal urine stream, poor growth) or with a positive family history of UTI or abnormal voiding patterns
6. Adolescents with pyelonephritis or after a second UTI with documented culture and no history of recent sexual activity

WHAT SHOULD BE DONE?

1. Renal and bladder ultrasonography: done initially in all children
2. Voiding cystourethrogram: done if ultrasound is abnormal, if child is <5 yr old, or if voiding dysfunction was present before UTI
3. Nuclear imaging scan: done to detect renal scars or parenchymal inflammation
4. Intravenous pyelogram: done if further definition of structure or function of the kidney is needed

WHEN SHOULD IT BE DONE?

1. Ultrasonography: during hospitalization or within 10 d in any child <5 yr old or with complicated UTI
2. VCUG: after urine has become sterile and the patient is asymptomatic. Some authorities recommend 4–6 wk after the diagnosis of UTI
3. As follow-up for pyelonephritis and vesicoureteral reflux

WHEN SHOULD PROPHYLAXIS BE USED?

1. After resolution of UTI and before radiological workup
2. To suppress recurrent UTI after radiological workup

T A B L E 30-7

Radiological Workup and Prophylaxis for Urinary Tract Infections
Continued

WHAT SHOULD BE USED FOR PROPHYLAXIS?

Approximately ⅓ to ½ the treatment dosage of antibiotic should be given at bedtime (Sheldon & Wacksman, 1995).

1. Nitrofurantoin (1 to 2 mg/kg qd or bid if >2 mo of age); expensive
2. TMP (2 mg/kg) + SMX (10 mg/kg) qd if >2 mo of age; TMP (1 mg/kg) + SMX (5 mg/kg) bid (can be used if bedwetting is a problem). A yearly CBC should be done to monitor for neutropenia
3. Sulfisoxazole (50 mg/kg bid if >2 mo of age)
4. Penicillin or ampicillin can be used for a newborn or premature infant

bid = twice daily; CBC = complete blood count; qd = every day; SMX = sulfamethoxazole; TMP = trimethoprim; UTI = urinary tract infection; VCUG = voiding cystourethrography.

for the diagnosis of UTI, and Figure 30-4 illustrates the management of a suspected UTI in children under 5 years of age.

Radiological workup of certain children with a UTI is recommended. Table 30-7 outlines these criteria.

REFERENCES

Boineau FG, Lewy JE: Evaluation of hematuria in children and adolescents. Pediatr Rev 11(4):101-107, 1989.

Cruz CC, Spitzer A: When you find protein or blood in the urine. Contemp Pediatr 15(9):89-109, 1998.

Dershewitz RA (ed): Ambulatory Pediatric Care, 3rd ed., Philadelphia, JB Lippincott, 1999.

Feld LG, Greenfield SP, Ogra PL: Urinary tract infections in infants and children. Pediatr Rev 11:72, 1989.

Feld LG, Waz WG, Perez LM, et al: Hematuria: An integrated medical and surgical approach. Pediatr Clin North Am 44(5):1191-1210, 1997.

Finberg L: Saunders Manual of Pediatric Practice. Philadelphia: WB Saunders, 1998.

Fitzwater PS, Wyatt RS: Hematuria. Pediatr Rev 15(3):102-108, 1994.

Heldrich FJ: UTI diagnosis: Getting it right the first time. Contemp Pediatr 12(2):110-133, 1995.

Hoberman A, Wald ER: UTI in young children: New light on old questions. Contemp Pediatr 14(11):140-156, 1997.

Opas LM: UTI: Burning issues (unpublished manuscript). Los Angeles, 1999.

Roy S: Hematuria. Pediatr Rev 19(6):209-212, 1998.

Rushton HG: UTI in children: Epidemiology, evaluation & management. Pediatr Clin North Am 44(5):1133-1169, 1997.

Sheldon CA, Wacksman J: Vesicoureteral reflux. Pediatr Rev 16(1):22-27, 1995.

Vogt BA: Identifying kidney disease: Simple steps can make a difference. Contemp Pediatr 14(3):115-127, 1997.

CHAPTER 31

Gynecological Conditions

Gynecological issues for pediatric patients range from normal developmental transitions to serious systemic diseases or abnormalities, providing the nurse practitioner with varied and interesting challenges. Establishing a rapport with children and adolescents as well as their parents during health care visits allows for open discussion of what are sometimes considered "personal" or "embarrassing" issues.

LABIAL ADHESIONS

One of the first gynecological conditions the nurse practitioner may see in younger children is labial adhesions or agglutination. Table 31-1 discusses the management of labial adhesions.

MENSTRUAL DISORDERS

As the child matures and reaches adolescence, menstrual disorders arise. Familiarity with the evaluation and treatment of mittelschmerz, dysmenorrhea, dysfunctional uterine bleeding, and endometriosis is essential. Table 31-2 discusses these conditions, and Table 31-3 gives common prostaglandin inhibitor dosages used in their management.

AMENORRHEA

Amenorrhea, although not seen as commonly as other menstrual disorders, has multiple etiologies and a complicated workup. Figure

Treatment of Labial Adhesions

DEGREE OF INVOLVEMENT	TREATMENT	PROGNOSIS
No urinary tract infection, no obstruction, no parental concern.	No treatment. Reassure and observe.	Resolution with puberty and estrogenization of tissue.
Opening ensures urinary and vaginal drainage, but treatment desired.	Apply ointment (e.g., A&D or Vaseline) nightly with cotton tipped swab with gentle pressure. Following separation, maintain good hygiene and mild ointment (e.g., Vaseline) nightly for 6–12 mo.	Separation within 8 wk. If not, double check technique to ensure gentle pressure is being applied. If persists, see use of estrogen cream below.
Urinary and vaginal drainage impaired.	Apply estrogen-containing 1% cream (e.g., Premarin) qd or bid, for 2–3 wk with cotton-tipped swab. Use gentle pressure until separation occurs. Following separation, use Vaseline nightly as outlined above. Alternate treatment is to use transdermal estrogen patch (Climara or FemPatch [change weekly], Alora or Vivelle [change twice a week], or Estraderm [cannot be cut]). Other patches may be cut to alter dosage. Apply near labial adhesions. Continue use for 1 mo following separation (Craighill, 1998).	Separation usually occurs within 8 wk (80–90%) (Emans et al., 1998). If not, check technique to ensure pressure is being applied. If unresponsive, may treat with 5% Xylocaine ointment or EMLA cream and gentle teasing of adhesions with a swab. Always avoid forceful separation.

TABLE 31-2

Evaluation and Treatment of Menstrual Disorders

	ETIOLOGY	HISTORY	PHYSICAL EXAMINATION & LABORATORY TESTS	MANAGEMENT
Mittelschmerz	Pain caused by rapid enlargement of dominant follicle before follicular rupture	Pain midway between cycles; dull, achy pain in lower abdomen lasting few minutes to several hours	Pain to palpation in either or both sides of lower abdomen overlying ovaries	Explain benign nature; heating pad; analgesics, especially PG inhibitors; follow up if pain changes
Dysmenorrhea	Primary: caused by exaggerated production of PGs Secondary: caused by infection, abnormality, or intrauterine device	Onset 6-24 mo after menarche; pain begins with menses, lasts less than 2 d; mild to severe cramping in lower midabdominal area radiating to back, thighs	Normal PE except for pain with examination of lower abdomen; may be pale	PG inhibitors at onset of menses for duration of pain; follow up by phone or if pain changes; refer for gynecological care if fails to respond after 6 mo

Table continued on following page

371

Evaluation and Treatment of Menstrual Disorders Continued

	ETIOLOGY	HISTORY	PHYSICAL EXAMINATION & LABORATORY TESTS	MANAGEMENT
Endometriosis	Bleeding from ectopic endometrial tissue outside pelvic cavity causes pain, irritation of nerve endings, and uterine contractions	Progressive dysmenorrhea; onset before menses continuing for several days; unresponsive to OC or PG inhibitors in moderate to severe forms; irregular or excessive bleeding; bowel and bladder dysfunction; chronic pelvic pain; first-degree relative with endometriosis	Small papules on labia, vagina clear to red; limited or fixed uterine mobility; enlarged ovaries; adnexal masses; pelvic tenderness; uterosacral ligament nodules or tenderness with movement	*Mild to moderate:* PG inhibitors, OC or progestin treatment; recheck 1–3 mo; refer if symptoms persist after 3–6 mo *Severe:* refer for laparoscopy
Dysfunctional uterine bleeding	Defect in the maturation of negative feedback system of estrogen and follicle-stimulating hormone causing disorderly endometrial shedding	Bleeding that may be excessive in quantity or duration, irregular in occurrence	Normal PE except pale if HgB is low; possible petechiae, bruising; observe for androgen excess, galactorrhea; rule out pregnancy, STD	*HgB > 12 g:* PG inhibitor or OC; iron supplement; menstrual calendar; reevaluate in 3 mo *HgB 10–12 g:* as above, OC preferred; folic acid supplement; reevaluate monthly

HgB = hemoglobin; OC = oral contraceptive; PE = physical examination; PG = prostaglandin; STD = sexually transmitted disease.

TABLE 31-3

Common Prostaglandin Inhibitors Used to Treat Adolescent Menstrual Disorders

Ibuprofen (Advil, Motrin), 400–800 mg q4–6h; loading dose of 800 mg
Naproxen, 500 mg at onset followed by 250–375 mg q6–8h
Naproxen sodium (Aleve, Anaprox), 550 mg at onset followed by 275 mg q6h; max dose 1375 mg per 24 hr
Mefenamic acid, 500 mg at onset followed by 250 mg q6h
Flurbiprofen, 50 mg q6h; 100 mg q8–12h
Meclofenamate, 100 mg initially; 50–100 mg q6h

31-1 provides an algorithm to evaluate adolescents with a normal genital tract for amenorrhea.

VAGINITIS

Vaginitis or vulvovaginitis is a common finding in prepubescent females due to lack of estrogen. In adolescent females, it is often (although not always) due to sexual contact. Table 31-4 outlines the evaluation and treatment of vaginitis. Table 31-5 lists general treatment measures.

SEXUALLY TRANSMITTED DISEASES

Multiple organisms are responsible for sexually transmitted diseases (STDs) in children and adolescents. Gonorrhea, syphilis, chlamydia, herpes, and human papillomavirus are the most common. Trichomonas (discussed in Table 31-4), hepatitis B, and human immunodeficiency virus (HIV) also are recognized as STDs. Chapter 19 discusses hepatitis B and HIV. STDs are considered epidemic, with the highest rates occurring in adolescents. Three million reported cases per year, or one in every eight 13- to 19-year-olds, have been documented. Table 31-6 discusses the evaluation and treatment of common STDs. Table 31-7 gives general treatment measures for STDs.

PELVIC INFLAMMATORY DISEASE

Pelvic inflammatory disease (PID) is considered a polymicrobial infection, with gonorrhea and chlamydia the two most common etiologic

Text continued on page 383

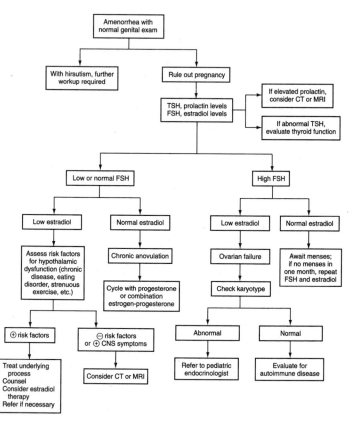

FIGURE 31–1
Amenorrhea with normal genital tract. (From Prose C, Ford C, Lovely L: Evaluating amenorrhea: The pediatrician's role. Contemp Pediatr 15(10):108, 1998.)

TABLE 31-4
Evaluation and Treatment of Vaginitis

	SIGNS AND SYMPTOMS	VAGINAL DISCHARGE	ETIOLOGY	LABORATORY DATA	TREATMENT
Nonspecific vaginitis	Itching; burning; dysuria; varied vulvitis	Scant to copious; brown to green; mucoid; foul smelling	Irritation from contact with various substances; poor hygiene	pH variable; no odor on whiff test; micro: leukocytes, bacteria, debris; normal UA	Refractory cases may need topical estrogen or antibiotics
Physiological leukorrhea	None or minimal itch or burn; minimal vulvitis; 6–12 mo before menarche; small hymenal opening; possible mild erythema	Scant to moderate; clear to white; odorless; nonirritating	Endogenous hormones 6–12 mo before menarche	pH < 4.5; no odor on whiff test; micro: epithelial cells, lactobacilli; normal UA	No treatment needed; explain and reassure
Chemical or mechanical	Itch, erythema, vulvar inflammation, dysuria	Scant amount yellow to white	Bubble bath, perfumed soap, lotion; tight-fitting clothes, sand or dirt from playground	pH < 4.5; no odor on whiff test; micro: leukocytes, epithelial cells	Remove irritant; topical steroids
Foreign body	Dysuria, discomfort, bleeding, minimal vulvar excoriation; history of foreign body in other orifices	Purulent, persistent, dark brown, foul smelling (18%), bloody (82%)	Toilet paper (prepubescent); tampons (adolescent); condoms or object used for masturbation	pH > 4.5; odd odor on whiff test; micro: WBCs, epithelial cells with bacteria and debris; UA normal	Remove foreign body with forceps or by irrigating with saline and small feeding tube; knee-chest position may work best

Table continued on following page

Evaluation and Treatment of Vaginitis Continued

	SIGNS AND SYMPTOMS	VAGINAL DISCHARGE	ETIOLOGY	LABORATORY DATA	TREATMENT
Bacterial	Acute respiratory, enteric, or skin infection	Green color, foul, copious with possible bleeding	*Streptococcus* (most common), *Escherichia coli*, *Enterococcus*, *Shigella*, *Staphylococcus*, or other bacteria	Strep test positive; culture positive	Penicillin, erythromycin, amoxicillin, broad-spectrum cephalosporin or other antibiotic as indicated
Candidiasis	Itching, burning, vulvar inflammation, dysuria, dyspareunia; history of antibiotic or steroid use	Thick, white, curdy cottage cheese adherent, odorless; vulva red, edematous with satellite lesions	Recent antibiotic or steroid use; diabetes or immunodeficiency; *Candida albicans*; pregnancy	pH < 4.5; no odor on whiff test; micro: fungal hyphae and buds or spores, culture positive for *Monilia*; UA with WBCs	Imidazoles or triazoles topically or intravaginally; ketoconazole orally
Pinworms	Recent exposure to pinworms; perineal itching especially at night; anal excoriation, erythema and lesions from scratching	No discharge	*Enterobius vermicularis* spread from anus	Normal UA; tape test reveals eggs	Mebendazole 100 mg once; repeated in 2 wk; treat family members

Condition	Symptoms	Discharge	Organism/Etiology	Diagnostic Findings	Treatment
Bacterial vaginosis (need 3 of 4* findings to diagnose)	Foul odor, especially after menses or intercourse; often asymptomatic; no inflammation; abdominal pain or irregular, prolonged bleeding	Homogenous, thin milky white discharge adherent to vaginal walls and pools in posterior fornix;* increased amount	*Gardnerella vaginalis* and anerobic bacteria; caused by replacement of normal vaginal flora; may or may not be sexually transmitted	pH > 4.5*; fishy odor on whiff test*; micro: clue cells,* few lactobacilli, gram-negative rods, no WBCs	May resolve without treatment. Treat only if symptomatic with metronidazole for 7 d or clindamycin; increased risk for PID
Trichomonas	Lower abdominal discomfort, dysuria, symptoms worse before and after menses; history of sexual contact; vulvar itching and erythema	White to yellow-grey, frothy, foul odor, profuse, purulent, slightly watery; vaginal mucosa erythematous, cervix friable with petechiae	*Trichomonas vaginalis,•* flagellated protozoa, primarily sexually transmitted	pH > 4.5, frequently has fishy odor on whiff test; micro: motile, flagellated organisms, WBC > 10/hpf on UA	Metronidazole for 7-10 d; prepubertal, 15 mg/kg in three divided doses or 40 mg/kg in single dose; postpubertal, 2 g in single dose

hpf = high-power field; micro = microscopic examination; PID = pelvic inflammatory disease; UA = urinalysis; WBC = white blood cell.

General Treatment Measures for Vaginitis

1. Hygiene
   - Wipe front to back
   - Change underwear every day
   - Wash hands frequently
   - Blow-dry perineal area with cool to warm air (especially if overweight)
2. Clothing
   - Wear absorbent white underwear, changing once or twice daily; do not wear underwear at night
   - Wear loose clothing—no pantyhose or tight jeans
   - Avoid spandex and sleeper pajamas
   - Change out of swimsuit after swimming
3. Comfort and healing measures
   - Take Sitz bath with thorough drying
   - Blow-dry for 10–15 min once or twice daily with cool to warm air or pat dry with towel
   - Apply hydrocortisone cream 1% once or twice daily for itching
   - Use oral diphenhydramine or hydroxyzine if itching is severe
4. Protective measures
   - Avoid bubble baths and perfumed lotions or powder
   - Use mild soap, e.g., Dove, Basis, Neutrogena
   - Avoid shampoo in bath water
   - Use protective ointment twice a day (e.g., Vaseline, A&D, Aquaphor)
   - Avoid bleach or fabric softener in wash; double rinse
   - Urinate with knees spread apart to minimize urinary reflux

Evaluation and Treatment of Sexually Transmitted Disease

	HISTORY	PHYSICAL EXAMINATION	ETIOLOGY	LABORATORY DATA	TREATMENT (See Table 31–7 and text for alternative treatment)
Gonorrhea (GC)	Often asymptomatic (33%); dysuria; vaginal discharge or bleeding; dyspareunia	Profuse, thick, green discharge, urethritis, cervicitis; Skene's or Bartholin's gland abscess; exudative pharyngitis	*Neisseria gonorrhoeae*; gram-negative diplococcus; often co-infected with chlamydia (15–20%) and other sexually transmitted diseases (STDs)	Gram's stain; culture; DNA probe for adolescent; rectal and pharyngeal swab if abuse suspected	Ceftriaxone 125 mg (IM) *plus* doxycycline 100 mg bid for 7 d; treat also for chlamydia; test for other STDs including HIV and hepatitis B; report to health department
Chlamydia	Often is asymptomatic (30–70%); spotting, vaginal discharge; dysuria, pyuria; mild abdominal pain or foreign body sensation in eyes possible	Clear to white or yellow discharge, mucopurulent cervicitis with edema, erythema, hypertrophy; Fitz-Hugh-Curtis syndrome (right upper quadrant pain); conjunctivitis	*Chlamydia trachomatis*; often co-infected with GC and other STDs; autoinoculation of eyes	Cell cultures; DNA probe in adolescent especially if part of high-prevalence population; direct fluorescent antibody (DFA) or enzyme immunoassays (EIA), polymerase chain reaction (PCR) or LCR, or TMA	Doxycycline 100 mg bid for 7 d or azithromycin 1 g single dose; test for other STDs; report to state health

Table continued on following page

TABLE 31-6

Evaluation and Treatment of Sexually Transmitted Disease Continued

	HISTORY	PHYSICAL EXAMINATION	ETIOLOGY	LABORATORY DATA	TREATMENT (See Table 31-7 and text for alternative treatment)
Syphilis	*Primary:* vaginal, anal, or oral chancre. *Secondary:* copper-penny rash especially on palms and soles, adenopathy, alopecia	Single painless papule with serous discharge, smooth base, raised edges; painless regional lymphadenopathy	*Treponema pallidum,* a motile spirochete	Dark-field microscopy, DFA; *nontreponemal tests:* venereal disease research laboratory (VDRL), rapid plasma reagin (RPR), automated reagin test (ART) to follow disease activity; *treponemal tests:* fluorescent treponemal anti-body resorption (FTA-ABS), micro-hemagglutination assay *Treponema pallidum* (MHA-TP) to confirm	Penicillin G IM 2.4 million units; refer if secondary or tertiary disease; follow with nontreponemal tests every 6–12 mo; test for other STDs; report to health department

Herpes simplex (HSV)	Painful rash, blisters and ulcers; HSV-1 of mouth and face; burning and irritation 24 hr before; dysuria; other systemic complaints	Clear to white to yellow discharge; vesicles on erythematous base that become ulcers in 1–3 d; extragenital lesions	HSV types 1 and 2, DNA virus from direct contact	Culture; Tzanck stain or DFA are presumptive	Acyclovir, famciclovir, or valacyclovir for 7–10 d; sitz bath, dry heat, lidocaine jelly 2%; candida often accompanies or follows
Human papillomavirus (HPV)	Asymptomatic or subclinical unrecognized; can be painful	Warts, friable and/or pruritic; moist, cauliflower-like anogenital and inguinal 4–6 wk after exposure	Small DNA virus, 20 types can infect genital tract; visible warts: types 6 and 11; anogenital warts; 16, 18, 31, 33, 35	Virapap; Papanicolaou smear (koilocytosis, squamous atypia, squamous intraepithelial lesions); biopsy rarely needed; DNA/PCR screen	*Patient applied:* podofilox or imiquimod; *Provider applied:* cryotherapy, podophyllin resin, trichloroacetic acid or bichloroacetic acid, or surgical removal

HIV = human immunodeficiency virus; LCR = ligase chain reduction; TMA = transcription mediated amplification.

T A B L E 31-7

General Treatment Measures for Sexually Transmitted Diseases

1. Have patient abstain from sexual intercourse until patient and partner are cured (treatment complete and symptoms resolved). Consequences of untreated sexually transmitted diseases (STDs) should be explained.
2. Test for other STDs, including human immunodeficiency virus, bacterial vaginosis, and trichomonas.
3. Notify, examine, and treat all partners of patient for any STD identified or suspected.
4. Report STDs (include gonorrhea and syphilis in every state, and chlamydia in most states). Check with the health department. Reporting to appropriate authorities is important to identify those at risk, recognize new strains, and assess extent of infection in community and the effect of prevention efforts.
5. Provide regular sex health assessment including Papanicolaou smears, vaginal examination, and testing for STDs.
6. Give hepatitis B vaccine if not done already.
7. Discuss safer sex practices including abstinence and use of condoms.
8. Educate and counsel about complications and transmission of STDs as well as perinatal consequences.

TABLE 31-8

Criteria for Diagnosing Pelvic Inflammatory Disease

Minimum criteria for treating pelvic inflammatory disease (PID) in sexually active adolescents with no other cause for illness identified:
  Lower abdominal tenderness
  Adnexal tenderness
  Cervical motion tenderness
Additional criteria that support a diagnosis of PID:
  Oral temperature > 101°F
  Abnormal cervical or vaginal discharge
  Elevated erythrocyte sedimentation rate
  Elevated C-reactive protein
  Laboratory documentation of cervical infection with gonorrhea or chlamydia
Definitive criteria for diagnosing PID, warranted in selected cases:
  Histopathological evidence of endometritis on endometrial biopsy
  Transvaginal sonography or other imaging techniques showing thickened fluid-filled tubes with or without free pelvic fluid or tubo-ovarian complex
  Laparoscopic abnormalities consistent with PID

Adapted from Centers for Disease Control and Prevention: Guidelines for treatment of sexually transmitted diseases. MMWR Morbid Mortal Wkly Rep 47(RR-1)i-116, 1998; and American Academy of Pediatrics Committee on Infectious Diseases: 1997 Red Book: Report of the Committee on Infectious Diseases, 24th ed. Elk Grove Village, IL, American Academy of Pediatrics, 1997.

agents. Diagnosis of PID requires a high index of suspicion, as it is often subtle in presentation and can go undiagnosed, thus contributing to its inflammatory sequelae. Table 31-8 lists criteria for the diagnosis of PID.

REFERENCES

American Academy of Pediatrics Committee on Infectious Diseases: 1997 Red Book: Report of the Committee on Infectious Diseases, 24th ed. Elk Grove Village, IL, American Academy of Pediatrics, 1997.

Centers for Disease Control and Prevention: Guidelines for treatment of sexually transmitted diseases. MMWR Morbid Mortal Wkly Rep 47(RR-1):i-116, 1998.

Craighill MC: Pediatric and adolescent gynecology for the primary care pediatrician. Pediatr Clin North Am 45(6):1659-1688, 1998.

Emans S, Lauter MR, Goldstein D: Pediatric and Adolescent Gynecology, 4th ed. Philadelphia, Lippincott-Raven, 1998.

Prose CC, Ford CA, Lovely LP: Evaluating amenorrhea: The pediatrician's role. Contemp Pediatr 15(10):83-110, 1998.

CHAPTER 32

Dermatological Diseases

ASSESSMENT OF THE SKIN

Disruptions of the skin account for 20 to 30% of all pediatric office visits. Important factors to consider in approaching a child with a dermatological condition are listed in Table 32–1. Proper description of the lesion is important in making a diagnosis, following a patient who is being treated, and facilitating communication between providers. Correct terminology is outlined in Table 32–2.

A few simple laboratory tests done on skin, nail scrapings, or hair roots are helpful in confirming dermatological conditions. These include:

- Potassium hydroxide (for hyphae or spores, fungal disorders)
- Gram's stain (for bacteria or herpes simplex virus or herpes zoster [giant cells])
- Tzanck smear (for herpes simplex, varicella, or herpes zoster)
- Culture (for bacteria, viruses, or fungi)

TABLE 32–1

Key Factors in Approaching a Child with a Dermatological Condition

- The three most common presenting complaints are pruritus, scaling, and cosmetic appearance (Weston, et al., 1996)
- Three questions to ask
  - How long have you had it, and how has it changed?
  - Does it itch?
  - What have you done to treat it?
- Key assessment is "Does the patient appear ill?" (differentiate few serious illnesses from the majority of remaining dermatological conditions)

T A B L E 32–2

Primary and Secondary Skin Changes and Vascular Lesions

Primary skin changes

Macule: flat, nonpalpable, discolored lesion ≤1 cm
Patch: macule >1 cm
Papule: solid, raised lesion of varied color with distinct borders ≤1 cm
Plaque: solid, raised, flat-topped lesion with distinct borders >1 cm
Nodule: raised, firm, movable lesion with indistinct borders and deep
palpable portion ≤2 cm
Tumor: large nodule, may be firm or soft
Wheal: fleeting, irregularly shaped, elevated, itchy lesion of varied size,
pale at center, slightly red at borders
Vesicle: blister filled with clear fluid
Bulla: vesicle >1 cm
Cyst: palpable lesion with definite borders filled with liquid or semisolid
material
Pustule: raised lesion filled with pus, often in hair follicle or sweat pore
Comedo: plugged, dilated pore; open (blackhead), closed (whitehead)

Secondary skin changes

Crusting: dried exudate or scab of varied color
Scaling: thin, flaking layers of epidermis
Desquamation: peeling sheets of scale
Lichenification: thickening of skin with deep visible furrows
Excoriation: abrasion or removal of epidermis, scratch
Fissure: linear, wedge-shaped cracks extending into dermis
Erosion: oozing or moist, depressed area with loss of superficial epidermis
Ulcer: deeper than erosion, open lesion extending into dermis
Atrophy: thinning skin, may appear translucent
Scar: healed lesion of connective tissue
Keloid: healed lesion of hypertrophied connective tissue
Striae: fine pink or silver lines in areas where skin has been stretched

Vascular skin lesions

Angioma or hemangioma: papule made of blood vessels
Ecchymosis: bruise, purple to brown in color, macular or papular, varied in
size
Hematoma: collection of blood from ruptured blood vessels >1 cm
Petechiae: pinpoint, pink to purple macular lesions 1–3 mm that do not
blanch
Purpura: purple macular lesion >1 cm
Telangiectasis: macular or raised, dilated capillaries

CARE AND TREATMENT OF THE SKIN

General management strategies include attention to hydration and lubrication (bathing, environment, fluid intake, skin care agents, and wet or occlusive dressings) as well as medications. Thought must be given to topical therapies that are used. Figure 32-1 describes various preparations or vehicles.

Topical steroid preparations, listed in Table 32-3, are frequently used to vasoconstrict, reduce inflammation, and decrease itching.

BACTERIAL, FUNGAL, AND VIRAL INFECTIONS

Rashes caused by bacterial, fungal, and viral infections are common in pediatrics. Impetigo, cellulitis, and folliculitis are common bacterial infections discussed in Table 32-4. Differentiation and management of common fungal infections are outlined in Table 32-5.

Viral infection is responsible for a multitude of rashes in children. Chapter 19 discusses some of these conditions. Diagnosis and management of herpes simplex and herpes zoster are discussed in Table 32-6, and treatment options for warts are listed in Table 32-7.

INFESTATIONS

Infestations with head lice and scabies are also common in pediatrics. Table 32-8 describes these conditions.

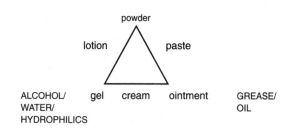

F I G U R E 32-1
Vehicles for dermatologic therapy.

T A B L E 32–3
Topical Steroid Preparations

DRUG (BRAND NAME)	DOSAGE FORM
LOW POTENCY	
Alclometasone dipropionate (Aclovate)	0.05% cream, ointment
Desonide (DesOwen, Tridesilon)	0.05% cream, ointment, lotion
Fluocinolone acetonide (Fluonid, Synalar)	0.01% solution
	0.5% cream, ointment
Hydrocortisone (Hytone, Nutracort, Cort-Dome, Synacort)	1% cream, ointment, lotion, solution
	2.5% cream, ointment
MODERATE POTENCY	
Betamethasone valerate (Valisone)	0.01% cream
	0.1% cream, ointment, lotion
Clocortolone pivalate (Cloderm)	0.1% cream
Desoximetasone (Topicort)	0.05% gel, cream
Fluocinolone acetonide (Synalar, Fluonid)	0.025% cream, ointment
	0.1% cream
Flurandrenolide (Cordran)	0.05% cream, lotion, ointment
Halcinonide (Halog)	0.025% cream
Hydrocortisone valerate (Westcort)	0.2% cream, ointment
Triamcinolone acetonide (Kenalog, Aristocort)	0.025%, 0.1% cream, ointment, lotion

Table continued on following page

TABLE 32-3

Topical Steroid Preparations Continued

DRUG (BRAND NAME)	DOSAGE FORM
HIGH POTENCY	
Amcinonide (Cyclocort)	0.1% cream, ointment
Betamethasone dipropionate (Diprosone)	0.05% cream, lotion, ointment, gel
Betamethasone dipropionate; clotrimazole (Lotrisone)	0.05% betamethasone; 1% clotrimazole cream
Desoximetasone (Topicort)	0.25% cream, ointment
Diflorasone diacetate (Florone)	0.05% cream, ointment
Fluocinolone acetonide (Synalar-HP)	0.2% cream
Fluocinonide (Lidex)	0.05% cream, solution, gel, ointment
Halcinonide (Halog)	0.1% cream, ointment, solution
Halobetasol propionate (Ultravate)	0.05% cream, ointment
Triamcinolone acetonide (Kenalog, Aristocort)	0.5% cream, ointment

T A B L E 32-4
Diagnosis and Treatment of Common Bacterial Infections

INFECTION	CAUSATIVE ORGANISM	PRESENTATION	AREA OF INVOLVEMENT	TREATMENT	PREVENTION
Impetigo	*Staphylococcus aureus* or *Streptococcus*	Honey-colored crust on erythematous base, or blisters that rupture, leaving varnish-like coat	Superficial layers of skin	Topical antibiotic if minor, oral antibiotics if more significant infection (cephalexin, dicloxacillin, cloxacillin, or erythromycin)	Moisturize skin; thorough cleansing of any break in skin
Cellulitis	Most commonly *Streptococcus*	Erythema, swelling, tenderness	Dermis and subcutaneous tissue	Oral antibiotic depending on likely organism; often penicillin or dicloxacillin	Same as above
Folliculitis	*Staphylococcus aureus*	Pruritus, erythematous papule or pustule at hair follicle	Hair follicle	Warm compresses, topical keratolytics, topical antibiotics, or antistaphylococcal antibiotic if severe	Same as above; good hygiene and antibacterial soap

Diagnosis and Treatment of Common Fungal Infections

INFECTION	CAUSATIVE ORGANISM	CLINICAL FINDINGS	MANAGEMENT	COMPLICATIONS
Candidiasis	Candida albicans	Moist, bright-red diaper rash with sharp borders, satellite lesions; associated white spots in mouth, mucous membranes, or corner of mouth	Topical or oral antifungal, generally nystatin; diaper area hygiene	Paronychia or onychomycosis
Tinea corporis	Trichophyton tonsurans, Microsporum canis, Epidermophyton floccosum	Pruritic, slightly erythematous circular lesion with a slightly raised border and central clearing; well demarcated	Topical antifungals; identify and treat source; exclude from day care until treated	Tinea incognita from steroid treatment
Tinea cruris	Same as for tinea corporis	Raised-border, scaly lesion on upper thighs and groin; penis and scrotum spared; symmetrical	Same as for tinea corporis; loose clothes, absorbent powder	Possible secondary infection

| Tinea pedis | Same as for tinea corporis | Vesicles and erosions on instep; fissure between toes with scaling and erythema; diffuse scaling on weight-bearing surfaces with exaggerated scaling in creases; pruritus | Same as for tinea corporis; absorbent powder; cotton socks; open-toed shoes; moisturize | Reinfection common |
| Tinea versicolor | *Malassezia furfur* or *Malassezia ovalis* | Multiple scaly, discrete oval macules on neck, shoulders, upper back, and chest; hypo- to hyperpigmented areas; fail to tan in summer | Selenium shampoo from face to knees overnight once a week × 4 wk or 10–30 min qd for 7–14 d or qd for 1 wk then wkly for 1 mo; topical imidazoles | 50% recurrence rate |

TABLE 32–6
Diagnosis and Treatment of Herpes Simplex (HS) and Herpes Zoster (HZ)

	PRESENTATION	CLINICAL FINDINGS	TREATMENT	EDUCATION
HS	Gingivostomatitis as primary infection; herpes labialis or herpes facialis as recurrent infection	Pharyngitis with erythematous vesicles on/in mouth; small, clear vesicles on erythematous base progressing to crusting	Burow's solution; acyclovir in primary case or underlying disorder; antibiotics if secondary infection; oral anesthetics; supportive care	Degree and duration of contagion; triggers to infection
HZ	Reactivation of latent varicella virus, especially after mild cases or in infants <1 yr of age or immuno-compromised host	2–3 clustered groups of vesicles on erythematous base, especially over thoracic or lumbosacral dermatomes	Burow's solution; antihistamine; drying lotions; possible acyclovir; silver sulfadiazine (Silvadene cream); antibiotics if secondary infection	New vesicles occur for up to 1 wk; takes 2–3 wk to resolve; contagious for varicella; vaccine to prevent varicella

T A B L E 32–7

Treatment Options for Warts

Keratolytics eliminate the wart by causing topical peeling and an inflammatory response. They are often available over the counter, cause little pain, and are low in cost and risk, but are slow to work.

Salicylic acid paints with a concentration of >20% are applied with a toothpick once or twice a day for 4–6 wk. On thick skin, a combination of 16.7% salicylic acid and 16.7% collodion is more effective. This method is useful for common or periungual warts and is not effective with warts >5 mm in diameter.

Salicylic acid plasters with 40% concentration are cut to size and taped in place for 3–5 d. After the plaster is taken off, the area should be soaked for 45 min and the dead epidermis removed. A new plaster is then applied. Treatment can last 3–6 wk. This method is useful for plantar warts.

Retinoic acid cream 0.025–0.05% applied once or twice daily brings resolution in 4–6 wk. This method is useful for flat warts, but does not work for common, plantar, or periungual warts.

Occlusion with tape for 6½ days, off ½ day followed by scraping of epidermis; painless, easy, and inexpensive (Siegfried, 1996).

Hyperthermia treatments (a 30-min water bath, 3 times a week at 45°C) has produced improvement within 3 wk (Siegfried, 1996).

Destructive agents eliminate the wart by causing necrosis and blister formation. Most techniques are painful and require patient cooperation.

Cryotherapy. Liquid nitrogen or CO_2 snow (dry ice) is applied for 10–30 sec after an area 1–3 mm beyond the wart turns white or patient complains of pain. This is the treatment of choice for common warts and an alternative for venereal warts. It should not be used with periungual or plantar warts, or in warts >7 mm in size, because of the chance of scarring. Retreatment is often necessary.

Cantharidin 0.7% applied directly to wart with a toothpick and covered with tape for 24 hr. This creates a blister in 2–3 d, which is sloughed after 7–14 d. This method is useful for periungual and some plantar warts.

Podophyllum 25% solution in alcohol applied to wart with a toothpick; may be repeated in 1 wk. Podofilox, available over the counter for home use, is applied twice a day for 3 d. After a 4-d rest period, the 3-d cycle may be repeated as necessary. This technique is useful for common or genital warts.

Surgery by snipping with scissors, not scalpel, is useful for filiform warts.

Electrocautery, CO_2 or pulsed laser, and bleomycin injections are other options but require anesthesia, are expensive, are more likely to scar, and often have recurrences.

Immunotherapy modalities stimulate an immune response to HPV. These newer treatment modalities do not have controlled studies evaluating their effectiveness.

Contact sensitization and interferon injection are methods used by dermatologists, usually in adult patients.

Cimetidine is a painless, low-risk, moderate-cost option with questionable efficacy used for common and plantar warts. A dose of 30–40 mg/kg/d orally in three divided doses for 2 mo has been used in clinical trials. This is usually used in conjunction with another method and often used for resistant cases (Friedlander, 1997; Siegfried, 1996).

HPV = human papillomavirus.

TABLE 32-8
Diagnosis and Treatment of Pediculosis and Scabies

	CLINICAL FINDINGS	TREATMENT
Pediculosis (head lice)	History of infestation; itchy scalp, scratches; postoccipital nodes; occasional visualization of mites or nits (small white oval cases), commonly on back of head, nape of neck, behind ears, possibly eyelashes	Key to treatment is proper technique! *First step* is pediculocide (permethrin or pyrethrin) *Second step* is removal of nits by combing hair with fine-toothed comb in 1-in sections with special attention to nape of neck and behind ears *Third step* is to cleanse the environment: check family, friends, day care/school contacts; clean sheets, towels, clothing, headgear; store other things in plastic for 2 wk; vacuum; soak brushes and combs; follow up in 2 wk with daily recheck at home; return to school after treatment
Scabies	*Key finding:* itching, worse at night, and complaints more significant than findings; fitful sleep, crankiness; curving burrows, especially in webs of fingers, sides of hands, folds of wrist, armpits, forearms, elbows, belt line, buttocks, proximal half of foot and heel; may be <10 lesions total; secondary excoriation; infants may have lesions on palms, soles, scalp, face, posterior auricle and axilla, folds, red-brown in color, dozens in number	Pharmacological treatment with permethrin 5%, repeated in 1 wk; antihistamine, hydrocortisone, nonsteroidal anti-inflammatory drugs for itching; simultaneously treat family members (even if asymptomatic), friends, school/day care contacts; cleanse environment: linens and clothing, vacuum, store anything else in plastic bags for 1 wk; rash and itch persist for up to 3 wk after treatment; return to school 24 hr after treatment

T A B L E 32-9
Treatment of Acne

TYPE OF ACNE	LESIONS	INITIAL TREATMENT	IF NOT IMPROVING
Comedonal	Open or closed comedones	Benzoyl peroxide 5% qd (if mild) or Tretinoin (Retin A) 0.025% cream qd (if moderate)	Combine benzoyl peroxide with tretinoin or Increase strength to 0.05%
Mild papulopustular	Red papules, few pustules	Benzoyl peroxide 5–10% qd or Azelaic acid bid (if mild) or Topical antibiotic bid or Erythromycin 3% with 5% benzoyl peroxide qd–bid (if moderate)	Increase benzoyl peroxide to bid or Combine benzoyl peroxide with tretinoin (for comedones) Substitute topical antibiotic bid (for inflammatory)
Moderate to severe papulopustular	Red papules, many pustules	Benzoyl peroxide 5% **and** tretinoin 0.025% or Azelaic acid (if comedonal) or Topical antibiotic bid (if no comedones) **and** oral antibiotic bid	Increase strength of treatment or Refer to dermatologist
Nodulocystic, scarring, or unresponsive	Red papules, pustules, cysts, and nodules	Oral antibiotics (tetracycline, erythromycin, minocin) bid and tretinoin 0.05% qd and benzoyl peroxide 10% gel bid (if comedonal)	Refer to dermatologist for oral isotretinoin

T A B L E 32–10

Diagnosis and Treatment of Diaper Dermatitis

TYPE	CAUSE	PRESENTATION AND LOCATION	OTHER CHARACTERISTICS	TREATMENT
Irritant contact dermatitis	Related to wearing diapers; contact with urine and feces	Chapped, shiny, erythematous, parchment-like skin with possible erosions on convex surfaces; creases spared	Peak at 9–12 mo; may progress to involve creases; skin may be dry	Frequent diaper changes, gentle cleansing; greasy lubricant; sitz bath, air-dry; hydrocortisone for inflammation
Candidiasis	Related to wearing diapers; a superinfection with Candida	Shallow pustules, fiery-red scaly plaques on convex surfaces, inguinal folds, labia, and scrotum	Satellite lesions, oral thrush; recent antibiotic or diarrhea; occurs at any age	Antifungal cream plus same measures as for contact dermatitis
Miliaria or intertrigo	Related to wearing diapers; due to heat and occlusion	Discrete vesicles or papules (miliaria); erythematous, scaly, maceration in folds of skin	Sweat retention or friction associated	Self-limited (miliaria); avoid precipitating factors; care as for contact dermatitis
Seborrhea	Exaggerated by wearing diapers; overgrowth of Malassezia yeast in areas of sebaceous gland activity	Greasy, erythematous scales, well circumscribed in creases of skin, groin; spared convex surfaces	Onset at 3–4 wk of age; also occurs on face or body; often superinfected with Candida	Topical ketoconazole is treatment of choice, or hydrocortisone

Atopic dermatitis (AD)	Exaggerated by wearing diapers; exact cause unknown	Increased number of lines in skin; areas of excoriation in folds and convex surfaces and buttocks; less widespread	AD in other areas; usually begins in first year of life; scratches skin with diaper change	Skin care as for contact dermatitis and as indicated for AD (see Chapter 21)
Psoriasis	Exaggerated by wearing diapers; psoriasis evolves as response to chronic trauma	Erythematous, well-defined sharp, scaly plaques on convex surfaces and inguinal folds; less widespread	Psoriasis affects other places; rare occurrence, if found, usually at 6–18 mo	Treatment often required for weeks or until toilet trained; steroids; topical ketoconazole if Candida present
Bacterial dermatitis	Usually due to staphylococcal or streptococcal infection	Red, denuded areas or fragile blisters; crusting and pustules in suprapubic area and periumbilicus	Usually in newborn, can occur anywhere	Econazole or ketoconazole cream if yeast present as well; mupirocin if minimal; cephalexin or oral erythromycin if extensive

T A B L E 32–11

Differentiating Drug Eruptions, Urticaria, and Erythema Multiforme

	ETIOLOGY	CLINICAL FINDINGS	TREATMENT
Drug eruption	Reaction to medication, especially penicillin, cephalexin, erythromycin, sulfa drugs, NSAIDs, barbiturates, isoniazid, carbamazepam, phenytoin	Symmetrical, macular, erythematous to papular, confluent morbilliform rash; intense itching; patches of normal skin throughout; begins on trunk, extends distally, including palms and soles; face with confluent erythema	Stop drug and label as allergen to the child; antihistamine, antipruritics, lubricate skin; prednisone if severe; rash can last 7–14 d; medical alert bracelet
Urticaria	Hypersensitive reaction; immunological antigen-antibody response to release of histamines; often unknown cause; possible reaction to food, drug, insect bite/sting, pollen; possible reaction to infection, especially streptococcal, sinus, mononucleosis, hepatitis	Family history of hives; rapid onset; possible atopy; intense itching; mild erythema, annular, raised wheals with pale centers; lesions scattered or coalesced; *Key finding:* appear suddenly, fade from 20 min to 24 hr; blanch with pressure; associated edema of eyelids, lips, tongue, hands, feet	Quick resolution; identify and remove or treat offending agent if possible; stop antibiotic; give oral antihistamines; topical antipruritics; epinephrine or prednisone if anaphylactic, angioedema, or refractory; refer if >6 wk duration

| Erythema multiforme (minor) | Immune-mediated hypersensitivity reaction often to infection, especially HSV, also to many other agents | History of infection, especially herpes labialis; variety of lesions on skin and mucous membranes—macules, papules, vesicles, early lesions like urticaria; *Key findings:* target or iris lesions; lesions fixed, symmetrical, typical distribution on hands, feet, elbows, knees, also face, neck, trunk; possible oral mucous membrane involvement | Identify, treat, discontinue trigger if possible; treat infection; supportive measures for hydration, prevention of secondary infection, relief of pain; oral antihistamines, cool compresses; oral lesions—mouthwash, topical anesthetics; lesions last 5–7 d, recur in batches over 2–4 wk, resolve without scarring or sequelae |

NSAIDs = nonsteroidal anti-inflammatory drugs; HSV = herpes simplex virus.

Diagnosis and Treatment of Other Less Common Skin Conditions

DIAGNOSIS	ETIOLOGY	CLINICAL FINDINGS	LABORATORY TESTS	TREATMENT	COMMENTS
Pityriasis rosea	• Probably viral, although specific organism unknown • Minimally contagious • Occurs most commonly in fall, early winter, and spring months in temperate climates • Greatest incidence 10–35 year olds (Hebert & Goller, 1996; Bloomfield, 1994)	• ± mild malaise and fever before eruption of rash • 1–10 mm solitary, ovoid, slightly erythematous herald spot 1–30 d before onset of papulosquamous rash that typically erupts on trunk and proximal extremities from neck to knees in a Christmas tree pattern, especially on back • Oval lesions of punctate hemorrhages, erosions, ulcerations, erythematous macules or annular plaques	• KOH of skin scraping to r/o tinea • VDRL to r/o secondary syphilis	• None • Patient education includes reassurance, spontaneous resolution in 4–12 wk, 2% chance of recurrence (Hebert & Goller, 1996), transient pigmentary changes can occur	• Is common, mild, and self-limited • 10–15% have atypical symptoms (urticaria, purpuric or lichenoid variants, absence of herald patch [Bloomfield, 1994]) • Differential diagnosis: psoriasis, scabies, tinea, syphilis, drug eruptions, viral exanthems

Psoriasis			
• History of recent streptococcal infection • Likely familial predisposition • Trauma, stress • Drug exposure (corticosteroids, lithium, NSAIDs)	• Chronic condition with spontaneous remissions and exacerbations • Discrete, initially erythematous, symmetrical becoming papular with silvery scales; commonly along hairline, external ears, elbows, knees, buttocks, ± face; in areas of trauma (genitalia, palms, soles) • Bleeding when scale removed • Nails show "ice pick" pits/ridges, (thick and discolored); splinter hemorrhages, can separate from nailbed	• r/o strep if gluttate pattern • KOH to r/o fungal infection • VDRL to r/o secondary syphilis	• Moderate sun exposure/UV treatment, avoiding sunburn • Topical steroids (moderate or strong) sometimes fluorinated tid • Tar or kerolytic shampoo • Mineral oil and warm towels to soak and remove plaques • Kerolytic agents (3% sulfur or 6% salicylic acid) to reduce unresponsive plaques • Tar preparation alone or combined with UV treatments • Anthralin for plaques resistant to steroids and tars • Vitamin D analog • Follow up every 2 wk until controlled • Refer to dermatologist if unresponsive to above treatments	Variations include • Acute guttate (teardrop) on trunk, proximal extremities, occasionally on face, rarely on palms or soles; less scaling than psoriasis vulgaris • Psoriasis vulgaris: silvery scales on elbows, knees, scalp, hairline, eyebrow, around ears, intergluteal folds, genital area • Napkin psoriasis: occurs in diaper area in infants • Differential diagnosis: pityriasis rosea, seborrhea, candida, contact dermatitis, atopic dermatitis, tinea, dyshidrosis, secondary syphilis

Table continued on following page

Diagnosis and Treatment of Other Less Common Skin Conditions Continued

DIAGNOSIS	ETIOLOGY	CLINICAL FINDINGS	LABORATORY TESTS	TREATMENT	COMMENTS
Traumatic alopecia	• Chemical • Thermal • Traction (hairstyling) • Friction (trichotillomania)	• Traumatic: incomplete hair loss with varying lengths • Traction: erythema and pustules, thins and breaks in certain areas, especially linear • Trichotillomania: circumscribed hair loss with irregular borders and broken hair of varied lengths, no erythema or scarring, especially frontal, parietal, or temporal	• Hair follicle culture and r/o tinea	• Traction: avoid hairstyles that precipitate; mild shampoo, gentle brushing; short course of antibiotics if pustules • Trichotillomania: discussion with parents, oil at night, counseling if entrenched, other interventions if significant	

KOH = potassium hydroxide; NSAID = nonsteroidal anti-inflammatory drug; r/o = rule out; tid = three times daily; UV = ultraviolet; VDRL = Venereal Disease Research Laboratory.

ALLERGIC AND INFLAMMATORY REACTIONS

There are a variety of allergic and inflammatory reactions seen in pediatrics, with acne and diaper dermatitis being the two most common. The severity of acne is determined by the quantity, type, and spread of lesions. Noninflammatory acne lesions (open comedo or blackhead and closed comedo or whitehead) and inflammatory acne lesions (papules, pustules, excoriations, nodules, cysts, scars, and sinus tracts) should be differentiated to determine appropriate treatment. Management of these conditions is discussed in Tables 32-9 and 32-10.

VASCULAR REACTIONS

Vascular reactions (drug eruptions, urticarias, erythema multiforme) are rashes that the nurse practitioner must often differentiate. Table 32-11 addresses these reactions.

PITYRIASIS ROSEA, PSORIASIS, AND TRAUMATIC ALOPECIA

There are a multitude of other dermatological conditions that the nurse practitioner may see in everyday practice, some relatively common, some quite rare. Pityriasis rosea, psoriasis, and traumatic alopecia are three of the more common ones discussed in Table 32-12.

REFERENCES

Bloomfield D: Pityriasis rosea. Pediatr Rev 15(4):159-160, 1994.

Friedlander SF: Pediatric Exanthems. Presented at the 55th Annual Meeting of the American Academy of Dermatologists, San Francisco, March 21-26, 1997.

Hebert AA, Goller MM: Papulosquamous disorders in the pediatric patient. Contemp Pediatr 13(2):69-88, 1996.

Siegfried EC: Warts on children: An approach to therapy. Pediatr Ann 25:75-90, 1996.

Weston WL, Lane AT, Morelli JG: Color Textbook of Pediatric Dermatology, 2nd ed. St. Louis, Mosby-Year Book, 1996.

CHAPTER 33

Musculoskeletal Disorders

INTRODUCTION

Because there are many normal variations in musculoskeletal development during the newborn period through early childhood, the nurse practitioner must be able to differentiate normal age-related musculoskeletal findings from those that represent pathological conditions. The nurse practitioner in a primary care setting also is likely to be involved in the assessment and management of musculoskeletal injuries (e.g., fractures, sprain, strains, and overuse syndromes) and common disorders. This chapter discusses these conditions and focuses on their early detection.

SPECIAL EXAMINATIONS OF THE MUSCULOSKELETAL SYSTEM

The physical examination is the key to diagnosing developmental dysplasia of the hip (Figs. 33-1 and 33-2), rotational problems of the hips and tibia (Figs. 33-3 and 33-4), scoliosis (Fig. 33-5), and metatarsus adductus (Fig. 33-6).

COMMON UPPER EXTREMITY PROBLEMS

Table 33-1 summarizes the assessment and management of brachial plexus injury and fractured clavicle, two upper extremity problems most commonly seen in the neonate.

BACK PROBLEMS: SCOLIOSIS, KYPHOSIS, AND LORDOSIS

Table 33-2 summarizes the characteristic findings and treatment of scoliosis, kyphosis, and lordosis. Early identification of scoliosis and referral to an orthopedic surgeon are important to prevent further lateral curvature of the spine (see Fig. 33-5).

MUSCULOSKELETAL PROBLEMS ASSOCIATED WITH LIMPING

Table 33-3 gives an overview of the significant orthopedic conditions and diseases that are associated with limping in children. These problems generally should be referred to an orthopedic surgeon for treatment. In addition to the initial assessment and referral, the nurse practitioner may be called on to help the family cope with issues of disability, deformity, and long-term care.

OVERUSE SYNDROMES

Overuse syndromes are due to repetitive movements that cause microtrauma. Treatment often involves rest, icing the joint or extremity, doing retraining and strengthening exercises, prescribing analgesics, and gradually reintroducing activities (Table 33-4).

ROTATIONAL CONCERNS AND PROBLEMS OF THE LOWER EXTREMITIES

Many rotational problems are just variants of normal in the growing child. Table 33-5 identifies typical rotational findings in normal and pathological conditions.

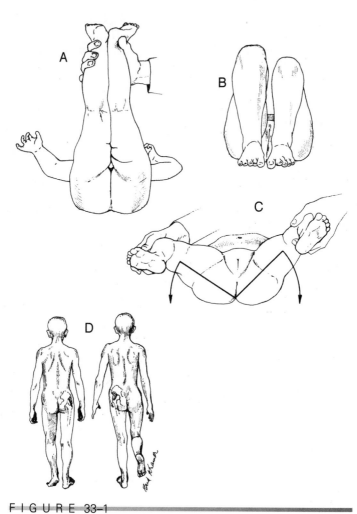

ABDUCTION TEST

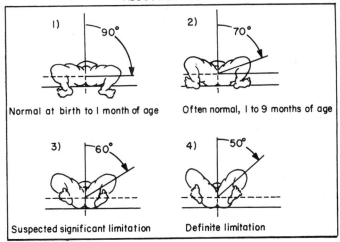

1) 90°

Normal at birth to 1 month of age

2) 70°

Often normal, 1 to 9 months of age

3) 60°

Suspected significant limitation

4) 50°

Definite limitation

FIGURE 33–2
Hip abduction test. Place the child supine, flex the hips 90 degrees, and fully abduct. Although the normal abduction range is quite broad, one can suspect hip disease in any patient who lacks more than 35–45 degrees of abduction. (From Chung SMK: Hip Disorders in Infants and Children. Philadelphia, Lea & Febiger, 1981.)

FIGURE 33–1
Physical findings in congenital hip dislocation. *A,* Thigh fold asymmetry is often present in infants with unilateral hip dislocation. An extra fold can be seen on the abnormal side. The finding is not diagnostic, however. It may be found in normal infants and may be absent in children with hip dislocation or dislocatability. *B,* Leg length inequality is a sign of unilateral hip dislocation. It is not reliable in children with dislocatable but not dislocated hips or in children with bilateral dislocation. *C,* Limitation of hip abduction is often present in older infants with hip dislocation. Abduction of greater than 60 degrees is usually possible in infants. Restriction or asymmetry indicates the need for careful radiological examination. *D,* Trendelenburg's sign. In single-leg stance, the abductor muscles of the normal hip support the pelvis. Dislocation of the hip functionally shortens and weakens these muscles. When the child attempts to stand on the dislocated hip, the opposite side of the pelvis drops. When bilateral dislocation is present, a wide-based Trendelenburg limp will result. (From Scoles P: Pediatric Orthopedics in Clinical Practice, 2nd ed. St. Louis, Mosby–Year Book, 1988.)

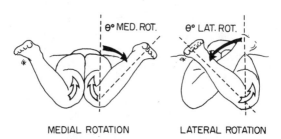

MEDIAL ROTATION   LATERAL ROTATION

F I G U R E 33–3

Medial and lateral rotation measurement. With the patient lying prone and the knees flexed 90 degrees, the femurs are examined for their range of motion at the hips in extension. (From Behrman R: Nelson Textbook of Pediatrics, 14th ed. Philadelphia, WB Saunders, 1992.)

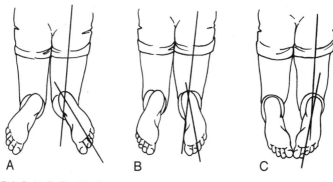

F I G U R E 33–4

Thigh-foot angle. With the child in the prone position and the knees flexed and approximated, the long axis of the foot can be compared with the long axis of the thigh. The long axis of the foot bisects the heel and the second toe or lies between the second and third toes. External tibial torsion *(A)* produces excessive outward rotation. Normal alignment *(B)* is characterized by slight external rotation. Internal tibial torsion produces inward rotation of the foot and is a negative angle *(C)*. (From Thompson GH: Gait disturbances. *In* Kliegman RM, Nieder ML, Super DM [eds]: Practical Strategies in Pediatric Diagnosis and Therapy. Philadelphia, WB Saunders, 1996.)

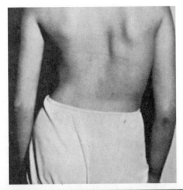

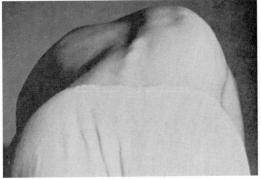

F I G U R E 33–5

Adam's position with rib hump of structural scoliosis. Lateral curvature of thoracic and lumbar segments of the spine, usually with some rotation of involved vertebral bodies.

Functional scoliosis is flexible; it is apparent with standing and disappears with forward bending. It may be compensatory for other abnormalities such as leg-length discrepancy.

Structural scoliosis is fixed; the curvature shows both on standing and on bending forward. Note rib hump with forward flexion. At greatest risk are females aged 10 through adolescence. (From Delp MH, Manning RT: Major's Physical Diagnosis: An Introduction to the Clinical Process, 9th ed. Philadelphia, WB Saunders, 1981.)

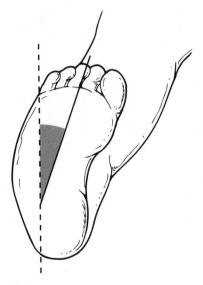

F I G U R E 33–6
Metatarsus adductus angle. An angle created by the intersecting lines that is greater than 15 degrees indicates metatarsus adductus. To determine the angle, draw a line from the middle of the heel through the second toe or between the second and third toes.

TABLE 33–1

Assessment and Management of Brachial Plexus Injury and Fractured Clavicle

	HISTORY	PHYSICAL FINDINGS	DIAGNOSTIC STUDIES	MANAGEMENT
Brachial plexus	Neck and shoulder stretched at birth	Erb palsy (C5 and C6): adducted limb; shoulder internal rotation; elbow flexed at wrists and fingers Klumpke palsy (C8 and T1): wrist and hand involved Erb-Duchenne-Klumpke palsy (C5, C6, C8, T1): flaccid extremity Phrenic nerve palsy (C3, C4, C5): involves diaphragm and respirations	Electromyography; radiographs of clavicle and spine as needed	Orthopedic referral; immobilize for 2 wk; PT for ROM; 80–90% resolve in first year
Fractured clavicle	Difficult delivery, often with shoulder dystocia; older child: fall or trauma	Pain with shoulder movement, decreased arm movement or absent Moro reflex; swelling and crepitus over fracture; may have associated Erb palsy	Usually not needed	Infant: move gently, no stress to arm until callus formation Older child: sling immobilization

PT = physical therapy; ROM = range of motion.

411

TABLE 33-2
Scoliosis, Kyphosis, and Lordosis

	CURVE	ETIOLOGY	CLINICAL FINDINGS	RADIOGRAMS	MANAGEMENT	PROGNOSIS
Scoliosis	Lateral	Classifications: idiopathic (most common); neuromuscular; constitutional; secondary; congenital; miscellaneous; functional (leg length discrepancy—not scoliosis)	Hx: Positive family hx; related to etiologies (classifications); painless curvature; PE: see Figure 33-5	AP and lateral standing views to identify degree of curve; >15° abnormal; may have 1 curve (C) or 2 curves (S); vertebrae show lateral deviation and rotation	Referral to orthopedic surgeon; brace or surgery; need to monitor progression of curve	Most curves do not increase after growth complete; females with idiopathic scoliosis more likely to have curve progress

Kyphosis	AP curve of thoracic spine	Familial (Scheuermann disease); secondary to tumor, trauma, etc.; congenital; postural: not true kyphosis	Postural round back	Narrow disc space and loss of normal anterior height of vertebrae	Postural: PT, dancing, and swimming can be helpful; if structural: refer to orthopedic surgeon for observation, bracing, or surgery
Lordosis	AP curve of lumbar spine	Due to hip contractures; physiological: family and racial groups, before puberty	Abdomen and buttock protuberant; if due to hip contractures, lordosis disappears when sitting	Standing lateral views	Lumbar spine flattens and lordosis disappears when child bends forward; it is physiological and no treatment; if fixed, refer to an orthopedist

AP = anteroposterior; Hx = history; PE = physical examination; PT = physical therapy.

T A B L E 33-3

Differential Diagnosis of Limping

CONDITION	AGE	PAIN +/−	HISTORICAL FINDINGS	CLINICAL FINDINGS	CAUSATIVE FACTORS	MANAGEMENT ISSUES
Developmental dysplasia of the hip	T, C, A	−	Breech delivery; metatarsus adductus; torticollis; poor treatment outcomes if not diagnosed at birth or shortly afterward	Limited abduction; + Trendelenburg; + radiography at 2–3 mo; shortening of leg; acetabular dysplasia; see Figs. 33–1 and 33–2	Familial; joint laxity, positioning, maternal hormones	Newborn: no triple diapers; Pavlik harness to hold hips in flexion—see weekly; after 6 mo, traction or open reduction; after 18 mo, osteotomy
Leg length inequality	T, C, A	−	None	Circumduction gait; joint contracture; >1 cm discrepancy in leg lengths	Congenital; neurogenic; vascular; tumor; trauma; infection	Shoe lifts; epiphysiodesis (fusion of growth plate to arrest growth of the opposite site), if discrepancy 2–6 cm
Neuromuscular (NM) disease	T, C, A	−	Depends on cause	Depends on cause; equinus or abductor gait	Cerebral palsy, muscular dystrophy, and other NM diseases	
Discitis	T, C, A	+	Varied: fever, malaise, unwilling to walk, backache	Stiff back, ↑ ESR; + x-ray 2–3 wk; early bone scan +	Bacterial infection in disc space (*Staphylococcus aureus*) or inflammatory response	Immobilization and antistaphylococcal antibiotic therapy

Table continued on following page

Septic arthritis	T, C, A	++	Moderate to high fever, malaise, arthralgias; irritability; progressive course	Redness, warmth, and swelling of joint—knee or hip; limited hip motion; ESR >25 mm/hr	S. aureus likely organism	Appropriate antibiotic coverage (7 d, IV; 3–4 wk total)
Osteomyelitis	T, C, A	+	Fever	Refusal to walk or move limb; point tenderness; 7–10 d to see radiographic bony changes	S. aureus likely organism	Appropriate antibiotic coverage (generally 7 d, IV; 4–6 wk total or until ESR normal)
Neoplastic	T, C, A	+	Depends on type of neoplasm	Varied	Neoplasm—benign or malignant	Referral to oncologist
Trauma	T, C, A	+	Depends on type (fractures, strains, sprains)	Varied	Varied	Rule out physical abuse if discrepancy related to developmental capabilities, injury history, and type of injury
Occult trauma: toddler fracture	T	+	Well child	Commonly spiral fracture of tibia; refusal to walk, mild soft tissue swelling; + radiograph	Trauma	See trauma above
Transient synovitis	3–8 yr	+	Mild to moderate fever, mild irritability; resolves within 1 wk	Limited hip motion; ESR <25 mm/hr	Inflammatory reaction; unknown etiology; often URI (50%) prior	Rest

TABLE 33-3
Differential Diagnosis of Limping Continued

CONDITION	AGE	PAIN +/-	HISTORICAL FINDINGS	CLINICAL FINDINGS	CAUSATIVE FACTORS	MANAGEMENT ISSUES
Juvenile arthritis (JA)	Childhood until 16 yr	+	Fever, rashes, ↑ WBC; some iritis; joint stiffness and swelling; S & S >3 mo	Mono/polyarticular arthropathy; +ANA (25–88%); ↑ ESR in moderate/severe JA	Unknown; genetic (HLA) or environmental	Treat with nonsteroidal anti-inflammatory agents initially; may need sulfasalazine, methotrexate; corticosteroids; joint replacements when older
Slipped capital femoral epiphysis	9–15 yr	+	>90 percentile weight; African-American; male	Limited abduction and extension; external rotation of thigh if hip flexed	Multifactorial: mechanical; endocrine; trauma; familial	Needs immediate surgery; non-weight-bearing crutches until admitted (sitting not advised); bilateral involvement does occur
Legg-Calvé-Perthes	4–8 yr	+	Acute/chronic onset; pain in hip, groin, knee; stiffness; male	+ Trendelenburg, shortening; ↓ abduction, internal rotation, hip extension; + radiographs but not early	Familial; breech birth; prior trauma (17%)	If in female, tends to be more serious problem; bedrest, traction, then PT; bracing and surgery may be needed; bilateral involvement does occur

T = toddler (1–3 yr); C = childhood (4–10 yr); A = adolescent (≥11 yr); ESR = erythrocyte sedimentation rate; IV = intravenous; PT = physical therapy; S & S = signs and symptoms; URI = upper respiratory infection; WBC = white blood cell; HLA = human leukocyte antigen; ANA = antinuclear antibody; ↑ = increased; ↓ = decreased.

Adapted from Behrman R, Kliegman RM, Arvin AM (eds): Nelson Textbook of Pediatrics, 15th ed. Philadelphia, WB Saunders, 1996; Staheli L: Fundamentals of Pediatric Orthopedics, 2nd ed. Philadelphia, Lippincott-Raven, 1998.

Overuse Injuries of Childhood: Characteristic Features and Their Treatment

CONDITION	CLINICAL FINDINGS	TREATMENT	COMMENTS
Osgood-Schlatter	Swelling and tenderness/pain over tibial tubercle	Nonsteroidal anti-inflammatory drugs (NSAIDs), knee pad, knee immobilizer if severe pain for 1–2 wk	Most resolve with time (12–18 mo), x-ray only if pain persists (soft tissue swelling and ossicle); pain persists, consider surgical incision of ossicle
Patellofemoral pain syndrome	Anterior knee pain	Rest, NSAIDs, retraining, and strengthening of quadriceps muscles	Arthroscopic surgery only if recurring problems
Proximal humeral epiphysiolysis, "Little League shoulder"	Shoulder pain—gradual onset; pain ↑ with throwing, especially curve ball	Modify activity; gradual restart but limit intensity and frequency of throwing with retraining	Seen in skeletally immature children; + radiographs—widening proximal humeral physis
Shin splints	Pain along medial border of tibia; child does prolonged running	NSAIDs; ice after running; retraining and muscle strengthening after inflammation ↓; gradual return to running	Associated with poor running technique, hard running surface, muscle weakness; inadequate running shoes; sudden increase in running; is an inflammatory response

Table continued on following page

417

Overuse Injuries of Childhood: Characteristic Features and Their Treatment *Continued*

CONDITION	CLINICAL FINDINGS	TREATMENT	COMMENTS
Stress fractures	Tenderness and swelling at site	Reduce or eliminate activity that caused injury for 10–14 d; may need to cast	Due to microtrauma; most commonly seen in active teens but can occur during childhood; proximal tibia most common site
Varus overload of the elbow, "Little League elbow"	Elbow pain with activity; locking and ↓ extension of elbow; medial humeral epicondyle tenderness	Rest; NSAIDs; ice; when pain-free, gradual return to activity with retraining; surgery if elbow instability	Leads to osteochondral lesions and stress fractures if severe; radiographs—widening proximal physis; also seen in gymnasts

↑ = increased; ↓ = decreased; + = positive.

Typical Cause of Intoeing and Out-Toeing Rotational Problems

	CAUSE	TYPICAL FINDING	AGE AT PRESENTATION
INTOEING	Equinovarus	Plantar foot flexion, forefoot adduction, and hindfoot varus	At birth
	Metatarsus adductus	Curved foot—refer if not flexible	Birth to 6 mo
	Abducted great toe	Searching toe—resolves spontaneously	Toddler period
	Medial tibial torsion	Refer if ~20 degree thigh-foot angle (TFA)	12–18 mo
	Medial femoral torsion	Refer if 70 degrees + medial and 10 degrees lateral hip rotation	2–5 yr
OUT-TOEING	Physiological infantile out-toeing	Feet may turn out when infant positioned upright—resolves spontaneously	Early infancy
	Lateral tibial torsion	Refer if TFA > +30 degrees	Late childhood
	Lateral femoral torsion	Refer if >2 SD of the mean	Late childhood

CHAPTER 34

Perinatal Conditions

The neonatal period is a highly vulnerable time for the infant. In the United States, two-thirds of all deaths in the first year of life occur among infants less than 28 days of age (Behrman et al., 1996). Mortality is the highest during the first 24 hours of life. Because serious health problems can arise for the infant in the hours after initial transition to extrauterine life, the nurse practitioner must be prepared to manage these problems while providing psychosocial support and education for the families. An understanding of the physiology of fetal development, risk factors for potential problems, and pertinent physical findings prepares the nurse practitioner to more effectively assist the newborn's transition to extrauterine life. Identification of high-risk pregnancies is the first step toward prevention of neonatal problems (Table 34-1).

NORMAL PHYSICAL TRANSITION AFTER BIRTH

A predictable series of changes or reactivities in vital signs and clinical appearance takes place after the delivery of most normal infants (Fig. 34-1). The first period of reactivity includes changes at the sympathetic as well as the parasympathetic level. After an interval of sleep, the infant enters a second period of reactivity. During this time, oral mucus again becomes evident, the heart rate becomes labile, the infant becomes more responsive to endogenous and exogenous stimuli, and meconium is often passed.

T A B L E 34–1

High-Risk Infants

DEMOGRAPHIC SOCIAL FACTORS

Maternal age <16 or >40 yr
Developmentally delayed mother
Illicit drug, alcohol, cigarette use
Poverty
Unmarried
Emotional or physical stress

PAST MEDICAL HISTORY

Diabetes mellitus
Hypertension
Asymptomatic bacteriuria
Rheumatological illness (SLE)
Chronic medication

PRIOR PREGNANCY

Intrauterine fetal demise
Neonatal death
Prematurity
Intrauterine growth retardation
Congenital malformation
Incompetent cervix
Blood group sensitization, neonatal jaundice
Neonatal thrombocytopenia
Hydrops
Inborn errors of metabolism

PRESENT PREGNANCY

Vaginal bleeding (abruptio placentae, placenta
   previa)
Sexually transmitted diseases (colonization:
   herpes simplex, group B streptococcus)
Multiple gestation
Preeclampsia
Premature rupture of membranes
Short interpregnancy time
Poly- or oligohydramnios
Acute medical or surgical illness
Inadequate prenatal care

LABOR AND DELIVERY

Premature labor (<37 wk)
Postdates (>42 wk)
Fetal distress
Immature L/S ratio: absent
   phosphatidylglycerol
Breech presentation
Meconium-stained fluid
Nuchal cord
Cesarean delivery
Forceps delivery
Apgar score <4 at 1 min

NEONATE

Birthweight <2500 or >4000 g
Birth before 37 or after 42 wk
   of gestation
SGA, LGA growth status
Tachypnea, cyanosis
Congenital malformation
Pallor, plethora, petechiae

SLE = systemic lupus erythematosus; SGA = small for gestational age; LGA = large for gestational age; L/S = lecithin-sphingomyelin ratio.

From Behrman RE, Kliegman RM, Arvin AM (eds): Nelson Textbook of Pediatrics, 15th ed. Philadelphia, WB Saunders, 1996, p 440.

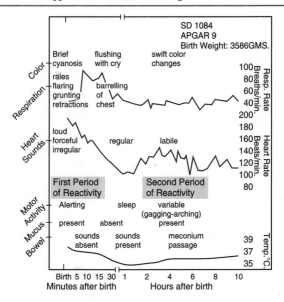

FIGURE 34–1

Summary of normal transition. (From Desmond MM, Rudolph AJ, Phitaksphraiwan P: The transition care nursery. Pediatr Clin North Am 13:651–668, 1966.)

NEWBORN SCREENING

All states require screening of infants for a variety of congenital abnormalities. The ideal timing of these tests is usually after the infant is older than 24 hours of age to ensure the baby's feeding and production of metabolites. Table 34-2 outlines guidelines for newborn screening.

EARLY DISCHARGE

Newborns are often discharged after a minimal time of observation. Guidelines for early discharge of normal, healthy newborns are listed in Table 34-3. Plans for follow-up care within 48 to 72 hours as well as for ongoing health maintenance should be confirmed before discharge. See Table 34-4 for guidelines for the 48- to 72-hour follow-

T A B L E   34–2

Newborn Screening

- All infants should be screened before discharge.
- All infants screened before 24 hr of age should be rescreened before 14 d of age.
- All infants should be tested before the 7th d of life.

1. For some diseases, such as phenylketonuria, the infant needs to be fed so that the intake or production of amino acids exceeds the infant's capacity to metabolize or excrete them.
2. Rescreening is now recommended in many states. Nurse practitioners need to be aware of the need for retesting, especially when infants are discharged early.
3. Cord blood is not acceptable for newborn screening because most metabolites accumulate after birth.
4. Filter papers should be used, preferably with 1 drop of blood filling the entire circle. Blood should not be added from the other side of the paper. If a capillary tube is used, it should not touch the paper. For sick infants, venous blood may be used, but care must be taken that no heparin or hyperalimentation components are included. To prevent hemolysis, the needle should not touch the paper.
5. The filter paper must not be contaminated in any way. The specimen should be dried while lying flat and not exposed to heat or sunlight. Remember that mailboxes may be hot in the summer!
6. Demographic data must be clearly written to ensure follow-up of abnormal results.
7. Specimens should be mailed within 24 hr of collection via first-class mail to avoid delays in reaching the laboratory.
8. Premature or sick infants should be screened by the 7th d of life.
9. Transfusions may temporarily affect results, so specimens should be collected before plasma or blood products are administered.

Adapted from Buist N, Tuerck J: The practitioner's role in newborn screening. Pediatr Clin North Am 39:199–211, 1992.

up visit of the healthy, normal newborn. Even newborns who are hospitalized longer need follow-up care within the first few days of life. All parents leaving the hospital with a newborn should have a confirmed time and place for follow-up as well as contacts in case of an emergency or questions.

▩ PREMATURE INFANTS

Premature infants have special needs that require follow-up after discharge (Table 34–5). Newborns with special needs owing to anoma-

T A B L E 34–3

Guidelines for Early Discharge of Normal, Healthy Newborns

Ante-, intra-, and postpartum course for baby and mother must be normal
Vaginal delivery
Single, appropriate for gestational age, term (38–42 wk) baby
Stable vital signs for at least 12 hr before discharge:
  Axillary temperature of 36.1–37°C in open crib
  Heart rate 100–160 bpm
  Respiratory rate < 60/min
  Passage of urine and stool
  Two successful feedings have been accomplished
  Normal physical examination
  No excessive bleeding at circumcision site for at least 2 hr
  No significant jaundice in first 24 hr
Mother knowledgeable in the care of the infant, including:
  Feeding
  Normal stool and urine frequency
  Skin, genital, and cord care
  Ability to identify illness (especially jaundice)
  Proper safety (car seat, sleeping position)
  Smoke alarms in the home
Social support and continuing health care identified
Infant laboratory data, including maternal syphilis and hepatitis B and infant
  blood type and Coombs' testing completed
Appropriately timed neonatal screening completed
Social situation adequate: include such areas as drug abuse, previous child
  abuse, mental illness, lack of social support, lack of permanent home,
  history of domestic violence, or teenage mother
Appropriate early follow-up care within 48 hr of discharge identified

Adapted from American Academy of Pediatrics: Hospital stay for healthy term newborns. Pediatrics 96(4):788–790, 1995; and National Association of Pediatric Nurse Associates and Practitioners: Newborn discharge and follow-up care. J Pediatr Health Care 11(3):147–148, 1997.

lies, disease states, social situation, or other variables also need arrangements made before discharge to provide support, education, and follow-up.

ERYTHEMA TOXICUM VS. HERPES SIMPLEX

Erythema toxicum, a common, benign rash of unknown etiology, is sometimes confused with the rash that occurs with herpes simplex. Table 34–6 provides a simple differentiation for these two rashes.

T A B L E 34-4

Guidelines for 48- to 72-Hour Follow-up Visit of the Normal, Healthy Newborn

1. Assess the infant's general health, hydration, and jaundice; identify any new problems; review feeding
2. Assess quality of bonding
3. Reinforce maternal and family education
4. Review outstanding laboratory data
5. Perform neonatal screen if indicated
6. Develop plan for health-care maintenance, including emergency care, preventive care, and periodic screenings

Adapted from American Academy of Pediatrics. Hospital stay for healthy term newborns. Pediatrics 96:788–790, 1995.

RESPIRATORY DISTRESS SYNDROME AND TRANSIENT TACHYPNEA OF THE NEWBORN

Respiratory distress syndrome due to atelectasis of the lungs is the most common pulmonary disease of the newborn. Transient tachypnea of the newborn occurs in full-term infants due to incomplete evacuation of fetal lung fluid in full-term infants. It is more common in infants born by cesarean delivery. Table 34-7 offers a clinical comparison of these two entities.

HYPOGLYCEMIA AND POLYCYTHEMIA

Hypoglycemia, defined as a blood glucose level below 30 mg/dl, and polycythemia, characterized by a central hematocrit of 65% or higher, are relatively common occurrences, especially in small-for-gestational age infants, infants of diabetic mothers, or infants affected by chronic in utero hypoxia, asphyxia at birth, or sepsis. Table 34-8 outlines characteristics and management of these conditions.

JAUNDICE

Jaundice becomes apparent when serum bilirubin levels exceed 5 to 7 mg/dl and advances in a pattern from the infant's head to toes. *Physiologic jaundice* is the most common type of jaundice in the newborn period, typically appearing after the first 24 hours of life.

Text continued on page 432

T A B L E 34–5

Guidelines for Discharge and Follow-up of the Premature Infant

DISCHARGE PLANNING

Identify all active medical or social problems through a review of the medical record and physical examination of infant

Ensure adequacy of immunizations based on infant's chronological age

Screen for anemia and begin iron or vitamins if necessary

Review with family member medications, feeding schedules, signs of illness, and appropriate response for infants with active medical conditions

Identify family and community resources if infant is to be discharged on home oxygen therapy

Ensure adequate training of family members in cardiopulmonary resuscitation and, if applicable, on home apnea monitor use

Counsel family in car seat adaptations for the premature infant

Consider need for visiting nurse, social service, respite care, support groups, or referral to the Women, Infants, and Children (WIC) Program

FOLLOW-UP PLANNING

Schedule audiograms (if not already done) for infants with:
  Craniofacial abnormalities
  In utero infections
  Birth weight <1500 g
  Meningitis
  Exchange transfusion for hyperbilirubinemia
  Use of ototoxic medications
  Apgar score of 0–4 at 1 min or 0–6 at 5 min
  Mechanical ventilation for ≥5 d
  Stigmata of syndrome associated with hearing loss
  Family history of deafness

Schedule at 4–6 wk chronological age a dilated indirect ophthalmoscopic examination for neonates with a birth weight ≤1500 g or with a gestational age of ≤28 wk as well as those infants >1500 g with an unstable clinical course thought to be at high risk for retinopathy of prematurity by their attending physician (AAP, AAPOS, and AAO, 1997)

Follow-up visits every 1–2 wk, especially if infant is receiving oxygen therapy

Growth and development should be of prime interest at each routine outpatient visit with referral for formal developmental assessment if any concerns are identified

T A B L E 34-6

Erythema Toxicum vs. Herpes Simplex Virus (HSV)

ERYTHEMA TOXICUM	HERPES SIMPLEX VIRUS
Benign, self-limited	Pathological, progressive
No specific maternal history	Frequently a history of maternal disease
Usually seen only in term infants	Can occur in infants of any gestational age
Begins on the 2nd or 3rd d of life, lasting as long as 1 wk	Often begins late in the 1st wk of life or early in the 2nd wk of life
Rash is evanescent, often involving the face, trunk, and extremities	Can be superficial and localized only to the presenting part (vertex or buttocks) or widespread and disseminated without cutaneous involvement
1- to 2-mm white papules or pustules on an erythematous base that occasionally may become vesicular	May present similar to sepsis without cutaneous findings, or as grouped vesicles on an erythematous base on the presenting part about 9–11 d of life
Wright or Giemsa stain of lesion scraping demonstrates large numbers of eosinophils and no organisms; cultures are sterile	Direct fluorescent antibody staining or enzyme-linked immunoassay detection of HSV antigens of vesicle scrapings, or growth of the organism from vesicle fluid are diagnostic
No specific therapy necessary	Acyclovir therapy

TABLE 34-7

Clinical Comparison of Transient Tachypnea of the Newborn and Respiratory Distress Syndrome (RDS)

TRANSIENT TACHYPNEA OF THE NEWBORN	RESPIRATORY DISTRESS SYNDROME
Seen only in infants delivered at or near term, often in infants born by cesarean delivery	Found only in premature infants, with the greatest incidence in infants weighing <1500 g
Increased respiratory rate is invariably present; grunting and intercostal retractions are not common	Usually, respiratory rate is increased, infants grunt at expiration, nasal flaring is noted, and sternal and intercostal retractions are commonly seen
Cyanosis is not a prominent feature	Cyanosis in room air is a prominent feature
Air exchange is good; rales and rhonchi are usually absent	Auscultation reveals diminished air entry
Begins at birth, usually resolving in the first 24-48 hr of life	Often begins late in the 1st wk of life or early in the 2nd wk of life
Chest radiograph shows central perihilar streaking with slightly enlarged heart	Chest radiograph demonstrates reticulogranular, ground-glass appearance and air bronchograms
Typical course involves gradual decrease in respiratory rate with resolution in the 1st 5 d of life	Course variable depending on infant's gestational weight and age; classically, RDS begins to improve after about 72 hr of symptoms
No specific therapy other than maintaining oxygenation is usually necessary	Artificial surfactant, as well as administration of steroids to the mother, can reduce the severity of this disease; mechanical ventilation is commonly needed

Management of Hypoglycemia, IDM, and Polycythemia in the Newborn

CONDITION	CLINICAL FINDINGS	WORKUP	TREATMENT	COMMENTS
Hypoglycemia	• Blood glucose <30 mg/dl • Infant with history of SGA; poorly controlled diabetic mother (IDDM); at risk for sepsis; asphyxia; erythroblastosis fetalis • Lethargy • Poor feeding and regurgitation • Apnea • Jitteriness • Pallor, sweating, cool extremities • Seizures	• Serum glucose—measure within 1 hr of birth, every 1–2 hr until 6–8 hr of life, then every 4–6 hr until 24 hr of life	• Give normoglycemic high-risk infants oral or gavage feedings with breast milk or formula at 1–3 hr of life and continue at every 2–3 hr intervals × 24–48 hr • Intravenous glucose at 4 mg/kg/min if serum glucose level low and oral feedings poorly tolerated	• Infants with symptomatic hypoglycemia (especially SGA and IDM, prolonged and severe hypoglycemia) are less likely to have normal intellectual development than asymptomatic infants

Table continued on following page

T A B L E 34-8

Management of Hypoglycemia, IDM, and Polycythemia in the Newborn Continued

CONDITION	CLINICAL FINDINGS	WORKUP	TREATMENT	COMMENTS
	• Infant of diabetic mother (IDM): large plump infant with large viscera; puffy facies; plethora; hyperactivity first 3 d; ± hypotonicity, lethargy, poor suck; ± cardiomegaly and murmurs	• Intensive observation and care • Serum glucose (as above)	• If clinically well and normoglycemic, initially give oral or gavage feedings with 5% glucose water or breast milk started within 2–3 hr of age and continued at 3-hr intervals • If infant is unable to tolerate oral feeding, discontinue feeding and give 10% glucose by peripheral intravenous infusion at a rate of 4–8 mg/kg/hr • Treat hypoglycemia, even in asymptomatic infants, with intravenous infusions of glucose to bring blood glucose to 30 mg	• IDM congenital anomalies increased threefold (cardiac malformation, lumbosacral agenesis most common); predisposition to childhood obesity • Avoid bolus injections of hypertonic glucose, as they cause further hyperinsulinemia and potentially produce rebound hypoglycemia

| Polycythemia | • Cyanosis, tachypnea, respiratory distress
• Hyperbilirubinemia
• Infant with history of diabetic mother, IUGR, exposure to chronic hypoxia; receipt of twin–twin transfusion; delayed clamping of umbilical cord; postmaturity; SGA
• Plethora
• Feeding disturbance | • Hct ≥65% | • Phlebotomy and replacement with saline or albumin, or partial exchange transfusion to reduce Hct to 50% | • Occurs in 1–5/100 births; 15–25% are asymptomatic
• Long-term problems include speech deficits, abnormal fine motor control, reduced IQ, and other neurological abnormalities |

Hct = hematocrit; IDDM = insulin-dependent diabetes mellitus; IDM = infants of diabetic mothers; IUGR = intrauterine growth retardation; SGA = small for gestational age.

The rate of rise in total bilirubin is less than 5 mg/dl/day, with the peak total bilirubin usually not exceeding 13 mg/dl and the direct bilirubin not exceeding 2 mg/dl. Physiologic jaundice does not persist beyond 1 week, and the infant shows no signs of illness.

Nonphysiologic (pathological) jaundice appears at less than 24 hours of age, lasts more than 8 days, or both. The rate of rise in total bilirubin is rapid, at greater than 0.5 mg/dl/hr. Total bilirubin levels are frequently greater than 12.5 mg/dl before 48 hours of age, or the direct bilirubin exceeds 1.5 to 2 mg/dl.

Early-onset breastfeeding jaundice can develop within 2 to 4 days of birth and is believed to occur as a result of infrequent breastfeeding and insufficient intake leading to decreased intestinal motility. *Late-onset breast milk jaundice* develops 4 to 7 days after birth, peaks at 10 to 15 days of life, and frequently persists for weeks. Jaundice is observed during the first week of life in approximately 60% of infants. Figure 34-2 and Table 34-9 outline the management of hyperbilirubinemia.

▰▰ SEPSIS

Risk factors for sepsis (systemic infection) in the newborn include early rupture of amniotic membranes followed by preterm labor, prolonged rupture of membranes, maternal fever, maternal diagnosis of chorioamnionitis, maternal tachycardia, fetal tachycardia, and malodorous amniotic fluid. The neonate with sepsis can be asymptomatic or have nonspecific symptoms or findings. Organisms quickly invade the systemic circulation, and significant deterioration can occur before sepsis is clinically recognized. Because of the serious nature of neonatal sepsis, newborns with significant risk factors or unstable neonates without perinatal risk factors should be carefully evaluated and appropriate antibiotics initiated (Table 34-10).

F I G U R E 34-2

Management of hyperbilirubinemia in the healthy term infant. D/C = discontinue. (Adapted from Banks et al: J Pediatr Health Care 10[5]:228–230, 1996; and the American Academy of Pediatrics: Practice parameter: Management of hyperbilirubinemia in the healthy term newborn. Pediatrics 94[4, Part 1]:558–565, 1994.)

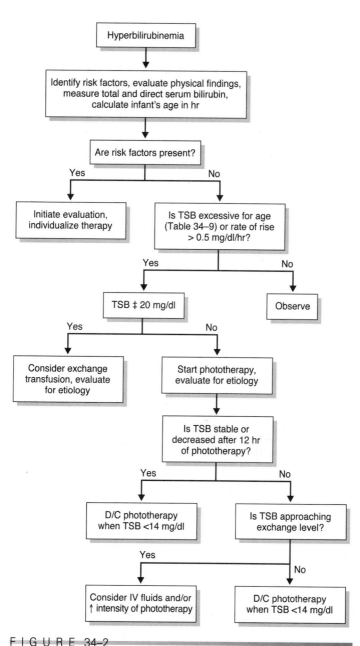

F I G U R E 34-2
See legend on opposite page

TABLE 34-9

Management of Hyperbilirubinemia in the Healthy Term Newborn

	TOTAL SERUM BILIRUBIN (TSB) LEVEL, mg/dl (μmol/l)			
AGE (hr)	Consider Phototherapy*	Phototherapy	Exchange Transfusion if Intensive Phototherapy Fails†	Exchange Transfusion and Intensive Phototherapy
≤24‡				
25–48	≥12 (205)	≥15 (260)	≥20 (340)	≥25 (430)
49–72	≥15 (260)	≥18 (310)	≥25 (430)	≥30 (510)
>72	≥17 (290)	≥20 (340)	≥25 (430)	≥30 (510)

*Phototherapy at these TSB levels is a clinical option, meaning that the intervention is available and may be used on the basis of individual clinical judgment.

†Intensive phototherapy should produce a decline of TSB of 1–2 mg/dl within 4–6 hr, and the TSB level should continue to fall and remain below the threshold level for exchange transfusion. If this does not occur, it is considered a failure of phototherapy.

‡Term infants who are clinically jaundiced at 24 hr are not considered healthy and require further evaluation.

Adapted from American Academy of Pediatrics: Practice parameter: Management of hyperbilirubinemia in the healthy term newborn. Pediatrics 94(4, pt1):560, 1994.

T A B L E 34–10

Neonatal Sepsis

HISTORY

Temperature instability
Jitteriness
Poor feeding, vomiting
Irritability or lethargy
Apnea
Bloody stools
Respiratory distress
Seizures

PHYSICAL EXAMINATION

Jaundice
Pallor
Petechiae or purpura
Rash
Hepatosplenomegaly
Poor tone and perfusion
Tachycardia or bradycardia
Cyanosis, grunting, flaring, retractions

LABORATORY EVALUATION

Blood for CBC with differential, platelet count, and culture—anemia; increase or decrease in WBC count with left shift; thrombocytopenia
Urine—urine culture usually not done in the 1st 72 hr of life because of low yield
CSF for protein, glucose, cell count, and culture—elevated protein and WBC count; depressed glucose often found in neonatal infections

MANAGEMENT

Combination broad-spectrum antibiotic coverage for gram-positive cocci, gram-negative bacilli, and *Listeria* is recommended. Consider adding coverage for herpes infection if this is a possibility. *Listeria* is treated with ampicillin; group B streptococci can be treated with the penicillins and the cephalosporins; gram-negative organisms are well-covered by aminoglycosides and some cephalosporins

CBC = complete blood count; WBC = white blood cell; CSF = cerebrospinal fluid.

REFERENCES

American Academy of Pediatrics: Practice parameter: Management of hyperbilirubinemia in the healthy term newborn. Pediatrics 94(4, Part 1):558-565, 1994.

American Academy of Pediatrics: Hospital stay for healthy term newborns. Pediatrics 96(4):788-790, 1995.

American Academy of Pediatrics (AAP), American Association for Pediatric Ophthalmology and Strabismus (AAPOS), and American Academy of Ophthalmology (AAO): Screening examination of premature infants for retinopathy of prematurity. Pediatrics 100:273, 1997.

Banks J, Montgomery D, Coody D, Yetman R: Hyperbilirubinemia in the term newborn. J Pediatr Health Care 10(5):228-230, 1996.

Behrman R, Kliegman RM, Arvin AM (eds): Nelson Textbook of Pediatrics, 15th ed. Philadelphia, WB Saunders, 1996.

Buist N, Tuerck J: The practitioner's role in newborn screening. Pediatr Clin North Am 39:199-211, 1992.

Desmond MM, Rudolph AJ, Phitaksphraiwan P: The transitional care nursery. Pediatr Clin North Am 13:651-668, 1966.

National Association of Pediatric Nurse Associates and Practitioners (NAPNAP): Newborn discharge and follow-up care. J Pediatr Health Care 11(3):147-148, 1997.

CHAPTER 35

Common Injuries

INTRODUCTION

Injuries are major pediatric health problems, with the type of trauma experienced most often related to the child's activities and developmental stage. This chapter focuses on the outpatient assessment and management of lacerations, burns, sprains and strains, anaphylaxis, and head injuries.

LACERATIONS

Lacerations are classified into three categories according to the degree of tissue loss, contamination, and depth of the wound (Table 35–1).

T A B L E 35–1

Classification of Lacerations

CLASSIFICATION	CHARACTERISTICS
1. Simple	No tissue loss, deep injury, or embedded debris
vs.	
Complex	Tissue loss, deep injury, and debris present
2. Clean	Injury done by a clean instrument directly onto skin
vs.	
Contaminated	Wound contains foreign debris, made through clothing or other material, or is associated with road or farm debris
3. Superficial	Skin and subcutaneous tissue involved
vs.	
Deep	Fascia, muscle, tendons, and/or nerves affected

Laceration management and suture removal are summarized in Table 35-2.

BURNS AND THEIR MANAGEMENT

The palm of the hand (including the digits) is approximately 1% of body surface area and can be used as a quick guide to estimate total body surface area in burn calculations. First-degree burns are not calculated in total body surface area estimations. For children, burns involving 10% or more of body surface or significant burns of the hands, feet, face, eyes, ears, and genitalia are considered major burns and require hospitalization or the expertise of a burn specialist (Hansbrough & Hansbrough, 1999).

The nurse practitioner should be familiar with the outpatient management of first- and second-degree or partial-thickness burns. As burns can be accidental or inflicted injuries, the nurse practitioner should obtain a detailed history to determine how the burn occurred, including agent of injury and length of time agent was in contact with skin and the circumstances surrounding injury. The key question the nurse practitioner should ask is whether the history is consistent with the type and degree of burn injury. Tables 35-3 and 35-4 identify burn characteristics and treatment of first- and second-degree burns, respectively.

CONTUSIONS, SPRAINS, STRAINS, AND FRACTURES AND DISLOCATIONS

General guidelines for the assessment and management of contusions, sprains, strains, and fractures and dislocations are summarized in Table 35-5. Remember that ankle ligaments are strong in children with open growth plates. Therefore, ankle fractures are more common than sprains in prepubertal children (Mankin & Zimbler, 1996).

ANAPHYLAXIS AND ITS TREATMENT

Allergic responses can range from mild to severe life-threatening anaphylactic reactions. Anaphylaxis is an IgE-mediated systemic reaction characterized by urticaria, angioedema, airway obstruction, and potential for cardiorespiratory arrest. Anaphylactoid reactions have the same

T A B L E 35–2

Management of Lacerations and Suture Removal

LACERATION MANAGEMENT
General Principles
- Cleanse wound (see Suturing) and cover with a saline-soaked gauze until ready to examine. Remember that adequate lighting is important.
- Wear gloves and a mask when examining and probing the wound.
- Administer local anesthesia before probing wound to determine depth, presence of debris, or involvement of deep tissue structures.
- Inspect for possible foreign body or debris.
- Evaluate range of motion and degree to which vascular and neurological structures are intact (in wound area and in distal area).
- Can shower 48 hr after sutures are in place.

Suturing
1. Soak wound in a mild antiseptic solution such as povidone-iodine for approximately 15 min. An alternative to soaking for wound cleaning is irrigation with a forced jet spray of tepid water, normal saline (NaCl), or povidone-iodine solution using a syringe or intravenous catheter (approximately 500 ml of irrigation is needed). Thoroughly rinse with NaCl after using povidone-iodine. Lip and eye wounds should be cleaned with only NaCl. Administration of local anesthesia is helpful.
2. Remove surface debris and blood.
3. Refer deep lacerations, complicated wounds, or wounds to the face to a surgeon.
4. Use a surgical scrub brush and forceps to remove foreign material.
5. Irrigate hematomas with saline.
6. Débride devitalized tissue, and trim ragged edges.
7. Suture wounds by primary closure unless the likelihood of infection is high (e.g., heavily contaminated wounds, animal bites, or wounds >12 hr old). Clean facial wounds can often be sutured as long as 12 hr after injury. Open wounds on other parts of the body (especially the lower extremities) have problems with bacterial growth ≤6 hr after injury.
8. Immediate suturing of animal bites is controversial. Some recommend that animal bites and deep punctures should not be immediately sutured (likelihood of infection) and delay primary closure for 4–5 d. Others close an animal bite if it is treated within 8 hr and does not appear infected.
9. Dress the wound using a nonadherent gauze for the first layer followed by a second layer of plain gauze if needed. Use elasticized gauze (tubular net bandage) to secure dressings.
10. Order tetanus booster or human tetanus immune globulin if indicated.
11. Antibiotic prophylaxis of clean wounds is not indicated; its use in contaminated wounds may be helpful, but careful wound cleaning and débridement are the most effective safeguards to prevent infection.

Table continued on following page

T A B L E 35-2

Management of Lacerations and Suture Removal Continued

SUTURE REMOVAL

Suture removal depends on location. Guidelines to use are as follows:
- Facial   3–4 d
- Upper extremity   7–10 d
- Trunk   10 d
- Lower extremity   14 d
- Over a joint   10–14 d

STERI-STRIPS AND TISSUE ADHESIVES

1. Steri-strips should be used only for small wounds whose edges are not far apart. Tissue adhesives are appropriate only for simple lacerations in relatively low-tension areas of the body. Do not use in hairy areas such as eyebrows or scalp due to risk of infection.
2. For adhesives, area must be dry to allow for proper polymerization.
3. The procedure for closing a wound with tissue adhesive is a three-step process:
   - Use forceps to approximate the edges together, or have assistant hold together.
   - Apply adhesive onto the skin surface as the edges are being held in close proximity with forceps—do not drip any adhesive into the wound.
   - Hold the wound closed for 20–30 sec until glue polymerizes.
4. A combination of subcutaneous suturing and application of tissue adhesive can be used for deeper wounds but obviates advantage of no sedation or restraint.
5. Use a nonocclusive bandage for wound coverage (Simon, 1997).

features but are non-IgE-mediated systemic reactions. Although the etiologies of these two reactions are different, it is appropriate to describe both types of reactions as anaphylaxis. Table 35-6 outlines the treatment of anaphylaxis.

HEAD INJURIES

Head injuries in children are classified as mild, moderate, and severe (Table 35-7). The level of consciousness is a key determinant of the child's prognosis. The following historical information should be obtained:

- Loss of consciousness or memory; confused, inappropriate behavior

T A B L E 35-3

Burn Characteristics and Treatment of First- and Second-Degree Burns

CATEGORY (DEGREE)	AREA	CHARACTERISTICS
First	Epidermis only	Reddened, slightly edematous, dry, painful, blanches with pressure, hypersensitive, no blisters or sloughing of epidermis
Second/partial-thickness	Dermis involved but viable	Erythematous, swollen, moist appearance, blisters or sloughing of the epidermis, sensitive, blanches with pressure, painful
Third/full-thickness	Extends to dermis, subcutaneous tissue exposed	White or blackened appearance, may be firm/leathery, swollen, dry surface, lack sensation, no blanching
Fourth	Extends to muscle fascia or bones	Rare

T A B L E 35–4

Primary Care Setting Management of First- and Second-Degree Burns

1. Nutrition: Maintain proper nutrition to enhance healing.
2. Superficial burns:
   - Apply cool compresses.
   - Administer analgesic (e.g., acetaminophen or ibuprofen).
3. Partial-thickness burns:
   - Monitor daily for the first few days; evaluate for healing and assess for infection.
   - Cleanse wound with dilute (1–5%) povidone-iodine solution.
   - Débride open blisters; remove devitalized tissue, proteinaceous material, or residue from prior dressing changes.
   - Rinse thoroughly with normal saline.
   - If burn involves ≤3% of TBSA, apply Xeroform gauze *in strips* to clean, débrided area, followed by a dry gauze outer dressing.
   - For burn wounds >3% of TBSA, apply silver sulfadiazine (SSD) after wound is cleansed unless known sulfa allergy.
   - Apply strips of fine-mesh gauze or nonstick telfa over wound. Do not wrap wound with gauze (wrapped gauze can impair circulation). Apply additional SSD to gauze strips.
   - Apply a tubular net bandage to hold gauze in place.
   - Administer adequate analgesic medication. Acetaminophen with codeine may be needed before wound care and during the day. Switch to acetaminophen as the pain subsides.
   - Use mittens to prevent scratching if itching occurs as the burn heals; if needed, use diphenhydramine.
4. If a second-degree burn involves an extremity, keep it elevated. Child with second-degree circumferential burns of an extremity may need hospitalization (compartment syndrome).
5. Postburn education:
   - Use sunscreen protection to prevent sunburn.
   - Reinforce safety issues/education.
   - Instruct that scars remain immature for first 12–18 mo and go through color and texture changes as child grows. Most scald injuries from hot liquids heal quickly with little or no scarring.
   - Protect newly healed burns from the sun for at least 12 mo. Healed burns remain sensitive to the sun and sunburn more severely than nonburned skin.

TBSA = total body surface area.

- Vomiting, especially how often
- Type of headache, presence of visual problems, irritability
- How injury occurred; if injury involved a fall, determine height from which child fell

Text continued on page 449

The Assessment and Management of Contusions, Sprains, Strains, and Fractures

INJURY	CLINICAL FINDINGS	DIAGNOSTIC STUDIES	MANAGEMENT
CONTUSION (bruise)	Swelling, discoloration, pain/tenderness, limited mobility depending on severity of the bruising	None needed	*Acute:* Ice or cold compresses for 20 min q4h for first 48–72 hr; pressure bandage; elevation; NSAIDs *After 24–48 hr:* warm compresses or soaks; stretching; ROM and strengthening exercises. Avoid exercise for 5–7 d that involves bruised area. Refer severe injuries
SPRAINS (stress to joint ligament)	May report "popping" sound or "knee gave way" *Grade I:* stable joint, minimal pain, tenderness, or swelling *Grade II:* little or no instability, wider area of tenderness, more swelling and discoloration, limited mobility *Grade III:* marked laxity, severe pain, swelling, marked loss of mobility, (may have numbness, tingling, weakness distal to injury)	Radiograph if suspect fracture or dislocation	*Acute:* RICE; ice immediately for 15–20 min, then q2–6h for 24–48 hr; no weight bearing until pain decreased; NSAIDs; heat after 24 hr if mild sprain *Nonacute/chronic:* Weight bearing as tolerated; brace unstable joint; PT, gradual exercises (isometric and strengthening); guidelines for return to activities: 1 wk for grade I, 2 wk for grade II; apply ice after exercise, no sports until pain free *Severe:* may need casting or surgery *Table continued on following page*

443

The Assessment and Management of Contusions, Sprains, Strains, and Fractures *Continued*

INJURY	CLINICAL FINDINGS	DIAGNOSTIC STUDIES	MANAGEMENT
STRAINS (injury to muscles and tendons)	*Grade I:* local tenderness, minimal swelling, little or no discoloration, no change in muscle mass *Grade II:* may report "popping sound"; small, palpable defect in muscle mass, moderate pain, swelling, discoloration *Grade III:* reports immediate and severe S & S; pain, complete rupture of fascia with large, palpable defect, swelling, marked discoloration (unless tendon alone is injured); may have hematoma and loss of mobility	Radiograph if suspect fracture or dislocation	RICE; NSAIDs; mild exercise after 1–2 d of rest and immobilization; strengthening exercises; prevention of future injury—warm-up and strength training

FRACTURE/ DISLOCATION	Point tenderness over site, generalized pain, deformity, misalignment of bone or joint, loss of function or mobility (especially in dislocation), muscle spasm, discoloration, swelling, lacerations (if open fracture) *Clinical pearl:* tenderness below the lateral malleolus is typically ankle sprain not fracture (Mankin & Zimbler, 1996); if excessive swelling or discoloration around the joint, suspect fracture or dislocation, especially of epiphysis	Lateral and AP radiographs; may need to repeat in 10–14 d as early and Salter I fractures may not appear on first films	Referral for casting or other orthopedic interventions
STRESS FRACTURE (repeated microtrauma)	Gradual onset of pain with activity that decreases with rest, point tenderness, local swelling; distal atrophy may be noted	Radiograph; if normal, bone scan/ ultrasonography	Rest and eliminate activity that caused microtrauma for 10–14 d; casting if complete fracture; retraining

AP = anteroposterior; NSAID = nonsteroidal anti-inflammatory drug; PT = physical therapy; RICE = rest, ice, compression, elevation; ROM = range of motion; S & S = signs and symptoms.

TABLE 35-6
Treatment of Anaphylaxis

I. PHARMACOTHERAPY*

DRUG	ROUTE	DOSAGE	FREQUENCY
Epinephrine (1:1000 aqueous)	SC	0.01 mg/kg or 0.01 ml/kg/dose (0.3 mg—child max; 0.5 mg—adult max)	15–20 min intervals for 2–3 doses
Antihistamines			
Diphenhydramine	IM or IV	1–2 mg/kg (50 mg max)	
Ranitidine	IV	1 mg/kg (50 mg max)	
Corticosteroids			
Methylprednisolone	IV	1–2 mg/kg	q4–6h
or			
Hydrocortisone	IV	5 mg/kg	q4–6h
Bronchodilators (if wheezing)			
Albuterol 0.5%	Inhalation	2.5 mg or 0.5 ml in 2–3 ml of NaCl	Intermittent nebulization q4–6h; may require more frequent doses

II. *INTRAVENOUS FLUIDS*

Administer if child is hypotensive

III. *OXYGEN*

Via nasal cannula/mask (100% at 4–6 L/min)

IV. *HOSPITALIZE*

As soon as possible via Emergency Medical Services

V. *FOLLOW-UP*

Refer to allergist for immunotherapy if known allergen or for evaluation of potential allergen
Education
Instruct in use of epinephrine pin (have kit readily available)
Avoidance of known allergen(s)/causal agents
Wear medical alert tag/bracelet

IM = intramuscular; IV = intravenous; SC = subcutaneous.
*Data from Boguniewicz & Leung (1999) and Taketomo et al. (1998).

T A B L E 35–7

Classification of Head Injuries Based on Key Characteristics

CLASSIFICATION	GLASGOW COMA SCALE*	NEUROLOGICAL FOCAL DEFICIT†	LOSS OF CONSCIOUSNESS	OTHER NEUROLOGICAL FINDINGS
Mild	13–15	No	No or brief loss (<30 min)	May have linear skull fracture
Moderate	9–12	Focal signs	Variable loss	May have depressed skull fracture or intracranial hematoma
Severe	≤8	Focal signs	Prolonged loss	Often have depressed skull fractures and intracranial hematoma

*Either initial or subsequent scores.
†Neurological focal deficit (e.g., hemiparesis, reflex asymmetry, Babinski sign, and/or abnormal cranial nerve findings).

General guidelines for ordering diagnostic studies (Coulter, 1998; Rosman, 1998) include

- Mild trauma—without focal signs or loss of consciousness and Glasgow Coma Scale (Table 35-8) scores of 13-15, usually do not need routine skull radiographs
- Moderate and severe trauma—need a cranial computed tomography (CT) scan and routine skull films (anteroposterior and lateral views of the skull) and other views if there also is a neck injury or depressed skull fracture

Indications for obtaining a CT include any of the following:

- History of loss of consciousness
- Depressed level of consciousness
- Focal neurological signs or deficit
- Depressed skull fracture
- Seizures
- Persistent vomiting

T A B L E 35-8
Glasgow Coma Scale

CATEGORY	BEST RESPONSE	SCORE*
Eye opening (E)	Spontaneous	4
	To speech (command)	3
	To pain	2
	None	1
Motor (M)	Obeys (command)	6
	Localizes	5
	Withdraws	4
	Abnormal flexion	3
	Extensor response	2
	None	1
Verbal (V)	Oriented	5
	Confused conversation	4
	Inappropriate words	3
	Incomprehensible sounds	2
	None	1

*Total score (E + M + V): Maximum 15; Minimum 3.
Coulter DL: Head trauma. *In* Finberg LL (ed): *Saunders Manual of Pediatric Practice.* Philadelphia: WB Saunders, 1998, pp 883–885.

Children who suffer a minor head injury with a brief period of loss of consciousness (no more than several minutes) can be monitored at home provided that

- The CT scan is normal
- There is a responsible, reliable parent or guardian who can follow home instructions and has transportation to return child immediately if problems develop
- The child is alert or with only a slight headache and dizziness and has no other injuries
- The neurological examination is normal (Rosman, 1998)

All parents or caregivers should receive a "head injury sheet" that addresses the need to do the following:

- Wake up the child every 2 to 4 hours for the first 24 hours
- Check that the child is moving his or her arms and legs normally
- Give only acetaminophen for headache or relief of pain of bumps and buises

REFERENCES

Boguniewicz M, Leung DY: Allergic disorders. *In* Hay WW, Hayward AR, Levin MJ, Sondheimer JM (eds): Current Pediatric Diagnosis and Treatment, 14th ed. Stamford, CT, Appleton & Lange, 1999, pp 917–942.

Coulter DL: Head trauma. *In* Finberg L (ed): Saunders Manual of Pediatric Practice. Philadelphia, WB Saunders, 1998, pp 883–885.

Hansbrough JF, Hansbrough W: Pediatric burns. Contemp Pediatr 20:117–124, 1999.

Mankin KP, Zimbler S: Foot and ankle injuries: Solving the diagnostic dilemmas. Contemp Pediatr 13(3):25–45, 1996.

Rosman NP: Head injury. *In* Finberg L (ed): Saunders Manual of Pediatric Practice. Philadelphia, WB Saunders, 1998, pp 431–436.

Simon HK: How good are tissue adhesives in repairing lacerations? Contemp Pediatr 14(11):90–96, 1997.

Taketomo CK, Hodding JH, Kraus DM: Pediatric Dosage Handbook, 5th ed. Hudson, OH, Lexi-Comp Inc., 1998.

CHAPTER 36

Genetic Disorders

INTRODUCTION

Genetic conditions are not specifically addressed in most pediatric health and illness visits. Genetics does, however, play an important role in the health of children. With the progress of the Human Genome Project and other research, much new knowledge is being gained so that genetics plays an increasingly large role in the work of primary care providers. This chapter includes some basic information for approaching and managing the child with a possible genetic condition. Keep in mind that genetics is a unique area of medicine in which the conditions are *family based,* so the *family,* as well as the identified patient, must be managed.

ASSESSMENT

Identification of children with genetic conditions is the first role of primary care clinicians. Table 36-1 provides a list of common minor malformations and variations of normal. If several of these variations are found in a child, suspect a genetic condition.

Table 36-2 lists features that are more strongly associated with genetic conditions. Finding any one of them in a child should raise suspicion of a genetic condition.

Finally, to complete the assessment, a genetic history provides important information to support the need for genetic studies, diagnostic studies that are often expensive, genetic counseling and other support for the family (Table 36-3).

T A B L E 36–1

Minor Malformations and Variations of Normal

Large fontanel
Epicanthal folds
Hair whorls
Widow's peak
Low posterior hairline
Preauricular tags or pits
Minor ear anomalies
Protruding ears
Rotated ears
Low-set ears
Darwinian tubercle (blunt point protruding from upper edge of helix)

Digital anomalies
Clinodactyly (curved finger)
Camptodactyly (bent finger)
Syndactyly (webbed finger)
Transverse palmar crease
Shawl scrotum
Redundant umbilicus
Widespread nipples
Supernumerary nipples

From Wardinsky T: Visual clues to diagnosis of birth defects and genetic disease. J Pediatr Health Care 8:63–73, 1994.

T A B L E 36–2

Features Suggesting a Genetic Disorder

Mental retardation/developmental delays
Seizures with mental retardation
Severe hypotonia in infancy
Loss of developmental milestones
Short stature
Failure to thrive/growth retardation
Microcephaly
Dysmorphic features
Two or more physical birth defects
Ambiguous genitalia
Pigmentary skin lesions
Ocular findings or blindness
Deafness

Adapted from Pacific Northwest Regional Genetics Group: Practical Genetics for Primary Care. Portland, OR, Oregon Health Sciences Center, Pacific Northwest Regional Genetics Group, 1996.

T A B L E 36-3

Genetic History Questions

TOPIC	SPECIFIC ITEMS OF HISTORY
Family history: Helps identify family members with conditions that may be genetically transmitted	1. The pedigree should focus on at least three generations and look for people with similar characteristics 2. Consanguinity of partners (closer than first cousins) is very important 3. Note the past and current health of each person listed on the pedigree 4. Note the age of onset for family members' illnesses 5. Note multiple miscarriages, stillbirths, and/or anomalies among families 6. Family members with learning disabilities or mental retardation are important to document
Environmental and occupational history	Exposure to environmental toxins, alcohol, cigarette smoke, drugs, or radiation that might affect offspring

Reproductive history: Helps identify malformations, genetic conditions, or infectious diseases transmitted from mother to child
1. Maternal medical history
2. Prenatal history
3. Pregnancy and delivery history
	1. Maternal medical history
	  • Uterine anomalies
	  • Maternal illnesses and diseases (e.g., phenylketonuria, diabetes)
	  • Immunization status
	2. Prenatal history. The reproductive history should list every pregnancy, stillbirth, and abortion. Fetuses with significant chromosomal disorders are often aborted, and 5–7% of stillbirths and perinatal deaths are related to genetic problems
	  • Recurrent miscarriages
	  • Parity
	  • Advanced maternal or paternal age
	  • Complications of pregnancy

Table continued on following page

TABLE 36-3
Genetic History Questions Continued

TOPIC	SPECIFIC ITEMS OF HISTORY
	• Polyhydramnios or oligohydramnios
	• Fetal movements
	• Fetal growth assessments
	• Prenatal screening results
	3. Pregnancy and delivery history
	• Breech position
	• Birth measurements
	• Gestational age
	• Results of newborn screening tests
	• Presence of three or more minor anomalies in neonate
	• Failure of neonate to adapt to extrauterine life
Dietary history: Helps identify infants with single-gene–related metabolic disorders	1. Infant feeding behavior
	2. Formula or food intolerance
	3. Temporal relation of symptoms to meals
	4. Relation of signs and symptoms to types of food
Medical history of affected child	Use routine past medical history questions—history and current status of illnesses, hospitalizations, surgeries, allergies, injuries, immunizations
	List all health-care providers involved with the child's care
Developmental history	1. Achievements of milestones
	2. Speech and language development
	3. School performance
	4. Developmental evaluations
	5. Growth

MANAGEMENT

Management of genetic conditions should include diagnostic, therapeutic, and educational components. The diagnostic components might include a karyotype, biochemical studies, or cytogenetic studies. Obtain a karyotype if a *chromosomal disorder* is a possible diagnosis. Remember that there are also single-gene defects, multifactorial problems, and mitochondrial DNA problems that are genetic but not apparent from a karyotype. Other types of DNA studies are also available. Table 36-4 lists indications for a karyotype.

Therapeutic management for primary care providers includes symptom monitoring and management and collaborating with a pediatric specialist who will manage specialty care. Case management by the primary care provider, including work with a variety of specialists, is an important role that supports the family's work with the child. Table 36-5 highlights some of the specific monitoring that can be done by primary care providers.

T A B L E 36-4

Indications for Karyotype Analysis

Suspected chromosomal problem
Two major malformations
One major and two minor malformations
Ambiguous genitalia
Congenital heart disease
Hypotonia
Malformed stillborns and normal stillborns when demise is of undetermined
  etiology
Mental retardation or developmental delay
Growth retardation or short stature
Couple with two or more miscarriages or infertility

Adapted from Pacific Northwest Regional Genetics Group: Practical Genetics for Primary Care. Portland, OR, Oregon Health Sciences Center, Pacific Northwest Regional Genetics Group, 1996.

T A B L E 36–5

Guidelines for Primary Care Management of Children with Common Genetic Conditions

All Children

- Use general health supervision guidelines as much as possible.
- Provide genetic counseling to all families.
- Provide family support and counseling services.
- Identify support groups that might be helpful for the family.
- Provide long-term planning.
- Address sexual and reproductive issues with the child approaching adolescence, including help for both the child and the parents.
- Evaluate school placement and educational progress at least annually.
- Coordinate care with a clinic specializing in services for children with the specific condition.
- Address developmental and behavioral issues with referrals made as needed.

DOWN SYNDROME

- Cardiac echocardiology: at diagnosis and follow-up as needed if defects identified (Toomey, 1996).
- Screen for mitral valve prolapse at adolescence (Vessey, 1996).
- Hearing: at 9 months (or sooner if concerns) and follow-up as needed (50–70% will have hearing loss) (Toomey, 1996).
- Ophthalmologic: at 4 mo (sooner if concerns), 12 mo, 24 mo, then every 2 yr and follow-up as needed (Toomey, 1996).
- Thyroid: newborn screen and every 6 mo to age 2 yr; yearly to age 5 yr; then as indicated (Toomey, 1996).
- Cervical spine for atlantoaxial instability: at 3 yr, 12 yr, and 18 yr (Toomey, 1996).
- Down (or multidisciplinary) clinic at 4 mo, 12 mo, and then annually to 6 yr; then biannually. (American Academy of Pediatrics, 1994).
- Early intervention services (American Academy of Pediatrics, 1994) for developmental delays.
- SSI referral (American Academy of Pediatrics, 1994).
- Use Down syndrome growth charts to evaluate shorter stature and increased weight (Vessey, 1996) and manage obesity.
- Screen for hip dislocation through age 10 yr (Vessey, 1996).

T A B L E 36–5

Guidelines for Primary Care Management of Children with Common Genetic Conditions *Continued*

NEUROFIBROMATOSIS

To be done at initial evaluation, with follow-up as indicated:
- Head and spine magnetic resonance imaging (MRI) at diagnosis (Toomey, 1996).
- Hearing (Toomey, 1996; American Academy of Pediatrics, 1995a).
- Blood pressure (Toomey, 1996; American Academy of Pediatrics, 1995a). (Renal artery stenosis, aortic stenosis, pheochromocytomas, adrenal tumors, and vascular hypertrophic lesions.)
- Imaging studies of identified affected areas as indicated (Toomey, 1996; American Academy of Pediatrics, 1995a).
- Vision screening (American Academy of Pediatrics, 1995a).
- Skin evaluations for new neurofibromas and progression of lesions (American Academy of Pediatrics, 1995a).
- Skeletal evaluations for scoliosis, limb abnormalities, localized hypertrophy (American Academy of Pediatrics, 1995a).

TURNER SYNDROME

To be done at initial evaluation, with follow-up as indicated:
- Cardiac (Toomey, 1996), echocardiography or MRI for aortic abnormalities (Rosenfeld et al., 1994).
- Renal sonogram (Toomey, 1996; Rosenfeld et al., 1994).
- Blood pressure because hypertension is common, even without cardiac or renal abnormalities (Rosenfeld et al., 1994).
- Hearing (Toomey, 1996; Rosenfeld et al., 1994).
- Karyotype (Toomey, 1996; Rosenfeld et al., 1994).
- Developmental assessment at 3 yr (or sooner if indicated) for mild learning disabilities (Toomey, 1996).
- Pelvic ultrasonography at time of referral to endocrinology prepubertally (Toomey, 1996).
- Possible referral for growth hormone therapy in mid to late childhood (Toomey, 1996).
- Thyroid function at diagnosis and every 1–2 yr because 10–30% have primary hypothyroidism (Rosenfeld et al., 1994).
- Vision screening because strabismus, amblyopia, and ptosis are common (Rosenfeld et al., 1994).
- Orthopedic evaluation of developmental dislocated hip and scoliosis (Rosenfeld et al., 1994).
- Obesity monitoring and management (Rosenfeld et al., 1994).
- Lymphedema monitoring and management (Rosenfeld et al., 1994).
- Short stature management, including growth hormone therapy if the girl drops below the 5th percentile for the normal female growth curve; estrogen therapy for induction of puberty and feminization (Rosenfeld et al., 1994).
- Fertility and family planning counseling because women with Turner syndrome can achieve pregnancy without ovarian function via donors (Rosenfeld et al., 1994).

TABLE 36–5

Guidelines for Primary Care Management of Children with Common Genetic Conditions Continued

ACHONDROPLASIA

- MRI of foramen magnum at diagnosis; if small, repeat at 3–6 mo and similarly thereafter; if normal, repeat at 1 yr (Toomey, 1996).
- Ultrasonography/computed tomography or MRI of brain at diagnosis; repeat if head growth exceeds achondroplasia growth curves or if symptoms of increased intracranial pressure are present (Toomey, 1996).
- Physical therapy to focus on gross and fine motor developmental motor skills (Toomey, 1996).
- Monitoring of upper airway restriction, obstructive sleep apnea, and potential for cor pulmonale (Toomey, 1996).
- Orthopedic evaluation if bowing of lower extremities progresses due to fibular overgrowth (Toomey, 1996).

HEMOPHILIA AND VON WILLEBRAND DISEASE

- Developmental screen as follow-up to head trauma (Dragone and Karp, 1996).
- Adequate protein and calcium intake for bone formation (Dragone and Karp, 1996).
- Safety: protective helmets, knee pads as needed (Dragone and Karp, 1996).
- ID bracelet with diagnosis, treatment product, blood type. Remember to update annually (Dragone and Karp, 1996).
- Noncontact sports participation (Dragone and Karp, 1996).
- Regular dental hygiene care. May need replacement products for dental extractions (Dragone and Karp, 1996).
- Annual hematocrit (Dragone and Karp, 1996).
- Annual screen for microscopic hematuria (Dragone and Karp, 1996).
- Hemophilia management through a hemophilia treatment center.

REFERENCES

American Academy of Pediatrics, Committee on Genetics: Health supervision for children with Down syndrome. Pediatrics 93:855–859, 1994.

American Academy of Pediatrics, Committee on Genetics: Health supervision for children with neurofibromatosis. Pediatrics 96:368–372, 1995a.

American Academy of Pediatrics, Committee on Genetics: Health supervision for children with achondroplasia. Pediatrics 95:443–451, 1995b.

American Academy of Pediatrics, Committee on Genetics: Health supervision for children with Turner syndrome. Pediatrics 96:1166–1173, 1995c.

Dragone M, Karp S: Bleeding disorders. In Jackson P, Vessey J (eds): Primary Care of the Child with a Chronic Condition, St. Louis, Mosby, 1996, pp. 145–171.

Rosenfeld R, Tesch L-G, Rodriguez-Rigau L, McCauley E, et al: Recommendations for diagnosis, treatment, and management of individuals with Turner syndrome. Endocrinologist 4:351–358, 1994.

Toomey K: Medical genetics for the practitioner. Pediatr Rev 17:163–174, 1996.

Vessey J: Down syndrome. In Jackson P, Vessey J (eds): Primary Care of the Child with a Chronic Condition, 2nd ed. St. Louis, Mosby, 1996, pp 371–399.

CHAPTER 37

Environmental Health Problems

The role of the environment in health status is becoming increasingly apparent. Children are especially vulnerable to environmental toxins for a number of reasons, including

- Small size (a smaller dose of toxins will have a greater effect)
- Rapid growth and rapid respiratory and cardiac rate in proportion to size (toxins are more readily absorbed in the body)
- Immaturity of organ systems (toxins are less efficiently or safely detoxified and/or excreted)
- Closer proximity to toxins (children play at ground level, chew on painted surfaces, and so forth)
- Developmental characteristics such as mouthing behavior (especially of infants and young children), high levels of curiosity and activity combined with limited knowledge and judgment (especially in toddlers and school-age children), and risk taking behaviors (of adolescents).

Table 37-1 identifies conditions or clinical signs and the toxins to which they may be related. The specific relationship between environmental factors and disease processes is not always clear, and most environmentally related diseases are probably influenced by multiple factors.

The health supervision visit should include an assessment of the child's risk of exposure to environmental health hazards. Table 37-2 outlines essential questions to include in this assessment, and Table 37-3 lists questions specific to screening for risk of lead poisoning.

Management of environmental health issues includes preventing exposure, reducing contamination or ingestion, and providing treatment appropriate to the organ systems affected and the toxins in-

Text continued on page 469

TABLE 37-1

Common Pediatric Toxicants and Relationship to Disease

SUBSTANCE	SOURCE	HEALTH EFFECTS	PREVENTION STRATEGIES
Lead	• Lead-based paint, caulk • Dust, soil, water (lead pipes) • Cosmetics • Leaded gasoline • Solder, ammunition • Bearings, fishing weights • Folk medicine remedies • Pottery, lead crystal • Some dyes used in paper, magazines, plastic wrappers • Lead-based insecticides • Industry that uses/processes lead (e.g., smelters, battery manufacturers)	• Abdominal pain • Anemia • Neurological: • Learning disabilities • Delayed growth and development • Hyperactivity or other behavior problems • Impaired hearing • Seizures, coma, and death	• Test blood for lead levels • Test soil, water, dust for lead • Use fresh, cold water from taps; when faucet has not been used for 2 hr or more, flush 30–60 sec until water is noticeably colder • Use lead-free paints, gasoline • Clean surfaces with high-phosphate cleaning solution • Keep children from chewing on painted surfaces • Keep children away from remodeling/demolition projects where lead dust could be released • Do not store or cook food in lead crystal or in old or imported pottery • If you reuse plastic bags, keep printing on the outside • Make sure diet has adequate iron and calcium • Be sure folk remedies are lead-free *Table continued on following page*

TABLE 37-1

Common Pediatric Toxicants and Relationship to Disease Continued

SUBSTANCE	SOURCE	HEALTH EFFECTS	PREVENTION STRATEGIES

Mercury	• Food chain; accumulated and concentrated in animals (especially fish) and grains and flour
	• Latex paints
	• Thermometers and thermostats
	• Button batteries
	• Folk medicine remedies or religious practices
		• Metallic taste in the mouth
		• Thirst
		• Fever
		• Gastrointestinal:
		  • Nausea and vomiting
		  • Pain
		  • Bloody diarrhea
		  • Splenomegaly
		• Neurological:
		  • Irritability
		  • Numbness or pain in extremities
		  • Hypotonia
		  • Tremors
		  • Ataxia
		  • Memory loss
		  • Impaired vision or hearing
		  • Photophobia
		  • Seizures, coma, and death
		• Renal:
		  • Necrosis and failure
		• Skin:
		  • Erythema of palms and soles
		  • Hyperkeratosis
		  • Vasodilation
		  • Scaly, pink rash
		  • Pruritis
		  • Edema
		  • Birth defects
			• Do not eat fish or other food sources suspected of being contaminated with mercury
			• Do not allow children to play with glass thermometers, electrical wires, paints, or other materials with mercury
			• Safely store and dispose of products containing mercury
			• Be sure folk remedies are mercury-free
			• Advise families from cultures that use elemental mercury in religious ceremonies of the danger, especially to children

Source	Description	Health effects	Interventions

Environmental tobacco smoke (ETS)	• Side-stream smoke from tobacco products being used by others
	• Second-hand smoke exhaled by smoker in child's environment
	• Smoking by child or adolescent
		• Acute and chronic respiratory conditions
		  • Bronchitis
		  • Pneumonia
		  • Asthma
		• Otitis media
		• Middle ear effusion
		• Premature coronary artery disease (especially white males)
		• Low birth weight (infant of mother exposed to ETS)
		• Sudden infant death syndrome (SIDS)
			• Create smoke-free environment
			  • Adults and siblings in child's environment stop smoking
			  • Enroll child in day care that is smoke-free
			  • Prevent child from starting smoking
			• Recommend smoking cessation programs
			• Health-care provider support of decision to stop smoking

Radon	• Air; concentrated in basements and low areas
	• Water
		• Lung cancer (recent research questions relationship between indoor radon exposure and lung cancer: Weinmann, 1996; Auvinen et al., 1996)	• Test air in basements and first floor of home for radon levels
			• Discourage children playing in basements of homes with radon
			• Reduce amount of radon in basements:
			  • Seal cracks in foundation of house
			  • Cover dirt crawl spaces with impermeable plastic
			  • Seal drains
			  • Pour concrete floors
			• Stop smoking, because tobacco smoke acts as a vehicle for radon to enter the body
			Table continued on following page

T A B L E 37-1

Common Pediatric Toxicants and Relationship to Disease Continued

SUBSTANCE	SOURCE	HEALTH EFFECTS	PREVENTION STRATEGIES

Particulate matter	• Outdoor:
	  • Industrial pollution
	  • Gasoline and diesel engines
	  • Woodburning stoves
	  • Natural phenomena
	    • Forest fires
	    • Volcanic activity
	• Indoor:
	  • Dust mites
	  • Animal dander
	  • Cockroach particles
	  • Molds
		• Acute and chronic respiratory conditions:
		  • Bronchitis
		  • Pneumonia
		  • Wheezing
		  • Decreased lung function
		  • Asthma (indoor particulate matter)
		• Cardiovascular conditions
			• When outdoor air pollution is high, keep children indoors, decrease outdoor playtime
			• Air condition the home
			• Check heating system to ensure it is clean
			• Cover mattresses, wash bedding frequently
			• Discard stuffed animals
			• Keep humidity low to decrease mold growth

Asbestos	• Construction materials (insulation, ceiling and floor tiles, and shingles)	• Lung irritation
		• Lung disease later in life with repeated exposure
			• Prevent exposure to asbestos products:
			  • If buildings that contain asbestos are in good repair, it may be best to leave it in place
			  • Use asbestos abatement measures as appropriate when renovating buildings
			  • If parents' workplace is a source of asbestos exposure, remove clothing and bathe before coming in contact with children

Molds	• Damp areas in the home (basements, ceilings, leaking roofs or faucets)
	• Plants
	• Dry leaves
	• Shower or bath steam
	• Wet clothes
		• Allergic reactions:
		  • Cough
		  • Wheezing or shortness of breath
		  • Sinus congestion
		  • Watery, itchy, light-sensitive eyes
		  • Sore throat
		  • Skin rash
		• Headaches, memory loss, mood changes
		• Aches and pains
		• Fever
			Maintain dry, clean environment:
			• Clean with hot water and detergent
			• Disinfect with bleach
			• If unable to thoroughly clean, discard moldy materials to prevent spores from being released when materials dry

Pesticides	• Food
	• Water
	• Direct contact with plants, grass, and other areas treated with pesticides, insecticides, herbicides, or fungicides
		• Death by poisoning
		• Skin rash
		• Increased risk of cancer
		• Neurological conditions:
		  • Developmental delay
		  • Neurotoxicity
		• May disrupt endocrine function
		• May contribute to immune dysfunction
			• Use few or no pesticides in the home; explore nonchemical treatments for pests
			• Follow directions for use carefully; use only amount recommended, for purpose stated
			• Protect skin from exposure when using; wash thoroughly after use
			• Do not inhale or use on a windy day
			• Keep children away from treated areas
			• Clean up any spills
			• Keep pesticides away from food or dishes
			• Store pesticides safely out of children's reach
			• Dispose of pesticides at a registered disposal site
			Table continued on following page

465

TABLE 37-1
Common Pediatric Toxicants and Relationship to Disease Continued

SUBSTANCE	SOURCE	HEALTH EFFECTS	PREVENTION STRATEGIES

			• Keep a copy of the label handy for reference if needed
			• Decrease pesticide exposure in foods:
			  • Vary kinds of fruits and vegetables children eat
			  • Grow own
			  • Buy organically grown products
			  • Wash and peel fruits and vegetables (many pesticides are in the product itself; washing and peeling will not remove it)
			  • Try to use in-season fruits and vegetables to avoid varieties sprayed for transport and preservation

Polychlorinated biphenyls (PCBs)	• Foods; PCBs accumulate in fatty tissues of animals • Prenatal exposure via maternal ingestion of contaminated food • Older electrical equipment or wiring	• Prenatal exposure contributes to problems of neurological and intellectual function in infants and young children • Growth delay • Developmental delay • Increased respiratory infections • Increased behavior problems • Smaller male genitalia • Chloracne, hyperpigmentation, and nail changes	• Avoid PCB-contaminated foods, especially prenatally • Avoid environmental exposure from electrical leakage

T A B L E 37-2

Environmental Health Assessment Questions

QUESTION	RATIONALE
How old is the home?	Homes built in the 1970s or earlier may contain lead paint
In what kind of environment does the child spend time (e.g., home, day care)?	Friable asbestos—basement risks Radon—basement and lower floors risk Formaldehyde—mobile home risk; new home risk
What is the source of heating?	Carbon monoxide (CO), air particulates, NO_2, polycyclic aromatic hydrocarbons
Is home renovation occurring or planned?	Lead dust, asbestos risk
Does the family use pesticides inside or outside the home?	Dermal absorption; respiratory absorption in children low to ground
Is the child exposed to asbestos or lead at school?	See lead and asbestos discussions; most schools are safe
Does the child or other family members have hobbies that involve toxic elements (e.g., model building, stained glass, cleaning guns)?	Lead in artists' paints, lead solder, toluene with model-building glues, lead with fishing weights and bullets
Is the family living near polluted areas, industry, commercial businesses, dumps?	Recent emissions, soil pollution, water pollution, air quality risks
Are there toxic plants in the child's play area? Wood preservatives on playground equipment? Asbestos in playground sand?	Risks in community play areas
What are the parents' occupations? Are children or adolescents employed? Workplace exposures? Safety hazards in the workplace? OSHA regulations followed at the workplace?	Take-home exposures have been documented and young people may be at increased risk in the workplace

Table continued on following page

T A B L E 37-2

Environmental Health Assessment Questions

QUESTION	RATIONALE
Are there cigarette smokers in the child's environment—home, school, day care, friends, car transport?	Environmental tobacco smoke is a risk factor for SIDS, asthma, other respiratory conditions, long-term effects
Is the child's diet a source of toxicants?	Ingested pesticides, lead, mercury, PCBs are all risks
Is the breastfeeding mother taking drugs or other medications, smoking, been exposed to toxicants?	
Is the water supply lead-free and pollution-free?	
Are fresh vegetables washed and prepared to reduce exposure?	
Are there lead poisoning risks (see Table 37-3)?	Lead is common in the environment and poses a lifelong risk
Does the home have safety items in place (smoke alarm, CO alarm, fire extinguisher, childproofed cabinets, electrical outlet covers, gates on stairs, barriers to fireplaces or woodstoves, edge guards for sharp corners, hot-water heater set at 125°F, fenced swimming pool with self-latching gates)?	Preventive measures for the most common accidents in the home
Do you think your child may be at risk from any exposures to toxins?	Families may have information or fears not addressed by the above questions

OSHA = Occupational Safety and Health Administration; SIDS = sudden infant death syndrome; PCBs = polychlorinated biphenyls.
Adapted from Balk SJ: The environmental history: Asking the right questions. Contemp Pediatr 13:19–36, 1996.

T A B L E 37-3

Lead Screening Criteria: Risk Assessment

Young children (1–2 yr) should be screened with a blood sample if they meet any of the criteria listed below. Children between 3 and 6 yr who have not been screened previously and who meet any of the criteria below should be screened at least once. Children in low-risk areas do not need to be screened routinely. Any child exhibiting signs of lead toxicity should be screened. If it is not possible to determine the child's risk, screening should be done.

An answer of "yes" or "don't know" to any of the following three questions:
   Does your child live in or regularly visit (e.g., a home/day care) a house built before 1950?
   Does your child live in or regularly visit a house built before 1978 with recent (within the last 6 mo) or ongoing renovations or remodeling?
   Does your child have a sibling or playmate who has or did have lead poisoning?

Is the child receiving public assistance services (e.g., Women, Infants, and Children Program, food stamps, Medicaid)?

Does the child live in a zip code area where ≥27% of housing was built before 1950? This information is available from the U.S. Census Bureau, but each state may have a listing as part of their inclusive planning process. Check with your state health department.

Data from Centers for Disease Control and Prevention: Screening Young Children for Lead Poisoning: Guidance for State and Local Public Health Officials. Atlanta, Centers for Disease Control and Prevention, 1997.

volved. Figure 37-1 can assist nurse practitioners as they make management decisions related to lead toxicity in children.

Table 37-4 includes information on syrup of ipecac, dosage, considerations, and contraindications.

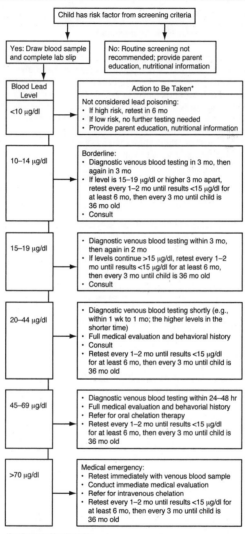

Child has risk factor from screening criteria

Yes: Draw blood sample and complete lab slip

No: Routine screening not recommended; provide parent education, nutritional information

Blood Lead Level	Action to Be Taken*
<10 μg/dl	Not considered lead poisoning: • If high risk, retest in 6 mo • If low risk, no further testing needed • Provide parent education, nutritional information
10–14 μg/dl	Borderline: • Diagnostic venous blood testing in 3 mo, then again in 3 mo • If level is 15–19 μg/dl or higher 3 mo apart, retest every 1–2 mo until results <15 μg/dl for at least 6 mo, then every 3 mo until child is 36 mo old • Consult
15–19 μg/dl	• Diagnostic venous blood testing within 3 mo, then again in 2 mo • If levels continue >15 μg/dl, retest every 1–2 mo until results <15 μg/dl for at least 6 mo, then every 3 mo until child is 36 mo old • Consult
20–44 μg/dl	• Diagnostic venous blood testing shortly (e.g., within 1 wk to 1 mo; the higher levels in the shorter time) • Full medical evaluation and behavioral history • Consult • Retest every 1–2 mo until results <15 μg/dl for at least 6 mo, then every 3 mo until child is 36 mo old
45–69 μg/dl	• Diagnostic venous blood testing within 24–48 hr • Full medical evaluation and behavorial history • Refer for oral chelation therapy • Retest every 1–2 mo until results <15 μg/dl for at least 6 mo, then every 3 mo until child is 36 mo old
>70 μg/dl	Medical emergency: • Retest immediately with venous blood sample • Conduct immediate medical evaluation • Refer for intravenous chelation • Retest every 1–2 mo until results <15 μg/dl for at least 6 mo, then every 3 mo until child is 36 mo old

*In *all* cases of lead toxicity:
• Provide parent education, nutritional information
• Remove child from source of lead if known
• Report to Public Health Department
• Initiate environmental investigation
• Encourage lead hazard control/abatement

F I G U R E 37–1
Lead screening protocol flow chart.

T A B L E 37–4

Considerations for Use of Syrup of Ipecac

AGE	DOSE	COMMENTS	CONTRAINDICATIONS (ALL AGES)
<10 mo		• Consult with poison control center or physician	• Stimulating emesis is not recommended in infants under 6 mo
10–12 mo	10 ml	• For all children under 1 yr, an emetic should be administered under supervision, in a health facility • Follow dose with 4–6 oz of water or clear liquid • Can repeat once if no emesis within 30 min	• Ingestion of acids, alkalis, or most hydrocarbons • Ingestion of seizure-inducing drugs or depressants • Ingestion of sharp objects • Diminished gag reflex
1–12 yr	15 ml	• Doses up to 30 ml have been found to stimulate more rapid emesis without increased adverse side effects • Follow dose with 8 oz of water or clear liquid • Can repeat once if no emesis within 30 min	• Altered level of consciousness • Coma
>12 yr (>90 lb)	30 ml	• Follow dose with 8 oz of water or clear liquid • Can repeat once if no emesis within 30 min	

Based on information from American Academy of Pediatrics: Handbook of Common Poisonings in Children. Elk Grove Village, IL, American Academy of Pediatrics, 1994.

REFERENCES

American Academy of Pediatrics: Handbook of Common Poisonings in Children. Elk Grove Village, IL, American Academy of Pediatrics, 1994.

Auvinen A, Makelainen I, Hakama M, et al: Indoor radon exposure and risk of lung cancer: A nested case-control study in Finland. J Natl Cancer Inst 88:966–972, 1996.

Balk SJ: The environmental history: Asking the right questions. Contemp Pediatr 13:19–36, 1996.

Centers for Disease Control and Prevention: Screening Young Children for Lead Poisoning: Guidance for State and Local Public Health Officials. Atlanta: Centers for Disease Control and Prevention, 1997.

Weinmann GG: An update on air pollution. Curr Opin Pulm Med 2:121–128, 1996.

CHAPTER 38

Complementary Therapies

There is an increasing trend for consumers of health care to seek medical therapies beyond those offered by practitioners of Western-style, allopathic medicine. In some areas of the United States, more than 50% of people (11% of children) may be integrating both conventional and nonconventional treatments—that is, using them to complement one another (Elder et al., 1997; Eisenberg et al., 1998; Spigelblatt, 1997).

Nurse practitioners should encourage the patient or family in a nonjudgmental manner to discuss their use of complementary therapies in order to help clarify the safety issues and explore how the products and services fit into the patient's management plan. The patient's medical history should be expanded to include

- Alternative products the patient may be taking, including herbs, "natural products," and homeopathic and nutritional supplements from a health food store
- Other practitioners the patient may be seeing
- Other kinds of activities engaged in to address a particular problem
- The perception of any benefit gained from the complementary treatment
- The patient's/family's philosophy and self-care approaches to wellness and illness.

Table 38-1 outlines herbal products that should not be used—or used with caution—in children.

The following safety issues are worthy of note:

- There are few documented reports of adverse reactions to herbal preparations; poisonings are rarely serious (Drew & Meyers, 1997; Fugh-Berman, 1997).

T A B L E 38–1

Herbals: General Precautions About Use in Children

Ephedra (ma huang)	*Not recommended*
Comfrey (*Symphytum*)	*Not recommended*
Borage (*Borago officinalis*)	*Not recommended*
Coltsfoot (*Tussilago farfara*) and species of *Crotalaria* and *Secacio* in herbal teas	*Not recommended*
Chaparral (*Larrea divaricata*)	*Not recommended*
Germander (*Teucrium chamaedrys*)	*Not recommended*
Jin bu huan	*Not recommended*
Monkshood/wolfsbane/aconite	*Not recommended*
Heliotropes	*Not recommended*
Rattlebox (Leguminosae)	*Not recommended*
Sassafras	*Not recommended*
Goldenseal/roots	Not for infants younger than 1 mo
Tea tree oil	Do not prescribe for internal use
Echinacea	Not for children younger than 2 yr
Pennyroyal	Do not prescribe for internal use

Data from Mack 1998; Castleman 1995; Fugh-Berman, 1997; Eisenberg 1997.

- Harmful side effects can occur with products taken in high doses, such as herbal or phytomedicinal products, megadose combination nutritional supplements, and colonics, or products taken in unconventional ways.
- Any treatment must be viewed as hazardous if its use delays the provision of proven, conventional care for a serious medical condition (Murray & Rubel, 1992; Nickerson & Silberman, 1992).
- Consistency of potency between batches of herbs may vary.
- Herbal products can lack standardization.
- Many herbs should be prescribed only by a knowledgeable herbalist or botanic professional.
- All herbs need to be respected; they are neither completely safe nor poisonous.
- Herbs can interact with other herbs or pharmaceutical drugs.
- Mind–body techniques (e.g., prayer, guided imagery, spiritual healing, relaxation) and acupuncture are unlikely to interact with conventional medications.

The nurse practitioner should not refer a patient to a complementary practitioner without having first completed a diagnostic evaluation. The following steps are useful when working with a patient who wishes to try a complementary treatment:

- Offer to assist in identifying a suitable, licensed practitioner.
- Provide the patient with questions to ask during the first consultative visit, including issues of safety and efficacy of any treatment.
- Follow-up with the patient to review the recommended treatment plan; encourage the patient to keep a symptom diary.
- Document all conversations with the patient.

It is suggested that the nurse practitioner who wants to inquire further, or who wishes to incorporate some complementary approaches into practice, use a good reference source that cites research and safety precautions. Chapter 43 in Burns et al. (2000) may serve as such a resource.

REFERENCES

Burns C, Brady M, Dunn A, et al: Pediatric Primary Care: A Handbook for Nurse Practitioners, 2nd ed. Philadelphia, WB Saunders, 2000.

Castleman M: The Healing Herbs: The Ultimate Guide to the Curative Power of Nature's Medicine. New York, Bantam, 1995.

Drew A, Myers S: Safety issues in herbal medicine: Implications for the health professions. Med J Aust 166(10):538-541, 1997.

Eisenberg D: Advising patients who seek alternative therapies. Ann Intern Med 127:61-69, 1997.

Eisenberg D, Davis R, Ettner S, et al: Trends in alternative medicine use in the United States, 1990-1997: Results of a follow-up national survey. JAMA 280(18):1569-1575, 1998.

Elder NC, Gillcrist A, Minz R: Use of alternative health care by family practice patients. Arch Fam Med 6:181-184, 1997.

Fugh-Berman A: Alternative Medicine: What Works. Baltimore, MD, Williams & Wilkins, 1997.

Mack R: "Something wicked this way comes"—herbs even witches should avoid. Contemp Pediatr 15(6):49-64, 1998.

Murray R, Rubel A: Physicians and healers—Unwitting partners in health care. N Engl J Med 326(1):61-64, 1992.

Nickerson J, Silberman T: Chiropractic manipulation in children. J Pediatr 12:172, 1992.

Spigelblatt L: Alternative medicine: A pediatric conundrum. Contemp Pediatr 14(8):51-64, 1997.

Medications

This is an abbreviated listing of medications used by the nurse practitioner. It is the responsibility of the reader/prescriber to seek detailed information and thoroughly investigate the drug being prescribed. The authors take no responsibility for any errors in prescribing.

NOTE: Some commonly used medications may be found in chapters in this text.

Medications

GENERIC/TRADE CLASSIFICATION	DOSE/INDICATIONS	SUPPLIED	REMARKS
Acetaminophen (Tylenol, Tempra) *Miscellaneous analgesic and antipyretic*	10–15 mg/kg/dose q4-6h PO (max. 5 doses) Adults: 325–650 mg q4-6h PO (max. 4 g/d) Treatment of mild to moderate pain and fever	80 mg/0.8 ml drops 160 mg/tsp elixir 80, 160 mg chewable 160, 325, 500 mg tab 80, 120, 325, 650 mg suppository	Drug interactions: barbiturates, carbamazepine, hydantoins, rifampin, sulfinpyrazone. Can cause severe hepatic toxicity with overdose.
Albuterol sulfate (Proventil, Ventolin) *Bronchodilator*	Treatment of bronchospasm: Children <5 yr: 0.1–0.2 mg/kg/dose PO tid (max. 2 mg tid) Children 6–11 yr: 2 mg PO tid-qid Nebulizer: 0.15 mg/kg/dose q4 hr prn MDI: Children >4 yr and adults: 2 inhalations q4-6h prn Adults: 2–4 mg PO q4-6h or 4–8 mg q12h Exercise induced bronchospasm: >12 yr: 2 inhalations 15 min before exercise	2 mg/5 ml syrup 2, 4 mg tab 4 mg sustained-release tab 5 mg/ml inhalation solution 90 µg/metered spray	Common side effects: tachycardia, tremor, palpitations. Do not administer with MAO inhibitors or tricyclic antidepressants.

Drug	Dosage/Indications	Available Forms	Comments
Amantadine HCl (Symmetrel) *Antiviral*	Prophylaxis or symptomatic relief of influenza A: Children 1–9 yr: 4.4–8.8 mg/kg/d PO divided bid-tid (max. 150 mg/d) Adults <64 yr and children >10 yr: 200 mg/d PO; continue 24–48 hr after symptoms disappear	50 mg/5 ml syrup 100 mg capsule	Not recommended for children age <1 yr. Do not administer with alcohol or stimulants.
Amoxicillin (Amoxil, Polymax, Trimox, Ultimox) *Penicillin*	Children: 40–90 mg/kg/d PO divided bid-tid Adults: 250–500 mg PO bid-tid (max. 2–3 g/d) Respiratory tract infections, sinusitis, skin, otitis, urinary tract, gonorrhea, streptococcal infections	50 mg/ml drops (#15, 30 ml) 125, 200, 250, 400 mg/tsp suspension 125, 200, 250, 400 mg chewable 250, 500, 875 mg capsule	Prophylaxis for otitis media with effusion: 20 mg/kg/d. Can cause a rash if given to a patient with mononucleosis. Side effects: GI.
Amoxicillin and clavulanate (Augmentin) *Penicillin, beta-lactamase inhibitor*	Children: 25–80 mg/kg/d PO divided bid-tid Adults: 250–500 mg PO tid (max. 2 g/d) or 875 mg bid Lower respiratory tract infections, otitis media, sinusitis, skin (periorbital cellulitis, human/animal bites)	125, 200, 250, 400 mg/tsp suspension (#75, 150 ml) 125, 200, 250, 400 mg chewable 250, 500, 875 mg tab (two 250 mg tabs do not equal one 500 mg tab)	Fewer side effects at bid dosing with 45 mg/kg/d. GI side effects—give with food. Peanut butter and cherry yogurt have been shown to decrease GI side effects.

Table continued on following page

Medications Continued

GENERIC/TRADE CLASSIFICATION	DOSE/INDICATIONS	SUPPLIED	REMARKS
Azithromycin (Zithromax) *Macrolide*	Children >6 mo: otitis media 10 mg/kg on day 1, 5 mg/kg on days 2–5. Give once daily Pharyngitis/tonsillitis > 2 yr: 12 mg/kg/d, days 1–5 Adults: 500 mg on day 1, then 250 mg days 2–5. Give once daily. Pharyngitis, pneumonia, skin and soft tissue disorders, gonococcal urethritis and cervicitis due to *Chlamydia trachomatis* (single dose); otitis media, sinusitis, pneumonia, streptococcal pharyngitis (5 d course); nontuberculous mycobacterial infections	250 mg tab 100 mg/tsp, 200 mg/tsp suspension 1 g single-dose packet	Food decreases bioavailability of capsules. Theophylline effect unknown. Alternative when erythromycin ethylsuccinate not tolerated. Some strains of *Streptococcus* are resistant to azithromycin. Drug interactions: Propulsid, digoxin, theophylline.

Drug	Dosage / Use	Comments
Beclomethasone dipropionate (Beclovent, Beconase, Vanceril, Vanceril DS, Vancenase-AQ) *Glucocorticoid, anti-inflammatory*	Children 6–12 yr (oral inhalation): 1 or 2 inhalations 3 or 4 times daily (max. 10 inhalations/d); DS 2 puffs bid Adults (oral inhalation): 2 inhalations 3 or 4 times daily (max. 20 inhalations/d) Adults (nasal): 1 spray to each nostril 2–4 times daily or 2 sprays/nostril bid Aqueous (AQ) solution: 1–2 sprays/nostril bid Used in the treatment of asthma, seasonal allergic rhinitis, and nasal polyps	Inhalation, oral, nasal: 42 μg/inhalation; 84 μg/inhalation AQ solution, nasal: 42 μg/inhalation	Contraindicated in patients with status asthmaticus. Use cautiously in patients with tuberculosis and those on oral steroids. Adverse reactions: hypothalamic-pituitary-adrenal axis suppression, oral candidiasis, headache, nasal irritation. Rinse mouth well following oral inhalation. When changing from oral to inhaled steroids, allow an overlap of at least 2 wk.
Benzoyl peroxide (2%, 5%, 10%) (Benzagel, Desquam-E, Desquam-X, Ersa-Gel) *Keratolytic agent*	Apply sparingly 1–3 times daily; effective alone or in conjunction with tretinoin or topical antibiotics Used in mild to moderate acne	5%, 10% gel 5%, 10% wash	Avoid contact with eyes, lips, mucous membranes. Adverse reactions: burning, swelling, peeling. Areas should be cleaned before application. Can bleach fabrics. Drug interactions: antacids. Do not crush tablets.
Bisacodyl (Dulcolax) *Stimulant laxative*	Children <3 yr: 5 mg rectally Children 3–12 yr: 5–10 mg or 0.3 mg/kg/d PO or 10 mg rectally Adults: 10–15 mg PO (max. 30 mg); 10 mg rectally Used to treat chronic constipation, bowel preparation	5 mg enteric-coated tablet 10 mg rectal suppository	

Table continued on following page

Medications Continued

GENERIC/TRADE CLASSIFICATION	DOSE/INDICATIONS	SUPPLIED	REMARKS
Brompheniramine maleate (Bromphen, Chlorphed, Codimal A, Conjec-B, Cophene-B, Dehist, Dimetone, Nasahist B, Oraminic II, Sinusol-B, Veltane) *Antihistamine*	0.5 mg/kg/d divided q6h, PO/IV/SC Children >6 yr: 2–4 mg PO tid-qid, or 8–12 mg q12h (max. 12–24 mg/d) Adults: 4–8 mg tid-qid PO/IV/SC (max. 24 mg/d)	2 mg/tsp 4 mg/tab 8, 12 mg time-released tab 10 mg/ml injection	Less drowsiness than with other antihistamines. Children <6 yr can experience hyperexcitability.
Budesonide (Pulmicort Turbuhaler) *Corticosteroid*	Children >6 yr and adults: 1 or 2 inhalations bid Maintenance and prophylactic therapy for asthma	Turbuhaler, 200 µg/dose, 200 doses	Drug interactions: ketoconazole. Side effects: dry mouth, oral candidiasis, HA, insomnia, GI disturbance.
Budesonide (Rhinocort) *Corticosteroid*	Children ≥ 6 yr and adults: 2 sprays per nostril bid or 4 sprays per nostril qd Allergic or perennial rhinitis	32 µg/spray Nasal inhaler, 200 metered doses per canister	Side effects: nasal irritation, epistaxis, pharyngitis, dry mouth.
Cefadroxil monohydrate (Duricef, Ultracef) *First-generation cephalosporin*	Children: 30 mg/kg/d PO qd or divided bid Adults: 500 mg PO bid Serious skin infections, urinary tract, bone and joint, streptococcal infections	125, 250, 500 mg/tsp (50, 100 ml) 500, 1000 mg tab	Can dose qd for streptococcal pharyngitis. Use cautiously in patients with serious penicillin hypersensitivity.

Drug	Indications and Dosage	Formulations	Comments
Cefixime (Suprax) *Third-generation cephalosporin*	Children: 8 mg/kg/d PO divided qd-bid (max. dose 400 mg) Adults: 200 mg bid or 400 mg qd PO Uncomplicated urinary tract infections, bronchitis, pharyngitis, tonsillitis, skin disorders (poor *Staphylococcus aureus* coverage), *Shigella* gastroenteritis, otitis media	100 mg/tsp (50, 100 ml) 200, 400 mg tab	Can be given as a single dose. Not indicated for infants <6 mo. Treat otitis media with suspension—gives higher therapeutic levels. GI symptoms common.
Cefprozil (Cefzil) *Second-generation cephalosporin*	Children: 30 mg/kg/d divided bid PO—otitis media, upper respiratory tract; 15 mg/kg/d divided bid PO—pharyngitis, skin, tonsillitis, lower respiratory tract Adults: 500 mg/d PO—pharyngitis, tonsillitis, lower respiratory tract, skin	125, 250 mg/tsp 250, 500 mg tab	Not indicated for infants <6 mo. Less efficacy against *Haemophilus influenzae* and *Moraxella catarrhalis* than other antibiotics.
Ceftriaxone (Rocephin) *Third-generation cephalosporin*	Children: 50–75 mg/kg/d divided 1–2 times daily, IV/IM Meningitis: 100 mg/kg/d IV/IM Adults: 1–2 g q12–24h IV/IM (max. 4 g/d) Skin, bone and joint, urinary tract, gynecological, respiratory tract, intraabdominal infections, bacteremia	0.25, 0.5, 1, 5, 10 g vial	GI side effects. Mix with lidocaine to prevent pain at IM injection site.

Table continued on following page

Medications Continued

GENERIC/TRADE CLASSIFICATION	DOSE/INDICATIONS	SUPPLIED	REMARKS
Cefuroxime axetil (Ceftin) *Second-generation cephalosporin*	Children: <2 yr: 30 mg/kg/d divided bid PO 2–12 yr: 250 mg bid PO Adults: 250–500 mg bid PO Pharyngitis, tonsillitis, skin, otitis media, lower respiratory tract, urinary tract, uncomplicated gonorrhea (single 1 g dose)	125, 250, 500 mg tab 125 mg/tsp suspension 250 mg/tsp suspension	Crushed tab has bitter taste.
Cephalexin monohydrate (Keflex, Keftab, Novolexin, Keflet) *First-generation cephalosporin*	Children: 25–50 mg/kg/d divided tid PO Adults: 250–1000 mg tid PO (max. 4 g/d) Skin, bone and joint, septicemia, respiratory tract, urinary tract, otitis media, pharyngitis	125, 250 mg/tsp 250, 500 mg tab 250, 500 mg and 1 g capsule	
Cetirizine (Zyrtec) *Antihistamine*	2–5 yr: 2.5 mg qd to max. of 5 mg qd or divided bid >6 yr: 5–10 mg qd Seasonal or perennial rhinitis, urticaria	10 mg tablets 5 mg/5 ml syrup	Drug interaction: large doses of theophylline. Side effects: fatigue, dry mouth, somnolence, HA.

Drug	Dosage	How Supplied	Comments
Chlorpheniramine maleate (Chlor-Trimeton) *Antihistamine*	Children: <2 yr: 0.35 mg/kg/d divided q4–6h PO 2–6 yr: 1 mg q4–6h, PO (max. 12 mg/d) 6–12 yr: 2 mg q4–6h PO Adults: 4 mg q4–6h PO (max. 24 mg/d) Allergic rhinitis, urticaria	2 mg/tsp syrup 2 mg chewable 4, 8, 12 mg tab 8, 12 mg timed-release tab, capsule	Used cautiously in patients with impaired renal or hepatic function. Adverse reactions: dizziness, confusion, headache. Drug interactions: diazepam, theophylline, propranolol, antacids, phenytoin, tricyclic antidepressants, oral contraceptives, warfarin.
Cimetidine (Tagamet) *Histamine-receptor antagonist*	Children: 20–40 mg/kg/d PO divided qid Adults: 300 mg PO qid before meals and qhs Used in the treatment of duodenal ulcer, hypersecretory conditions, gastroesophageal reflux	300 mg/tsp liquid 200, 300, 400, 800 mg tab	
Ciprofloxacin hydrochloride & hydrocortisone (Cipro HC Otic) *Antibiotic and steroid*	Adults and children >1 yr: 3 drops to affected ear bid for 7 d Otitis externa	Otic suspension, 10 ml bottle	Do not use if TM is perforated. Side effects: HA, pruritus, rash.
Clemastine fumarate (OTC) (Tavist) *Antihistamine*	Children 6–12 yr: 0.67–1.34 mg PO bid (max. 4.02 mg/d) Adults: 1.34–2.68 mg PO bid (max. 8.04 mg/d) Allergic rhinitis urticaria, allergies	0.67 mg/tsp syrup 1.34, 2.68 mg tab	Indicated for treatment of urticaria at doses of 2.68 mg.

Table continued on following page

Medications Continued

GENERIC/TRADE CLASSIFICATION	DOSE/INDICATIONS	SUPPLIED	REMARKS
Clotrimazole (OTC) (Mycelex troches, Lotrimin, Gyne-Lotrimin) *Local anti-infective, antifungal*	Oral candidiasis: Children >3 yr and adults: 10 mg troche PO—dissolve slowly, 5 times daily for 2 wk Vaginal candidiasis: 1 applicator or 1 vaginal tab qhs for 1–2 wk Tinea pedis, tinea cruris, tinea corporis, or tinea versicolor: topical application of cream bid for 1–8 wk	10 mg troche 1% cream, solution, lotion 100, 500 mg vaginal tab	Adverse reactions: nausea, vomiting, abnormal liver function tests.
Codeine *Opiate agonist, antitussive*	Children: Analgesic: 0.5–1 mg/kg/dose q4–6h PO, IM, SC (max. 60 mg/dose) Antitussive: 2–6 yr: 2.5–5 mg q4–6h PO (max. 30 mg/d); 7–12 yr: 5–10 mg q4–6h PO (max. 60 mg/d) Adults: 10–20 mg/dose q4–6h (max. 120 mg/d)	15 mg/tsp solution 15, 30, 60 mg tab 30, 60 mg/ml injection	

Drug	Dosage/Indications	Preparations	Comments
Cromolyn sodium (Intal, Nasalcrom) *Mast cell stabilizer*	Children >2 yr (oral inhalation): 20 mg qid Adults and children >5 yr (oral inhalation): 2 inhalations qid by metered-dose inhaler or 20 mg, oral or nebulizer qid; 1 spray, intranasally, 3 or 4 times daily Used as prophylaxis in treatment of allergic disorders and asthma; used for exercise-induced bronchospasm	Solution: 20 mg/2 ml for nebulization Solution, nasal: 40 mg/ml Aerosol: 800 μg/metered spray	Not to be used to treat acute asthmatic attacks. Adverse reactions: HA, bronchospasm, urticaria, cough, throat irritation. Do not withdraw drug abruptly.
Cyproheptadine HCl (Periactin) *Antihistamine*	2–6 yr: 2 mg q8–12h PO (max. 12 mg/d) 7–14 yr: 4 mg q8–12h PO (max. 16 mg/d) Adults: 12–16 mg/d divided q8h (max. 0.5 mg/kg/d) Allergic rhinitis, urticaria, allergic conjunctivitis, vascular cluster headaches Experimentally used to stimulate appetite and increase weight gain in children	2 mg/tsp syrup 4 mg tab	Can cause weight gain. In some patients, sedative effect disappears within 3–4 d.

Table continued on following page

TABLE A-1
Medications *Continued*

GENERIC/TRADE CLASSIFICATION	DOSE/INDICATIONS	SUPPLIED	REMARKS
Dexamethasone (Decadron) *Glucocorticoid, anti-inflammatory*	Children (anti-inflammatory): 0.03–0.15 mg/kg/d PO, IV, or IM divided 2–4 times daily Adults (anti-inflammatory, other uses): 0.5–9 mg/d PO, IV, or IM divided 2–3 times daily Used in the treatment of chronic inflammatory disorders, cerebral edema, shock, allergies, and hematological disorders	0.5 mg/5 ml elixir 1 mg/ml oral solution 0.5, 0.75, 1, 1.5, 2, 4, 6 mg tab	Contraindicated in patients with systemic fungal infections. Use cautiously in patients with untreated viral or bacterial infections, renal disease, heart disease, tuberculosis, ulcerative colitis, hypothyroidism, diabetes. Do not give live vaccines to patients taking Decadron. Can mask signs and symptoms of infection. Drug interactions: oral anticoagulants, oral contraceptives, rifampin, phenytoin, barbiturates, hypoglycemics
Dextroamphetamine saccharate; dextroamphetamine sulfate; amphetamine aspartate; amphetamine sulfate (Adderall) *Amphetamine, CNS stimulant*	3–5 yr: 2.5 mg qd Increases of 2.5 mg/per wk >6 yr: 5 mg qd Increases of 5 mg/wk Max. 40 mg/d in divided doses, at intervals of 4–6 hr Used in the treatment of ADHD/ADD	5, 10, 20, 30 mg tablets. All tablets are double scored	Drug interactions: MAO inhibitors, tricyclic antidepressants, antihypertensives, phenobarbital, meperidine, phenytoin. Abuse potential. Side effects: HTN, anorexia, dry mouth, GI disturbance. Can exacerbate tics and Tourette syndrome.

Dextroamphetamine sulfate (Dexedrine) *Amphetamine, CNS stimulant*	Narcolepsy: Children 6–12 yr: 5 mg initially; may increase by 5 mg/d at weekly intervals (max. 60 mg/d) Adults: 10 mg initially; increase by 10 mg/d at weekly intervals (max. 60 mg/d); give in divided doses or use long-acting forms ADHD: Children 3–5 yr: 2.5 mg/d initially; increase by 2.5 mg/d weekly; usual dose 0.1–0.5 mg/kg/d, given in the AM (max. 40 mg/d) Children >6 yr: 5 mg/d initially given qd or divided bid; increase by 5 mg/d weekly; usual dose 0.1–0.5 mg/kg/d, given in the AM (max. 40 mg/d) Used in the treatment of ADHD and narcolepsy	5, 10, 15 mg capsule (spansule), sustained release 5, 10 mg tab 5 mg/tsp elixir	Contraindicated in patients with hypertension, hyperthyroidism, glaucoma, or cardiovascular disease. Drug interactions: MAO inhibitors, tricyclic antidepressants, phenobarbital, phenytoin; insulin requirements may be altered. Do not give within 6 hr of bedtime. Adverse reactions: GI disturbances, dry mouth, anorexia, hypertension, tremor, tachycardia. Avoid caffeine.

Table continued on following page

Medications Continued

GENERIC/TRADE CLASSIFICATION	DOSE/INDICATIONS	SUPPLIED	REMARKS
Dextromethorphan hydrobromide (Benylin DM, Delsym, Hold, Robitussin DM, Sucrets Cough) *Non-narcotic antitussive*	Children: 2–5 yr: 2.5–5 mg q4h PO (max. 30 mg/d) >6 yr: 5–10 mg q4h PO (max. 60 mg/d) Adults: 10–20 mg q4h PO (max. 120 mg/d) Cough suppression	5, 7.5, 10, 15 mg/tsp syrup 5 mg lozenge 15 mg chewable 30 mg/tsp extended-release syrup	
Dicloxacillin monohydrate (Dycill, Dynapen, Pathocil) *Penicillinase-resistant penicillin*	Children <40 kg: 12–50 mg/kg/d PO divided q6h Children >40 kg and adults: 125–500 mg PO q6h Sinusitis, skin, bone and joint, respiratory tract (infections caused by penicillinase-producing *Staphylococcus*)	62.5 mg/tsp suspension 125, 250, 500 mg capsule	Drug interactions: warfarin, rifampin, aminoglycosides. Food decreases absorption.

Drug	Dosage	Preparations	Comments
Diphenhydramine hydrochloride (OTC) (Benadryl) *Antihistamine*	Children: 1.0 mg/kg/dose q6-8h PO/IM/IV (max. 300 mg/d) Adults: 25-50 mg/dose q4-6h PO/IM/IV Allergic rhinitis, urticaria, allergic reaction to blood or plasma, motion sickness, vertigo, cough, insomnia, control of dyskinetic movement	6.25 and 12.5 mg/tsp syrup, elixir 12.5 mg chewable 25-50 mg tab, capsule 10, 50 mg/ml injection 1%, 2% cream, lotion	Can cause respiratory suppression.
Docusate sodium (Colace) *Laxative*	Children 3-6 yr: 20-60 mg/d PO Children 6-12 yr: 40-120 mg/d PO Adults: 50-400 mg/d PO divided 1-4 times daily Stool softener	10 mg/ml liquid 50, 100 mg capsule	Drug interactions: mineral oil. Mix liquid with fruit juice or milk to mask taste.
Epinephrine (Asthma-Nefrin, Bronkaid Mist, EpiPen, EpiPen Jr., Sus-Phrine) *Bronchodilator, vasopressor, cardiac stimulant*	Children: 0.01 mg/kg SC repeat q15 min for 2 doses, then q4h prn (max. 0.5 mg/dose) Adults: 0.2-0.5 mg SC q20 min-4 hr (max. 1 mg/dose) Inhalation: 1 or 2 inhalations of 1:100 or 2.25% Bronchodilation; anaphylactic reactions	1:1000 (1 mg/ml) injection 1%, 1.25%, 2.25% nebulizer inhaler 160, 200, 250 μg/metered spray	Inhaled beta$_2$-agonist preferred. Rotate injection sites. Adverse effects: ECG changes, restlessness, tremor, nausea, vomiting.

Table continued on following page

Medications *Continued*

GENERIC/TRADE CLASSIFICATION	DOSE/INDICATIONS	SUPPLIED	REMARKS
Erythromycin (E-Mycin, ERYC, Ery-Tab, PCE Dispertabs)	All 3 preparations dosed as follows:	125 mg pellets in capsule	Most prescribe tid. GI upset common. Give with food to decrease side effects. Drug interactions: theophylline, carbamazepine, cyclosporine, digoxin, terfenadine, warfarin. Useful in patients allergic to penicillin.
Erythromycin estolate (Iliosone)	Children: 30–50 mg/kg/d PO divided q6h	250, 333 mg tab; 250 mg capsule 100 mg/ml drops; 125, 250 mg/tsp 125, 250 mg chewable	
Erythromycin ethylsuccinate (EES) (E.E.S., EryPed, Wyamycin E)	Adults: 250–500 mg PO qid Upper and lower respiratory tract, otitis media, pharyngitis, syphilis, gonorrhea, skin, gynecological disorders, and Legionnaires' disease	250, 500 mg tab 200, 400 mg/tsp 200 mg chewable; 400 mg tab	
EES and sulfisoxazole (Pediazole, Eryzole) *Erythromycin and sulfonamide*	Children >2 mo: 40–50 mg/kg/d PO divided q6h (max. 2 g erythromycin, 6 g sulfisoxazole/d) Upper and lower respiratory tract disorders, otitis media	EES 200 mg and sulfisoxazole 600 mg/ tsp (100, 150, 200, 250 ml)	Most prescribe tid. Drug interactions as with erythromycin.

Drug	Dosage	Notes
Ferrous sulfate (OTC) (Feosol, Fer-In-Sol, Fer-Iron) *Oral iron supplement*	Children (elemental iron): 1–2 mg/kg/d to 15 mg/d for prophylaxis; 3–6 mg/kg/d in divided doses for treatment of iron deficiency Adults (ferrous sulfate): 300 mg/d for prophylaxis; 300 mg bid to 300 mg qid for iron deficiency Used in the prevention and treatment of iron deficiency anemia	Fer-In-Sol drops: 15 mg/0.6 ml elemental iron Fer-In-Sol elixir: 18 mg/tsp elemental iron Feosol elixir: 44 mg/tsp elemental iron Tab: 300 mg ferrous sulfate Contraindicated in patients with enteritis, ulcers, ulcerative colitis, hemochromatosis, hemolytic anemia, hepatitis. Drug interactions: tetracycline, vitamin C, antacids, chloramphenicol. Adverse reactions: GI symptoms, staining of teeth, dark stools. Overdosage can be fatal, at levels >300 µg/ml.
Fexofenadine HCl (Allegra) *Antihistamine*	>12 yr: 60 mg bid; 60 mg qd if decreased renal function Treatment of seasonal allergic rhinitis	60 mg capsules Allegra-D has 120 mg of pseudoephedrine in each capsule for extended release. Drug interactions: MAO inhibitors, antihypertensives. Side effects: HA, GI upset, insomnia, dry mouth.
Fluconazole (Diflucan) *Antifungal*	Oral candidiasis: >2 wk of age: 6 mg/kg on day 1, then 3 mg/kg/d for 2 wk Adults: 200 mg on day 1, then 100 mg/d for 2 wk Vaginal candidiasis: Adults: 150 mg PO once Used for oral, esophageal, systemic candidiasis	10 mg/ml; 40 mg/ml 50, 100, 150, 200 mg tab Monitor renal and liver function with long-term therapy. Can cause nausea, HA, rash, vomiting, abdominal pain, diarrhea. Drug interactions: warfarin, theophylline, oral hypoglycemics, phenytoin, cyclosporine, rifampin, hydrochlorothiazide, propulsid, astemizole.

Table continued on following page

T A B L E A–1

Medications Continued

GENERIC/TRADE CLASSIFICATION	DOSE/INDICATIONS	SUPPLIED	REMARKS
Flunisolide (AeroBid, Nasalide, Nasarel) *Glucocorticoid, anti-inflammatory*	Children 6–14 yr: 1 inhalation or 1 spray each nostril bid (max. 4 inhalations or sprays daily) Adults: 2 inhalations or 2 sprays each nostril bid (max. 8 inhalations or sprays daily) Used in the treatment of asthma requiring chronic steroid use; nasal solution used to treat seasonal allergic rhinitis	250 µg/metered spray oral inhalant 25 µg/metered spray nasal inhalant	Rinse mouth following oral inhalation. Contraindicated in patients with fungal, untreated bacterial, or viral infections. Not to be used to treat acute asthmatic attacks. Adverse reactions: oral candidal infections, nasal irritation, adrenal suppression, headache. Do not stop drug abruptly. Use caution when transferring from systemic steroids to inhaled steroids.

Fluoride (many preparations) *Mineral supplement*	Osteoporosis: Children: 0.5 mg/kg/d in divided doses Adults: 30–100 mg/d in divided doses Nutritional supplement: <0.3 ppm fluoride content of water: 6 mo–3 yr: 0.25 mg PO daily 3–6 yr: 0.5 mg PO daily 6–16 yr: 1 mg PO daily 0.3–0.6 ppm fluoride content of water: 6 mo–3 yr: no supplement required 3–6 yr: 0.25 mg PO daily 6–16 yr: 0.5 mg PO daily Used to prevent dental caries and in treatment of osteoporosis	Drops calibrated by fluoride ion Luride drops: 0.125 mg/drop Pediaflor drops: 0.5 mg/ml Tri-Vi-Flor drops: 0.25, 0.5 mg/ml Oral solution: 1 mg/ml fluoride ion Chewable tab: 0.25, 0.5 mg fluoride ion Tab: 0.25 mg fluoride ion	Do not give if fluoride content of water >0.6 ppm. Do not give with milk products. Adverse reactions: GI upset; do not swallow rinse or gel. Dental fluorosis can occur if supplements are given unnecessarily. Infants <6 mo should not receive fluoride supplements. This includes those exclusively breastfed.
Fluticasone propionate (Flovent, Flonase) *Steroid*	>4 yr: 50 μg bid to maximum of 100 μg bid when using rotadisk 1 spray per nostril to maximum of 2 sprays per nostril when using nasal spray Treatment of seasonal or perennial allergic rhinitis and as asthma therapy	50, 100, 250 μg rotadisk Nasal spray, 16 g, 120 sprays 44 μg/inhalation, 110 μg/inhalation inhalers	Side effects: nasal irritation, HA, candidiasis, pharyngitis. If exposed to varicella, consider prophylactic therapy to prevent varicella. Rinse mouth following use.

Table continued on following page

Medications *Continued*

GENERIC/TRADE CLASSIFICATION	DOSE/INDICATIONS	SUPPLIED	REMARKS
Griseofulvin (Fulvicin, Grifulvin, Grisactin, Gris-PEG) *Penicillium griseofulvum derivative*	Children: 10 mg/kg/d (microsize) or 5 mg/kg/d (ultra-microsize) Adults: 500–1000 mg qd (microsize), 125–165 mg bid (ultra-microsize), or 250–330 mg qd For treatment of tinea corporis, tinea pedis, tinea capitis, tinea unguium, tinea cruris	Microsize: 125 mg/tsp suspension 125, 250 mg capsule 250, 500 mg tab Ultra-microsize: 125, 165, 250, 330 mg tab	Give with fatty foods to increase absorption. Use with caution in penicillin-sensitive patients. Adverse reactions: blood dyscrasias, nausea, vomiting, photosensitivity. Drug interactions: alcohol, barbiturates, warfarin, anticoagulants.
Hydroxyzine hydrochloride (Atarax, Vistaril) *Miscellaneous anxiolytics, sedative, hypnotic, antihistamine*	Children: 0.6 mg/kg/dose q6h PO; 1 mg/kg/dose q4–6h IM Adults: Antiemetic: 25–100 mg IM Anxiety: 50–100 mg qid PO (max. 600 mg) Preop: 50–100 mg PO, 25–100 mg IM Pruritus: 25 mg q6–8h PO	10 mg/tsp syrup (Atarax) 25 mg/tsp suspension (Vistaril) 10, 25, 50 mg tab (Atarax) 25, 50, 100 mg capsule (Vistaril) 25, 50 mg/ml injection	

Drug	Dosage	Supplied	Comments
Ibuprofen (Advil, Motrin, Nuprin) *Nonsteroidal anti-inflammatory*	Children >6 mo: Antipyretic: 5–10 mg/kg/dose q6–8h PO: maximum dose 40 mg/kg/dose Juvenile arthritis: 30–70 mg/kg/d PO divided tid Analgesic: 4–10 mg/kg/dose PO divided tid Adults: 200–800 mg/dose tid-qid Management of inflammatory disorders: analgesic for mild/moderate pain: antipyretic: dysmenorrhea	40 mg/ml, 100 mg/tsp 100 mg chewable 200 mg tab (OTC) 300, 400, 600, 800 mg tab (Rx)	Drug interactions: digoxin, methotrexate. Can cause GI upset. Contraindicated in patients with aspirin sensitivities or bleeding disorders.
Imipramine (Tofranil, Tofranil-PM) *Tricyclic antidepressant*	Children >6 yr (enuresis): 25 mg PO initially qhs: increase by 10–25 mg/dose increments weekly (max. 2.5–5.0 mg/kg/d or 75 mg qhs) Adults (depression): 50–100 mg/d PO initially divided tid; increase by 25–50 mg to max. of 300 mg/d Used in the treatment of childhood enuresis and depression	10, 25, 50 mg tab 75, 100, 125, 150 mg capsule—Tofranil-PM (imipramine pamoate)	Use with caution in patients with cardiac disease, glaucoma, seizure disorders, diabetes. Drug interactions: MAO inhibitors (if given within 14 d), warfarin, CNS depressants, antihypertensive agents. Adverse reactions: drowsiness, dry mouth, GI upset, photosensitivity, arrhythmias. Can take 2–4 wk to see full effects of therapy. *Table continued on following page*

Medications *Continued*

GENERIC/TRADE CLASSIFICATION	DOSE/INDICATIONS	SUPPLIED	REMARKS
Isoniazid (INH, Laniazid) *Antituberculosis agent*	Children: 10–20 mg/kg/d PO divided bid Prophylaxis: 10 mg/kg/d (max. 300 mg/d) Adults: 5 mg/kg/d PO qd (usual dose 300 mg/d) Disseminated disease: 10 mg/kg/d divided bid Prophylaxis: 300 mg/d Following 1–2 mo of treatment for tuberculosis: Children: 20–40 mg/kg/dose (max. 900 mg) biweekly Adults: 15 mg/kg/dose (max. 900 mg) biweekly	50 mg/tsp 100, 300 mg tab	Take on empty stomach. Avoid food containing tyramine. Avoid alcohol. Drug interactions: phenytoin, diazepam, carbamazepine. Adverse reactions: peripheral neuritis, seizures, ataxia, stupor, tinnitus, diarrhea.

Ketoconazole (Nizoral) *Antifungal*	Systemic candidiasis, histoplasmosis, blastomycosis, chromomycosis Children <2 yr: 3.3–6.6 mg/kg/d PO Adults and children >40 kg: Initially 200 mg PO qd: may increase to 400 mg qd if no response to lower dose Minimum treatment for candidiasis is 7–14 d; for other systemic fungal infections, use for 6 mo Topical treatment of tinea corporis, tinea cruris, tinea versicolor Adults and children: apply 1 or 2 times daily for 2 wk	100 mg/tsp suspension 200 mg tab (scored) 2% cream (15, 30, 60 g)	Adverse reactions: hepatotoxicity, nausea, vomiting. Most effective oral antifungal. Drug interactions: phenytoin, cimetidine, ranitidine, rifampin, terfenadine.
Levalbuterol HCl (Xopenex) *Bronchodilator*	>12 yr: 0.63 mg tid (6–8 h). 1.25 mg may be used in more severe asthma or in patients not responding to 0.63 mg Prevention and treatment of bronchospasm	0.63 mg/3 ml unit dose, 1.25 mg/3 ml inhalation solution	Drug interactions: β-blockers, diuretics, digoxin, MAO inhibitors or tricyclic antidepressants Side effects: tachycardia, tremor, nervousness, pain, flu-syndrome. *Table continued on following page*

497

TABLE A-1
Medications Continued

GENERIC/TRADE CLASSIFICATION	DOSE/INDICATIONS	SUPPLIED	REMARKS
Lindane (Kwell, Kwildane, Scabene) *Scabicide, pediculicide*	Scabies: Adults and children: apply thin layer, massage, moving from neck to toes; shower after 8–12 h; treatment can be repeated in 1 wk Lice: Adults and children: apply to hairy areas and adjacent areas, wash off in 8–12 h; for scalp, shampoo well for 4–5 min, rinse, and comb hair to remove nits	1% cream, lotion, shampoo	Avoid contact with eyes, mucous membranes, face, and urethral meatus. Not recommended for infants or young children. Body should be clean and dry before application. Do not apply to broken or inflamed skin. Itching may continue for 4–6 wk.
Loratadine (Claritin) *Antihistamine*	Children >6 yr: 5–10 mg qd Adults and children >12 yr: 10 mg qd PO Nasal and non-nasal symptoms of seasonal allergic rhinitis	10 mg tab 10 mg redi-tab 10 mg/10 ml syrup	Give on empty stomach. Possible interaction with macrolide antibiotics, ketoconazole, cimetidine, ranitidine, or theophylline.

Drug	Dosage/Form	Indications/Dosing	Comments
Mebendazole (Vermox) *Anthelmintic*	100 mg tab (chewable)	Pinworms: Adults and children >2 yr: 100 mg PO as single dose; can repeat in 2–3 wk if infection persists Roundworms, whipworms, hookworms: Adults and children >2 yr: 100 mg PO bid for 3 d; can repeat in 3 wk	Few side effects at low doses. Occasional abdominal pain and diarrhea. Can swallow tablets.
Mefenamic acid (Ponstel) *Nonsteroidal anti-inflammatory*	250 mg tab	>14 yr: 500 mg, then 250 mg q4–6 hr—not to exceed 1 wk Mild to moderate pain, dysmenorrhea, inflammatory disease	Adverse reactions: blood dyscrasias. Drug interactions: anticoagulants, phenytoin, sulfonamides, corticosteroids.
Methylphenidate (Ritalin) *CNS stimulant*	5, 10, 20 mg tab (scored) 20 mg sustained-release tab	Children >6 yr (ADHD): 5 mg PO 1 or 2 times daily initially; increase by 5–10 mg weekly; usual dose 0.3–0.7 mg/kg/dose given 2 or 3 times daily Adults (narcolepsy): 10 mg PO 2 or 3 times daily, up to 60 mg/d; give before meals Used for the treatment of narcolepsy and ADHD	Contraindicated in patients with hyperthyroidism, cardiovascular disease, glaucoma, hypertension. Cautious use in patients with tics or Tourette syndrome. Drug interactions: MAO inhibitors, tricyclic antidepressants, anticonvulsants. Adverse reactions: anorexia, insomnia, nausea. *Table continued on following page*

T A B L E A–1
Medications Continued

GENERIC/TRADE CLASSIFICATION	DOSE/INDICATIONS	SUPPLIED	REMARKS
Metronidazole (Flagyl) *Anti-infective* (miscellaneous)	Children (PO): Amebiasis: 35–50 mg/kg/d divided tid Other parasites: 15–30 mg/kg/d divided tid Anaerobic: 30 mg/kg/d divided q6h *Clostridium difficile* (antibiotic-associated colitis): 20 mg/kg/d divided q6h (max. 2 g/d) Adults (PO): Amebiasis: 500–750 mg q8h for 5–10 d Other parasites: 250 mg q8h or 2 g as single dose Anaerobic: 30 mg/kg/d divided q6h Antibiotic-associated colitis: 250 mg qid for 10–14 d	50 mg/ml 250, 500 mg tab	Adverse reactions: HA, metallic taste, nausea, diarrhea, dizziness, dry mouth. Avoid alcohol. Drug interactions: warfarin, phenobarbital, cimetidine.

Drug	Dosage	Formulation	Notes
Miconazole nitrate (Micatin, Monistat-Derm, Monistat 7) *Local antifungal*	Topical treatment of tinea pedis, tinea cruris, tinea corporis, tinea versicolor: Children >2 yr and adults: apply bid for 2–4 wk Vaginal or vulvar candidiasis: 1 application or vaginal suppository qhs for 1 wk	2% cream, lotion, spray, powder 100, 200 mg vaginal suppository	
Mineral oil (OTC) (Agoral) *Laxative*	Children: 1–2 ml/kg/dose bid PO Adults: 15–60 ml/d PO as single dose; retention enema, 60–150 ml	Sterile liquid Fleet enema—133 ml	Contraindicated in children <4 yr due to aspiration potential. Enema form not for use in children <2 yr. Give on empty stomach.
Minocycline HCl (Minocin) *Tetracycline*	>8 yr: 4 mg/kg/d PO divided bid Adults: Carriers: 200 mg initially, then 100 mg bid for 5 d Acne: 50 mg 1–3 times daily Syphilis/gonorrhea: 200 mg initially, then 100 mg q12h for 10–15 d Other indications: *Mycoplasma, Chlamydia, Rickettsia,* neisserial meningitis carriers	50 mg/tsp 50, 100 mg tab and capsule	Photosensitivity. Outdated products can be toxic.

Table continued on following page

Medications *Continued*

GENERIC/ TRADE CLASSIFICATION	DOSE/INDICATIONS	SUPPLIED	REMARKS
Montelukast sodium (Singulair) *Leukotriene receptor antagonist*	Children 6–14 yr: 5 mg qhs Adults and children >15 yr: 10 mg qhs Prophylaxis and chronic treatment of asthma	5 mg chewable tablet 10 mg tablet	Drug interactions: phenobarbital, rifampin. Side effects: asthenia/fatigue, abdominal pain, HA, cough.
Mupirocin (Bactroban) *Topical antibiotic*	Apply 3 times daily Useful in the treatment of impetigo due to *Staphylococcus, Streptococcus*	2% ointment or cream (15 g)	
Naproxen (Naprosyn) *Nonsteroidal anti-inflammatory*	Children >2 yr: 10–20 mg/kg/d in 2 divided doses Juvenile arthritis: 10–15 mg/kg/d (max. 1000 mg/d) Analgesic: 5–7 mg/kg/dose q8–12h Adults: Rheumatoid arthritis: 500–1000 mg/d Analgesia: 250 mg q6–8h (max. 1250 mg/d)	125 mg/tsp suspension 250, 375, 500 mg tab	Use cautiously in patients with impaired renal function or burns. Take with milk, antacids, or food. Drug interactions: warfarin, methotrexate.

Drug (classification)	Dosage/Use	Preparation	Nursing Considerations
Nedocromil sodium (Tilade) *Nonsteroidal anti-inflammatory*	Adults and children >6 yr (inhalation): 2 inhalations, qid. Adults and children >2 yr (nebulizer): 1 ampule qid. Used as prophylaxis in treatment of asthma	175 µg/metered spray oral inhalant; 0.5% nebulizer solution; 11 mg/2.2 ml ampules	Not to be used for acute asthma attacks. Not approved for children <6 yr. Adverse reactions: bad taste, HA.
Neomycin, polymyxin B, hydrocortisone (Pediotic) *Antibiotic, anti-inflammatory*	3–4 drops 3–4 times daily until symptoms are relieved. Used for treatment of superficial bacterial infections of the external ear	Otic suspension	A wick can be used to instill drops—saturate cotton with drops and leave in ear canal. The wick should be replaced q24h.
Nitrofurantoin (Furadantin, Macrodantin) *Urinary anti-infective*	Children: 5–7 mg/kg/d PO divided q6h. Chronic therapy: 1–5 mg/kg/d divided bid (max. 400 mg/d). Adults: 50–100 mg/dose PO q6h. Prophylaxis: 50–100 mg/dose qhs. Prevention and treatment of urinary tract infections; *Pseudomonas, Serratia,* and *Proteus* are resistant to this drug	25 mg/tsp; 50, 100 mg tab (scored); Macrodantin—25, 50, 100 mg capsule	Can cause discoloration of urine. Do not crush tab. Rinse mouth following administration of suspension to prevent staining of teeth.

Table continued on following page

T A B L E A-1
Medications Continued

GENERIC/ TRADE CLASSIFICATION	DOSE/INDICATIONS	SUPPLIED	REMARKS
Nystatin (Mycostatin, Nilstat, Nystex, O-V Statin) *Antifungal*	Oral *Monilia:* Neonates: 100,000 U qid Infants: 200,000 U qid Children and adults: 500,000 U qid Gastrointestinal infections: Adults: 500,000–1 million U as tab qid Cutaneous and mucocutaneous candidal infections: Topical: apply 2 or 3 times daily Vaginal: 1–2 tabs qhs for 2 wk	100,000 U/ml suspension 500,000 U tab 100,000 U vaginal tab 100,000 U/g cream, ointment, powder	Vaginal tabs can be used by pregnant women up to 6 wk before term. Paint oral suspension in infant's mouth to coat lesions. Vaginal tabs can be used orally by immuno-suppressed patients to provide prolonged drug contact with oral mucosa.

Drug	Dose	How supplied	Comments
Penicillin G benzathine (Bicillin) *Penicillin*	Children (IM): Streptococcal pharyngitis: 25,000 U/kg for 1 dose (max. 1.2 million U) Prophylaxis of rheumatic fever: 25,000 U/kg q3–4 wk (max. 1.2 million U/dose) Syphilis: 50,000 U/kg for 1 dose (max. 2.4 million U) Adult (IM): Streptococcal pharyngitis: 1.2 million U for 1 dose Prophylaxis of rheumatic fever: 1.2 million U q3–4w or 600,000 U bimonthly Syphilis: 2.4 million U for 1 dose	200,000 U tab 300,000, 600,000 or 1,200,000 U/ml injection	Give deep IM in upper, outer quadrant of buttocks. Give midlateral thigh in infants and small children. Adverse reactions: hypersensitivity, pain at injection site.
Penicillin V potassium (Pen-Vee K, Veetids) *Penicillin*	Children: 25–50 mg/kg/d PO divided tid-qid Prophylaxis of pneumococcal infection: <5 yr: 125 mg bid >5 yr: 250 mg bid Other indications: skin and soft tissue disorders, streptococcal pharyngitis	125, 250 mg/tsp drops and solution 125, 250, 500 mg tab	Food interferes with absorption. Drug interactions: tetracycline. Suspension has unpleasant taste.

Table continued on following page

Medications *Continued*

GENERIC/TRADE CLASSIFICATION	DOSE/INDICATIONS	SUPPLIED	REMARKS
Permethrin (OTC) (Nix) *Pediculicide*	Head lice and their eggs: Adults and children >2 yr: apply to hair, leave on for 10 min, then rinse; can repeat treatment in 7 d if lice are observed	1% lotion	Not recommended for children <2 yr. Thorough combing to remove nits is required as well as cleansing of the equipment.
Prednisolone (Delta-Cortef, Pediapred, Prelone) *Glucocorticoid, anti-inflammatory*	Children: Anti-inflammatory: 0.1–2 mg/kg/d PO divided 1–4 times daily Asthma: 1–2 mg/kg/d divided 1–2 times daily for 3–5 d Adults: 5–60 mg/d PO Used in the treatment of inflammatory disorders of respiratory and GI tracts, allergic disorders, and rheumatic disease	Oral solution: 5 mg/5 ml, 15 mg/5 ml	Contraindicated in patients with active, untreated infections, including varicella. Can mask symptoms of infections. Do not abruptly stop drug. Adverse reactions: growth suppression, fractures, GI discomfort, vertigo, acne.

Prednisone (Deltasone, Liquid Pred, Orasone) *Glucocorticoid, anti-inflammatory*	Children: 0.1–2 mg/kg/d PO in 1–4 divided doses Adults: 5–60 mg/d PO divided in 1–4 doses Used in the treatment of inflammatory disorders, allergic disorders, and hematological diseases	Solution: 5 mg/ml, 15 mg/5 ml 1, 2.5, 5, 10, 20, 50 mg tab	See contraindications and side effects for prednisolone.
Promethazine HCl (Phenergan) *Antiemetic, antivertigo*	Children: 0.25–0.5 mg/kg q4–6h PO, IM, IV, rectally Adults: 12.5–25 mg q4–6h PO, IM, IV, rectally Used to treat vertigo, nausea, vomiting	6.25, 25 mg/tsp syrup 12.5, 25, 50 mg tab 12.5, 25, 50 mg suppository 25, 50 mg/ml injection	Drug interactions: MAO inhibitors, CNS depressants. Adverse reactions: confusion, dry mouth, dizziness, drowsiness, blurred vision.
Pyrethrins (OTC) (A-200 Pyrinate, Pyrinyl, Pronton, RID) *Pediculicide*	Pediculosis: Apply to hair and affected body areas, leave on 10 min, rinse; can repeat in 7–10 d; do not repeat in <24 hr	Available as gel, shampoo, liquid	Avoid contact with eyes, face.

Table continued on following page

T A B L E A–1
Medications Continued

GENERIC/TRADE CLASSIFICATION	DOSE/INDICATIONS	SUPPLIED	REMARKS
Ranitidine HCl (Zantac) *Antiulcer agent*	Children: Oral: 1.5–2.3 mg/kg/dose q12h IM, IV: 0.1–0.8 mg/kg/dose q6–8h Adults: 150 mg bid or 300 mg qhs Short-term treatment of active duodenal ulcers and benign gastric ulcers; long-term prophylaxis of duodenal ulcer and gastric hypersecretion; gastroesophageal reflux	25 mg/ml injection 15 mg/ml syrup 150, 300 mg tab	Use with caution if liver and renal impairment. Adverse reactions: HA, dizziness, sedation, malaise, mental confusion, nausea, vomiting, constipation, rash, arthralgia, bradycardia, or tachycardia.
Salmeterol xinafoate (Serevent) *Bronchodilator*	Adults and children >12 yr: 2 inhalations q12h (max. 4 inhalations daily) Children >4 yr: use diskus inhalation q12h Used as maintenance therapy in the treatment of asthma	21 µg/inhalation metered-dose inhaler 50 µg/inhalation diskus	Not used as treatment for acute asthma attack. Use cautiously (high incidence of overuse). Patient education is very important. Drug interactions: MAO inhibitors, tricyclic antidepressants.

Drug	Dosage/Indications	Supplied/Strength	Comments
Sodium citrate and citric acid (Bicitra) *Alkalinizing agent*	Infants and children: 2–3 mEq/kg/d PO divided tid–qid Children: 5–15 ml PO diluted, after meals and qhs Adults: 15–30 ml PO diluted in water or juice, after meals and qhs Used in the management of metabolic acidosis and in conditions requiring alkaline urine	Solution: sodium citrate 500 mg and citric acid 334 mg/5 ml 1 mEq of sodium and 1 mEq of bicarbonate in each 1 ml of Bicitra	Contraindicated in patients with renal insufficiency and in those with a sodium restriction. Drug interactions: antihypertensives. Adverse reactions: hypernatremia, metabolic alkalosis, diarrhea.
Sodium sulfacetamide (Bleph-10, Isopto, Cetamide) *Sulfonamide*	Solution: 1–2 drops 3–4 times daily for 7–10 d; ointment is used 1–4 times daily Used for treatment of ocular infections	Ophthalmic solution 10%, 15% Ophthalmic ointment 10%	Solution will burn with instillation. Do not use in children <2 mo. Eyes should be cleansed before instillation—inactivated by purulent discharge.
Sulfisoxazole (Gantrisin) *Sulfonamide*	Urinary tract infections: >2 mo: 50–60 mg/kg/d dose initially, then 25–30 mg/kg bid (max. 75 mg/kg/d) Adults: 2 g initially, then 1 g bid–tid Otitis media with effusion prophylaxis: 50–75 mg/d	500 mg/tsp 500 mg tab	Not indicated for infants <2 mo. Take on empty stomach.

Table continued on following page

509

Medications Continued

GENERIC/TRADE CLASSIFICATION	DOSE/INDICATIONS	SUPPLIED	REMARKS
Sumatriptan (Imitrex) *5-HT₁ receptor agonist*	>18 yr: 6 mg SC; repeat in 1 hr to maximum of 2 doses per 24 hr Tablets: 25–100 mg once; repeat dose at 2 hr intervals to maximum of 200 mg/d Nasal spray: 5, 10 or 20 mg intranasally; can repeat once; maximum 40 mg or 4 uses/ month Acute treatment of migraine HA	6 mg/0.5 ml SC injection 25, 50 mg tablet 5, 20 mg spray	Drug interactions: MAO inhibitors, SSRIs. Contraindicated in patients with ischemic heart disease or HTN. Side effects: increased blood pressure, flushing, nausea, drowsiness, sweating; local reactions with spray and injection.
Terbutaline (Brethaire, Brethine, Bricanyl) *Bronchodilator*	Children <12 yr: 0.05 mg/kg/dose PO tid (max. 0.15 mg/kg/dose tid or 5 mg/d); 0.01 mg/kg/dose SC (max. 0.3 mg/dose q15–20 min for 2 doses) Adults and children >12 yr: 2.5 mg/dose PO tid; maintenance dose: 5 mg/dose or 0.075 mg/ kg PO 3 or 4 times a day Used in asthma and COPD	2.5, 5 mg tab 0.2 mg/dose aerosol 1 mg/ml injection	Drug interactions: MAO inhibitors, tricyclic antidepressants, β-blockers. Can cause tachycardia, tremor, hypertension, HA, palpitations.

Drug	Dosage	Formulation	Notes
Tetracycline (Achromycin, Sumycin) *Tetracycline*	>8 yr: 25–50 mg/kg/d PO divided qid Adults: 250–500 mg PO qid *Mycoplasma, Chlamydia*, rickettsia, acne, exacerbation of bronchitis, gonorrhea, syphilis (in patients sensitive to penicillin)	125 mg/tsp 250, 500 mg capsule	Take on empty stomach. Photosensitivity. Outdated drugs may be toxic. Drug interactions: antacids, milk, zinc, iron.
Triamcinolone acetonide (Azmacort, Nasacort AQ) *Glucocorticoid, anti-inflammatory*	Children >6 yr: 1–2 oral inhalations 3–4 times daily (max. 12 inhalations daily); 1 spray/nostril qd Adults: 2 oral inhalations 3–4 times daily (max. 16 inhalations daily); 2 sprays/nostril qd Used in the treatment of steroid-dependent asthma; seasonal and perennial allergic rhinitis	100 μg/metered dose, oral inhalation 55 μg/nasal spray	See contraindications and side effects for flunisolide.

Table continued on following page

511

GENERIC/TRADE CLASSIFICATION	DOSE/INDICATIONS	SUPPLIED	REMARKS
Trimethoprim (TMP)-sulfamethoxazole (SMX) (Co-trimoxazole, Bactrim, Bactrim DS, Septra, Septra DS, Sulfatrim, TMS) *Sulfonamide*	Children >2 mo: 6–10 mg TMP/kg/d PO divided bid or 1 ml/kg/d divided bid Adults: 1 DS tab PO bid Urinary tract infections, bronchitis in adults, otitis media, shigellosis, traveler's diarrhea, *Pneumocystis carinii* infection, typhoid fever	TMP 40 mg and SMX 200 mg/tsp TMP 80 mg and SMX 400 mg/tab TMP 160 mg and SMX 800 mg/DS tab	Adverse reactions: Stevens-Johnson syndrome. GI side effects minimal. Not effective against streptococcal infections. Drug interactions: warfarin, methotrexate, phenytoin.
Zafirlukast (Accolate) *Leukotriene receptor antagonist*	>12 yr: 20 mg bid Prophylactic treatment for mild persistent asthma	20 mg tab	Drug interactions: warfarin, erythromycin, theophylline, aspirin. Cautious use with cisapride, calcium channel blockers, cyclosporine, astemizole. Side effects: HA, GI disturbances, dizziness.

Key to abbreviations:

ADD = attention deficit disorder
ADHD = attention deficit with hyperactivity disorder
bid = twice daily
CBC = complete blood count
CNS = central nervous system
COPD = chronic obstructive pulmonary disease
ECG = electrocardiogram
GI = gastrointestinal
GU = genitourinary
HA = headache
HSV = herpes simplex virus
HTN = hypertension
IM = intramuscular
IV = intravenous
LFT = liver function test
MAO = monoamine oxidase
max. = maximum
MDI = metered dose inhaler
OTC = over the counter
PO = by mouth

prn = as needed
q = every
qam = every morning
qd = every day
qhs = bedtime
qid = four times daily
qod = every other day
qwk = every week
RSV = respiratory syncytial virus
Rx = prescription
SC = subcutaneous
SGOT = serum glutamic-oxaloacetic transaminase
SL = sublingual
SSRIs = selective serotonin uptake inhibitors
tab(s) = tablet(s)
tid = three times daily
TM = tympanic membrane
tsp = teaspoon
U = units
URI = upper respiratory infection
wk = week

TABLE A-2
Topical Steroid Preparations

DRUG	DOSAGE FORM
LOW POTENCY	
Alclometasone dipropionate (Aclovate)	0.05% cream, ointment
Desonide (DesOwen, Tridesilon)	0.05% cream, ointment, lotion
Fluocinolone acetonide (Fluonid, Synalar)	0.01% solution, cream
	0.5% cream, ointment
Hydrocortisone (Hytone, Nutracort, Cort-Dome, Synacort)	1% cream, ointment, lotion, solution
	2.5% cream, ointment
MODERATE POTENCY	
Betamethasone valerate (Valisone)	0.01% cream
	0.1% cream, ointment, lotion
Clocortolone pivalate (Cloderm)	0.1% cream
Desoximetasone (Topicort)	0.05% gel
Fluocinolone acetonide (Synalar, Fluonid)	0.025% cream, ointment
	0.1% cream
Flurandrenolide (Cordran)	0.05% cream, lotion, ointment
Fluticasone propionate	0.005% ointment
	0.05% cream
Halcinonide (Halog)	0.025% cream, ointment
Hydrocortisone valerate (Westcort)	0.2% cream, ointment
Mometasone furoate	0.1% cream, lotion, ointment
Triamcinolone acetonide (Kenalog, Aristocort)	0.025%, 0.1% cream, ointment, lotion

HIGH POTENCY

Amcinonide (Cyclocort)	0.1% cream, ointment
Betamethasone dipropionate (Diprosone)	0.05% cream, lotion, ointment, gel
Betamethasone dipropionate, clotrimazole (Lotrisone)	0.25% cream, ointment, emollient cream
Desoximetasone (Topicort)	0.05% cream, ointment
	0.25% cream, ointment
Diflorasone diacetate (Florone, Psorcan)	0.2% cream
	0.05% cream, ointment
Fluocinolone acetonide (Synalar-HP)	0.05% cream, solution, gel, ointment
Fluocinonide (Lidex)	0.1% cream, ointment, solution
Halcinonide (Halog)	0.05% cream, ointment
	0.1% cream, ointment, solution
Halobetasol propionate (Ultravate)	0.05% cream with 1% clotrimazole
Triamcinolone acetonide (Kenalog, Aristocort)	0.5% cream, ointment

REFERENCES

Murphy J (ed): Nurse Practitioner's Prescribing Reference. New York, Prescribing Reference, Inc., 1999.

Physicians' Desk Reference, 53rd ed. Montvale, NJ, Medical Economics Data Production Company, 1999.

Staible SA (ed): Formulary and Drug Dosing Handbook, 2nd ed. The Children's Hospital, Denver, CO., Hudson, OH: Lexi-Comp, 1996.

Growth Grids

REFERENCES

Donovan EF, Tyson JE, et al: Inaccuracy of Ballard scores before 28 weeks' gestation. J Pediatr 135:147–152, 1999.

Sanders M, Allen M, Alexander GR, et al: Gestational age assessment in preterm neonates weighing less than 1500 grams. Pediatrics 88:542–546, 1991.

T A B L E B-1

Weight for Age: Girls 0 to 36 Months

CDC Growth Charts: United States

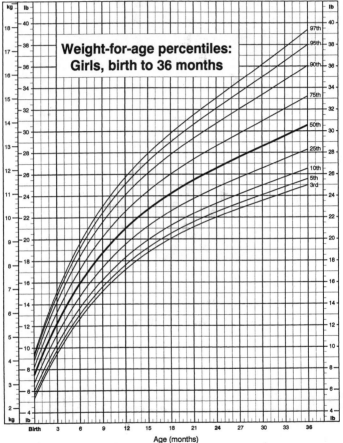

Weight-for-age percentiles: Girls, birth to 36 months

Age (months)

SOURCE: Developed by the National Center for Health Statistics in collaboration with the National Center for Chronic Disease Prevention and Health Promotion (2000).

TABLE B-2

Length for Age: Girls 0 to 36 Months

CDC Growth Charts: United States

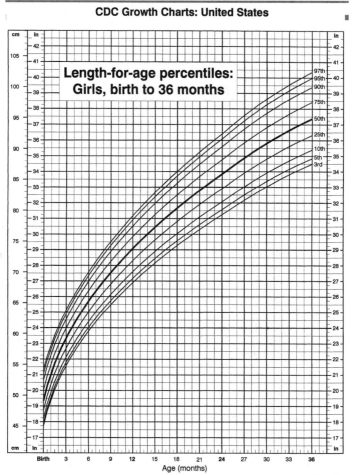

Length-for-age percentiles:
Girls, birth to 36 months

SOURCE: Developed by the National Center for Health Statistics in collaboration with the National Center for Chronic Disease Prevention and Health Promotion (2000).

T A B L E B–3

Weight for Length: Girls 0 to 36 Months

CDC Growth Charts: United States

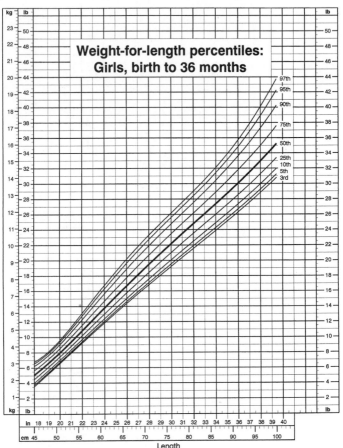

Weight-for-length percentiles:
Girls, birth to 36 months

Length

SOURCE: Developed by the National Center for Health Statistics in collaboration with the National Center for Chronic Disease Prevention and Health Promotion (2000).

T A B L E B–4

Weight for Age: Girls 2 to 20 Years

CDC Growth Charts: United States

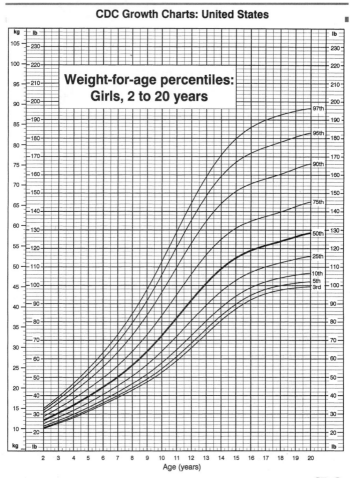

Weight-for-age percentiles:
Girls, 2 to 20 years

Age (years)

SOURCE: Developed by the National Center for Health Statistics in collaboration with
the National Center for Chronic Disease Prevention and Health Promotion (2000).

TABLE B-5

Stature for Age: Girls 2 to 20 Years

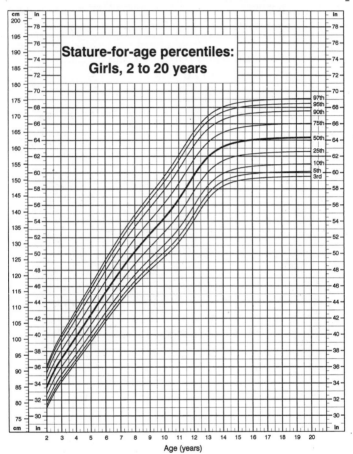

CDC Growth Charts: United States

Stature-for-age percentiles:
Girls, 2 to 20 years

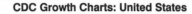

SOURCE: Developed by the National Center for Health Statistics in collaboration with the National Center for Chronic Disease Prevention and Health Promotion (2000).

T A B L E B–6

Weight for Stature: Girls

CDC Growth Charts: United States

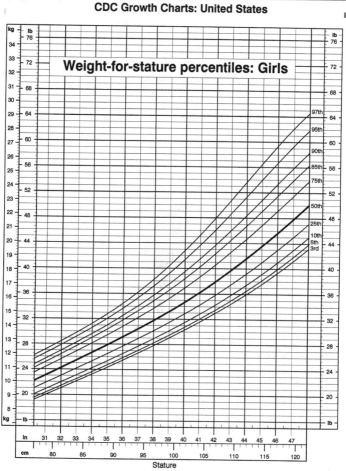

SOURCE: Developed by the National Center for Health Statistics in collaboration with
the National Center for Chronic Disease Prevention and Health Promotion (2000).

T A B L E B–7

Body Mass Index for Age: Girls 2 to 20 Years

CDC Growth Charts: United States

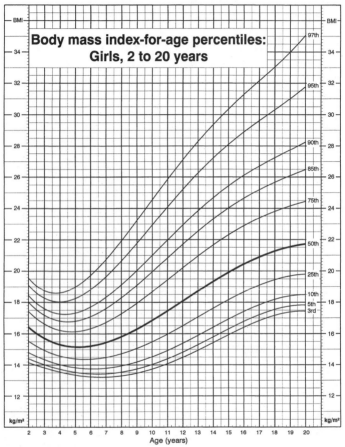

Body mass index-for-age percentiles:
Girls, 2 to 20 years

Age (years)

SOURCE: Developed by the National Center for Health Statistics in collaboration with the National Center for Chronic Disease Prevention and Health Promotion (2000).

T A B L E B–8

Weight for Age: Boys 0 to 36 Months

CDC Growth Charts: United States

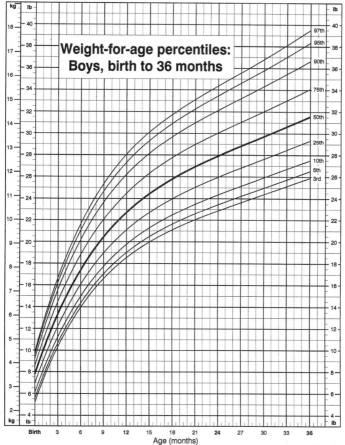

**Weight-for-age percentiles:
Boys, birth to 36 months**

SOURCE: Developed by the National Center for Health Statistics in collaboration with
the National Center for Chronic Disease Prevention and Health Promotion (2000).

TABLE B-9

Length for Age: Boys 0 to 36 Months

CDC Growth Charts: United States

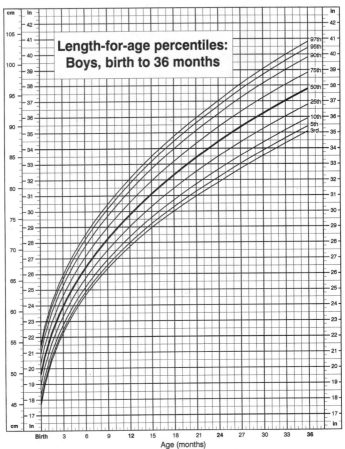

Length-for-age percentiles:
Boys, birth to 36 months

SOURCE: Developed by the National Center for Health Statistics in collaboration with the National Center for Chronic Disease Prevention and Health Promotion (2000).

T A B L E B–10

Weight for Length: Boys 0 to 36 Months

CDC Growth Charts: United States

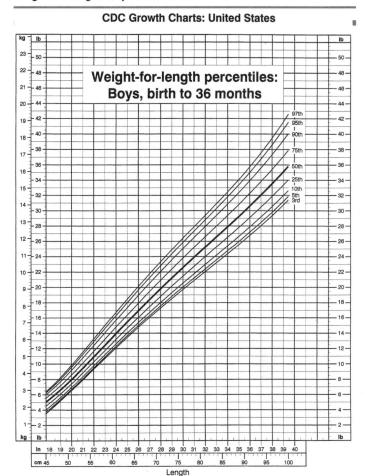

Weight-for-length percentiles: Boys, birth to 36 months

Length

SOURCE: Developed by the National Center for Health Statistics in collaboration with the National Center for Chronic Disease Prevention and Health Promotion (2000).

TABLE B–11

Weight for Age: Boys 2 to 20 Years

CDC Growth Charts: United States

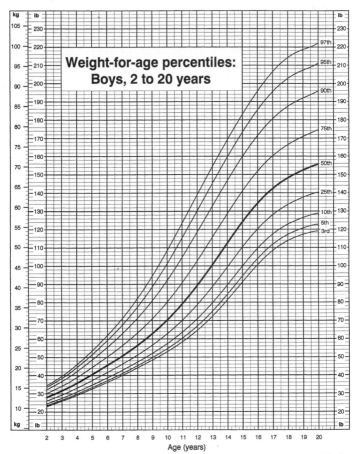

Weight-for-age percentiles: Boys, 2 to 20 years

Age (years)

SOURCE: Developed by the National Center for Health Statistics in collaboration with the National Center for Chronic Disease Prevention and Health Promotion (2000).

T A B L E B–12

Stature for Age: Boys 2 to 20 Years

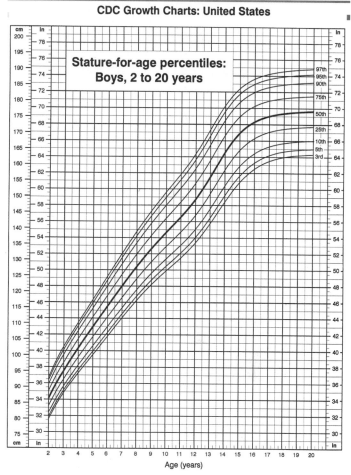

CDC Growth Charts: United States

Stature-for-age percentiles:
Boys, 2 to 20 years

Age (years)

SOURCE: Developed by the National Center for Health Statistics in collaboration with
the National Center for Chronic Disease Prevention and Health Promotion (2000).

T A B L E B–13

Weight for Stature: Boys

CDC Growth Charts: United States

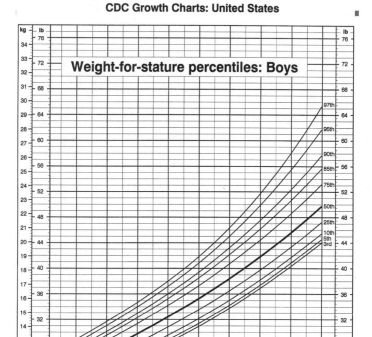

Weight-for-stature percentiles: Boys

SOURCE: Developed by the National Center for Health Statistics in collaboration with the National Center for Chronic Disease Prevention and Health Promotion (2000).

TABLE B-14

Body Mass Index for Age: Boys 2 to 20 Years

CDC Growth Charts: United States

Body mass index-for-age percentiles: Boys, 2 to 20 years

97th
95th
90th
85th
75th
50th
25th
10th
5th
3rd

Age (years)

SOURCE: Developed by the National Center for Health Statistics in collaboration with the National Center for Chronic Disease Prevention and Health Promotion (2000).

T A B L E B–15

Head Circumference Chart (Girls)

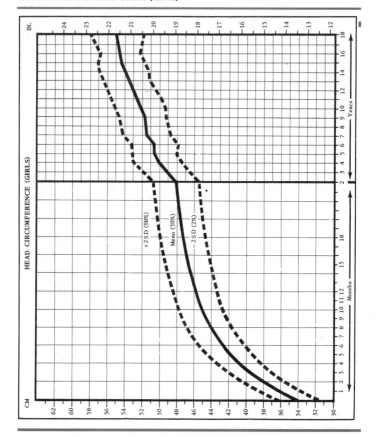

Nellhaus G: Head circumference from birth to eighteen years. Practical composite international and interracial graphs. Pediatrics 41:106–114, 1968.

T A B L E B–16

Head Circumference Chart (Boys)

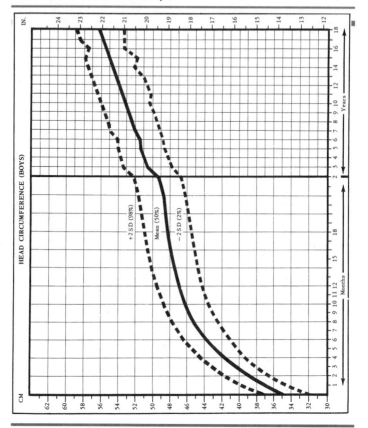

Nellhaus G: Head circumference from birth to eighteen years. Practical composite international and interracial graphs. Pediatrics 41:106–114, 1968.

T A B L E B–17

Growth Record for Premature Infants in Relation to Gestational Age and Fetal and Infant Norms

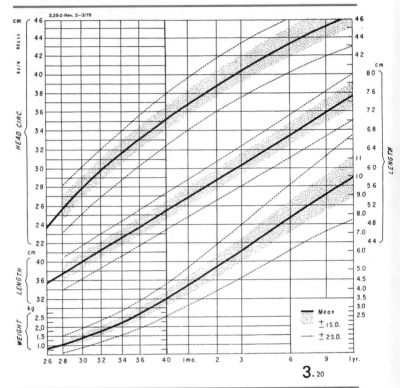

3.20

Babson S, Benda G: Growth graphs for the clinical assessment of infants of varying gestational age. J Pediatr 89:814–820, 1976.

MATURATIONAL ASSESSMENT OF GESTATIONAL AGE (New Ballard Score)

NAME _____   SEX _____

HOSPITAL NO. _____   BIRTH WEIGHT _____

RACE _____   LENGTH _____

DATE/TIME OF BIRTH _____   HEAD CIRC. _____

DATE/TIME OF EXAM _____   EXAMINER _____

AGE WHEN EXAMINED _____

APGAR SCORE: 1 MINUTE _____ 5 MINUTES _____ 10 MINUTES _____

NEUROMUSCULAR MATURITY

NEUROMUSCULAR MATURITY SIGN	SCORE							RECORD SCORE HERE
	-1	0	1	2	3	4	5	
POSTURE								
SQUARE WINDOW (Wrist)	>90°	90°	60°	45°	30°	0°		
ARM RECOIL		180°	140°-180°	110°-140°	90°-110°	<90°		
POPLITEAL ANGLE	180°	160°	140°	120°	100°	90°	<90°	
SCARF SIGN								
HEEL TO EAR								

TOTAL NEUROMUSCULAR MATURITY SCORE

PHYSICAL MATURITY

PHYSICAL MATURITY SIGN	SCORE							RECORD SCORE HERE
SKIN	sticky friable transparent	gelatinous red translucent	smooth pink visible veins	superficial peeling &/or rash, few veins	cracking pale areas rare veins	parchment deep cracking no vessels	leathery cracked wrinkled	
LANUGO	none	sparse	abundant	thinning	bald areas	mostly bald		
PLANTAR SURFACE	heel-toe 40-50 mm:-1 <40 mm:-2	>50 mm no crease	faint red marks	anterior transverse crease only	creases ant. 2/3	creases over entire sole		
BREAST	imperceptible	barely perceptible	flat areola no bud	stippled areola 1-2 mm bud	raised areola 3-4 mm bud	full areola 5-10 mm bud		
EYE/EAR	lids fused loosely: -1 tightly: -2	lids open pinna flat stays folded	sl. curved pinna; soft; slow recoil	well-curved pinna; soft but ready recoil	formed & firm instant recoil	thick cartilage ear stiff		
GENITALS (Male)	scrotum flat, smooth	scrotum empty faint rugae	testes in upper canal rare rugae	testes descending few rugae	testes down good rugae	testes pendulous deep rugae		
GENITALS (Female)	clitoris prominent & labia flat	prominent clitoris & small labia minora	prominent clitoris & enlarging minora	majora & minora equally prominent	majora large minora small	majora cover clitoris & minora		

Reference
Ballard JL, Khoury JC, Wedig K, et al: New Ballard Score, expanded to include extremely premature infants. *J Pediatr* 1991; 119:417-423. Reprinted by permission of Dr Ballard and Mosby–Year Book, Inc.

TOTAL PHYSICAL MATURITY SCORE

SCORE

Neuromuscular _____

Physical _____

Total _____

MATURITY RATING

SCORE	weeks
-10	20
-5	22
0	24
5	26
10	28
15	30
20	32
25	34
30	36
35	38
40	40
45	42
50	44

GESTATIONAL AGE (weeks)

By dates _____

By ultrasound _____

By exam _____

FIGURE B-1

Classification of newborns by intrauterine growth and gestational age. (From Ballard JL, Khoury JC, Wedig K, et al: New Ballard Score, expanded to include extremely premature infants. J Pediatr 119: 417-423, 1991.) Note: Although used routinely by neonatal care providers, the Ballard scale may not accurately reflect actual gestational age in preterm infants (Donovan et al., 1999; Sanders et al., 1991). If accurate dates are available based on ultrasonography or date of last menstrual period, those also should be used to assess gestational age.

Normal Laboratory Values

A limited selection of blood chemistry, urine, and hematological values is presented as the most common laboratory screening tests requested. The authors recognize that the nurse practitioner may have the need for more complex tests, for example, cerebrospinal fluid studies, immunoglobulins, and therapeutic drug levels. The reader is directed to seek the source of these values with the performing laboratory and its respective standards in comparison with control specimens. Some pediatric specimens need to be sent to a special laboratory for appropriate testing.

Laboratories employ a variety of analytical methods to determine biochemical and hematological values. The normal values for laboratory tests vary depending on the procedure employed. Normal ranges reflect a combination of the population served, individual biological differences, specimen collection and handling techniques, and intrinsic laboratory variation. Given this variability, if any questions arise, it is recommended that the reader consult with the reference laboratory for its methods and the established normal range of values for the methods employed.

Interpretation of laboratory values can be a complex diagnostic exercise. In Table C-1 the comments in the Interpretation column are intended to offer the reader general ideas about each test and its common use. The skilled clinician uses laboratory data with other clinical data to make decisions, sometimes combining several tests to best understand the physiological status of the client.

TABLE C-1

Normal Laboratory Values for Infants, Children, and Adolescents

TEST NAME	REFERENCE RANGE		INTERPRETATION
BLOOD CHEMISTRY (from serum)			
Alanine aminotransferase (ALT, SGPT) (U/L)	Newborn/infant	13–45	Liver, heart, and skeletal muscle have significant levels. High levels are associated with hepatic cell damage
	Adult M	10–40	
	F	7–35	
Amylase (U/L)	Newborn	5–65	Marked rise generally indicates acute pancreatitis
	Adult	27–131	
Aspartate aminotransferase (AST, SGOT) (U/L)	Newborn	25–175	Elevated levels occur with heart, liver, and muscle disease
	Infant	15–60	
	Adult	8–20	
Bilirubin, total (mg/dl)	Premature cord blood	<2.0	Elevated levels occur with increased destruction of RBCs or impairment of liver excretory function
	0–1 d	<8.0	
	1–2 d	<12.0	
	3–5 d	<16.0	
	Full-term		
	Cord blood	<2.0	
	0–1 d	1.4–8.7	
	1–2 d	3.4–11.5	
	3–5 d	1.5–12.0	
	Adult	0.3–1.2	

Table continued on following page

T A B L E C-1

Normal Laboratory Values for Infants, Children, and Adolescents *Continued*

TEST NAME	REFERENCE RANGE		INTERPRETATION
BLOOD CHEMISTRY (from serum)			
Chloride (mmol/L)	Cord blood	96–104	Values increase in metabolic acidosis and other conditions.
	0–30 d	98–113	Decreased values occur with diuresis, GI losses, and
	>30 d	98–107	other conditions
Cholesterol (5th–95th percentile, mg/dl)	Cord blood		Elevated levels indicate disorders of blood lipids
	M	44–103	
	F	50–108	
	0–4 yr		
	M	114–203	
	F	112–200	
	5–9 yr		
	M	121–203	
	F	126–205	
	10–14 yr		
	M	119–202	
	F	124–201	
	15–19 yr		
	M	113–197	
	F	119–200	
	20–24 yr		
	M	124–218	
	F	122–216	

Creatinine (mg/dl)	Cord blood	0.6–1.2	Elevated levels indicate impaired renal function, muscle disease, congestive heart failure, shock, dehydration, and other conditions
	Newborn	0.3–1.0	
	Infant	0.2–0.4	
	Child	0.3–0.7	
	Adolescent	0.5–1.0	
	Adult		
	M	0.7–1.3	
	F	0.6–1.1	
Ferritin (ng/ml)	Newborn	25–200	Ferritin is a more sensitive indicator than iron or TIBC for diagnosing iron deficiency or overload
	1 mo	200–600	
	2–5 mo	50–200	
	6 mo–15 yr	7–140	
	Adult		
	M	15–200	
	F	12–150	
Glucose (fasting) (mg/dl)	Cord blood	45–96	Fasting low levels may indicate a physiological response or a disorder in glucose metabolism. Increased fasting levels may indicate diabetes mellitus, pancreatic disorders, endocrine diseases, drugs, and other conditions
	Premature	20–60	
	Neonate	30–60	
	Newborn		
	1 d	40–60	
	>1 d	50–80	
	Child	60–100	
	Adult	74–106	

Table continued on following page

TABLE C-1

Normal Laboratory Values for Infants, Children, and Adolescents *Continued*

TEST NAME	REFERENCE RANGE		INTERPRETATION
BLOOD CHEMISTRY (from serum)			
Iron (µg/dl)	Newborn	100–250	Decreased levels occur with iron deficiency, blood loss, and other conditions. Elevated levels occur with hemolytic anemias; iron intoxication, hepatitis, and other conditions
	Infant	40–100	
	Child	50–120	
	Thereafter		
	M	50–160	
	F	50–170	
	Intoxicated child	280–2550	
	Fatally poisoned child	>1800	
Lead (whole blood specimen) (µg/dl)	Child	<10	Increased levels indicate lead toxicity
	Adult	<40	
	Lethal dose	≥100 (variable)	
Potassium (mEq/L)	Newborn	3.7–5.9	Decreased levels may indicate shifting of potassium into cells, GI loss, biliary loss, renal loss, and reduced uptake. Increased levels occur with shifts to intracellular fluid, decreased excretion, or increased uptake
	Infant	4.1–5.3	
	Child	3.4–4.7	
	Thereafter	3.5–5.1	
Sodium (mEq/L)	Newborn	133–146	Decreased levels indicate sodium loss or water excess (caused by numerous conditions). Increased levels may occur with an increase in sodium or an excessive loss of water (caused by numerous conditions)
	Infant	139–146	
	Child	138–145	
	Thereafter	136–145	

Thyrotropin (thyroid-stimulating hormone, TSH) (μU/ml)	Newborn	3–18	Decreased levels are associated with hyperthyroidism. Increased levels are associated with hypothyroidism
	Thereafter	2–10	
Thyroxine, free (FT$_4$) (μg/dl)	Newborn	2.6–6.3	Decreased levels are associated with hypothyroidism or overproduction of T$_3$. Increased levels are associated with Graves' disease and thyrotoxicosis from overproduction of T$_4$
	Adult	0.8–2.7	
Thyroxine, total (T$_4$) (μg/dl)	1–3 d	11.8–22.6	T$_4$ serves as a good index of thyroid function only if binding globulin (TBG) is normal
	1–2 wk	9.8–16.6	
	1–4 mo	7.2–14.4	
	4–12 mo	7.8–16.5	
	1–5 yr	7.3–15.0	
	5–10 yr	6.4–13.3	
	10–15 yr	5.5–11.7	
	Adult		
	M	4.6–10.5	
	F	5.5–11.0	
Urea nitrogen (BUN) (mg/dl)	Premature (1 wk)	3–25	Measures glomerular function and production/excretion of urea. Decreased with liver failure, malnutrition, and other conditions. Increased with impaired renal function, congestive heart failure, salt/water depletion, shock, and other conditions
	Newborn	4–12	
	Infant/child	5–18	
	Adult	6–20	

Table continued on following page

TABLE C-1
Normal Laboratory Values for Infants, Children, and Adolescents *Continued*

TEST NAME	REFERENCE RANGE	INTERPRETATION
HEMATOLOGY (whole blood specimens)		
Erythrocyte count (RBC) (millions of cells/mm^3)	1–3 d (capillary) 4.0–6.6	Measures total number of RBCs. Decreased with anemia, cell destruction, and decreased production. Increased with increased RBC production, renal disease, tumors, altitude, pulmonary disease, cardiovascular diseases, and other conditions. A relative increase may occur with dehydration
	1 wk 3.9–6.3	
	2 wk 3.6–6.2	
	1 mo 3.0–5.4	
	2 mo 2.7–4.9	
	3–6 mo 3.1–4.5	
	0.5–2 yr 3.7–5.3	
	2–6 yr 3.9–5.3	
	6–12 yr 4.0–5.2	
	12–18 yr	
	M 4.5–5.3	
	F 4.1–5.1	
	18–49 yr	
	M 4.5–5.9	
	F 4.0–5.2	

Erythrocyte sedimentation rate (ESR, sed rate) (mm/hr)	Westergren, modified		Not diagnostic, but indicates a disease process. Increases occur with collagen diseases, infections, inflammatory conditions, neoplasms, heavy metal poisoning, tissue destruction, and other conditions
	Child	0–10	
	Adult		
	M <50 yr	0–15	
	F <50 yr	0–20	
	Wintrobe		
	Child	0–13	
	Adult		
	M	0–9	
	F	0–20	
Hematocrit (HCT, Hct) (% packed erythrocyte volume [erythrocyte volume/whole blood × 100])	1 d	48–69	Low values indicate blood loss or inadequate production or excess destruction of RBCs. High values indicate erythrocytosis, severe dehydration, shock, and other conditions
	2 d	48–75	
	3 d	44–72	
	2 mo	28–42	
	6–12 yr	35–45	
	12–18 yr		
	M	37–49	
	F	36–46	
	18–49 yr		
	M	41–53	
	F	36–46	

Table continued on following page

543

T A B L E C–1

Normal Laboratory Values for Infants, Children, and Adolescents *Continued*

TEST NAME	REFERENCE RANGE		INTERPRETATION
HEMATOLOGY (whole blood specimens)			
Hemoglobin, total (Hb) (g/dl)	1–3 d	14.5–22.5	Decreased levels are found with anemia, hyperthyroidism, cirrhosis, severe hemorrhage, hemolysis, and systemic diseases. Very low values may lead to heart failure and death
	2 mo	9.0–14.0	
	6–12 yr	11.5–15.5	
	12–18 yr		
	M	13.0–16.0	
	F	12.0–16.0	
	18–49 yr		
	M	13.5–17.5	
	F	12.0–16.0	
Leukocyte count (white blood cell count, WBC) ($\times$ 1000 cells/ mm³)	Birth	9.0–30.0	Indicates total WBC count circulating in the blood. With some infections, WBCs increase as cells are transported. A low count may occur in overwhelming bacterial infection (sepsis) or with the use of immunosuppressive agents. Elevated levels may occur in response to an underlying disease, a primary cellular disorder (leukemia), pregnancy, corticosteroid treatment, strenuous exercise, and other conditions
	24 hr	9.4–34.0	
	1 mo	5.0–19.5	
	1–3 y	6.0–17.5	
	4–7 y	5.5–15.5	
	8–13 y	4.5–13.5	
	Adult	4.5–11.0	

Test	Subcategory	Value	Description
Leukocyte differential (%)	Myelocytes	0	Describes the proportion of the types of WBCs. Used in conjunction with the total leukocyte count to determine absolute cell counts
	Neutrophils—"bands"	3–5	Neutrophils: Usually increased during bacterial infections. May be decreased in viral infections. Composed of bands and segmented types
	Neutrophils—"segs"	54–62	
	Lymphocytes	25–33	Eosinophils: Increased during allergic responses and parasitic infections
	Monocytes	3–7	Basophils: Increased in allergic reactions, hematological disorders, and other conditions
	Eosinophils	1–3	Lymphocytes: Increased in viral infections
	Basophils	0–0.75	Monocytes: Increased in severe and recovery stages of infections (phagocytosis)
			Myelocytes: Involved in the early maturation of neutrophils, eosinophils, basophils, and monocytes
Platelet count (thrombocyte count)	Newborn	84–478 × 10³/mm³	Decreased platelet counts occur with anemias, some infections, congestive heart failure, bone marrow lesions, and other conditions. Increases occur with malignancies, splenectomy, collagen diseases, some anemias, and other conditions
	1 wk–adult	150–400 × 10³/mm³	
Reticulocyte count (%)	1 d	0.4–6.0	Provides an estimate of the rate of RBC production. The percentage may be used to calculate the absolute value. An elevated count with normal hemoglobin indicates RBC loss with bone marrow compensation. A normal reticulocyte count with a low hemoglobin level indicates an inadequate response to anemia
	7 d	<0.1–1.3	
	1–4 wk	<1.0–1.2	
	5–6 wk	<0.1–2.4	
	7–8 wk	0.1–2.9	
	9–10 wk	<0.1–2.6	
	11–12 wk	0.1–1.3	
	Adult	0.5–1.5	

Table continued on following page

T A B L E C-1

Normal Laboratory Values for Infants, Children, and Adolescents *Continued*

URINE

TEST NAME	REFERENCE RANGE	INTERPRETATION
Urine, macroscopic Bilirubin	All ages Negative	Increased in hepatocellular disease or intrahepatic/ extrahepatic biliary obstruction
Blood, occult	Negative	RBCs increased in acute glomerulonephritis, acute infections, renal calculi, trauma, and other conditions
Glucose, qualitative	Negative	Increased when blood glucose level exceeds the reabsorption capacity of the renal tubes (pathological or benign)
Hemoglobin	Negative	Hemoglobinuria may occur in intravascular hemolysis and other conditions
Ketones	Negative	Increased with adequate carbohydrate intake or a defect in carbohydrate metabolism. Especially significant with diabetes mellitus
Leukocyte esterase	Negative	Measures WBCs. Increase indicates inflammation and/or infection. Associated with certain renal diseases and diseases of the urinary tract or vaginitis
Nitrite	Negative	Increase associated with urinary tract infection
pH	4.6–8.0	Indication of acid-base balance
Protein, qualitative	Negative	Increased in pathological or physiological conditions (e.g., fever, stress, strenuous exercises)

		Value	Description
Specific gravity		1.001–1.030	Measures the concentrating and diluting ability of the kidney. Associated with tubular damage
Urobilinogen		0.2–1.0 mg/dl	Increased in liver disease. Decreased in obstruction of bile ducts and other conditions
Urine, microscopic			
Casts			
Hyaline		0–1/lpf	Hyaline casts: Increased in pathological or physiological conditions. Implies damage to the glomerular capillary membrane permitting leakage of proteins through the glomerular filtrate
Other		None	Other casts: Involved in a variety of conditions depending on type of cast. Involved in tubular epithelial damage (epithelial cell cast), renal infection (WBC cast), vascular disorder (RBC cast), renal disease (granular cast), chronic renal condition (waxy cast), severe renal disease (broad cast), degenerative tubular disease (fatty cast)
Red blood cells		0–2/hpf	RBCs: Denotes bleeding into the urinary system
White blood cells	M	0–3/hpf	WBCs: Associated with an inflammatory process
	F and children	0–5/hpf	
Urine volume (ml/24 hr)	Newborn	50–300	Decreased in dehydration, renal ischemia, renal disease, obstruction, and other conditions. Increased in diabetes insipidus, diabetes mellitus, chronic progressive renal failure, and other conditions
	Infant	350–550	
	Child	500–1000	
	Adolescent	700–1400	
	Thereafter		
	M	800–1800	
	F	600–1600	

BUN = blood urea nitrogen; GI = gastrointestinal; hpf = high-power field; lpf = low-power field; RBC = red blood cell; T_3 = triiodothyronine; TBG = thyroxin-binding globulin; TIBC = total iron-binding capacity; WBC = white blood cell.

REFERENCES

Behrman R, Kliegman R, Arvin A (ed): Nelson Textbook of Pediatrics, 14th ed. Philadelphia, WB Saunders, 1996.

Burtis C, Ashwood E: Tietz Textbook of Clinical Chemistry. Philadelphia, WB Saunders, 1999.

Fishbach F: A Manual of Laboratory and Diagnostic Tests, 5th ed. Philadelphia, JB Lippincott, 1996.

Free HM: (ed): Modern Urine Chemistry. Elkhart, IN: Miles, Inc., 1991.

INDEX

Note: Page numbers in *italics* indicate figures; those with a t indicate tables.